Exercise Cardiopulmonary Function in Cardiac Patients

Michael S. Sagiv

Exercise Cardiopulmonary Function in Cardiac Patients

Springer

Michael S. Sagiv, Ph.D.
Wingate College
Wingate, Netanya
Israel

ISBN 978-1-4471-2887-8 ISBN 978-1-4471-2888-5 (eBook)
DOI 10.1007/978-1-4471-2888-5
Springer Dordrecht Heidelberg New York London

Library of Congress Control Number: 2012937363

Printed on acid-free paper

Springer is part of Springer Science+Business Media (www.springer.com)

This book is dedicated to the memory of my parents Judith and Jacob Samama

Foreword

It is quite obvious nowadays that exercise training in heart disease patients is changing fast and noticeably. For the last half century, the attention of exercise physiologists in general has been largely directed to maintain a healthy heart, thus keeping heart disease at bay. Exercise has a beneficial effect on the heart. Regular physical activity is one of the best ways to improve exercise capacity and to reduce morbidity and mortality. The myocardium is a muscle and without proper exercises it will weaken. A weakened heart muscle does not pump blood as efficiently and therefore becomes disease prone. However, just like any skeletal muscle myocardial functional capacity will significantly improve with a concomitant reduction in heart rate and increased contractility, at rest, and at peak exercise following some moderate exercise for at least 30 min every day and up to 60 min if overweight. A slower heart rate is a more efficient heart and a stronger one. That is why an athlete has a slower heart rate than a sedentary individual at the same absolute workload. By exercising regularly, cardiac disease or heart disease may be prevented. It is the one thing we all should strive to do. Exercising is crucial for our health and there is no need to be an athlete to attain the benefits.

Within this setting, the author Professor Michael S. Sagiv has undertaken to write a book that, in my opinion, is incomparable in its approach. It covers comprehensively a wide range of exercise physiology issues and in a way that combines the exercise physiologist approach and the clinical cardiologist approach as well. The text contains mainly physiological changes during exercise in health and disease including aging with a small portion devoted to physiology at rest. The textbook is for medical and graduate students, physicians, exercise scientists, sports medicine specialists, athletic trainers, and sport physical therapists. It will undoubtedly serve in courses dealing in depth with work capacity of the cardiopulmonary system in cardiac patients and healthy subjects. The text is research oriented but also deductive.

I am impressed with the author's ability to provide deep understanding of the cardiovascular function in health and disease during exercise. This text is comprehensive and provides an excellent understanding on the role of the different modes of exercise toward alleviation of cardiac symptoms. I compliment the author. His work is a significant contribution to the cardiac exercise physiology literature.

Professor Ehud Goldhammer, M.D., FESC
Heart Institute, Bnei-Zion Medical Center
and the Faculty of Medicine,
The Technion Institute of Technology,
Haifa, Israel

Preface

This book represents an extended and thoroughly revised literature on the Exercise Cardiopulmonary Function in Cardiac Patients and Healthy Subjects. The key idea, which enables to deal with a wide range of complex cardiac problems in easy-to-check conditions and which also provides generally good solutions, is based on the fact that a large part of the book deals with exercise influences on the cardiopulmonary system and a very minor portion is devoted to cardiopulmonary physiology. This approach is based on the assumption that the reader is acquainted with medical physiology, especially of the cardiopulmonary system.

A substantial proportion of the figures is original and has been prepared specifically for this book; none was taken from published articles or books. Discussions are partially driven from articles by leading authors and partially (marginal portion) from exercise physiology books.

The material presented in the book can be used for courses taught to understand cardiac problems and solutions through physical activity. By-product of the book is a cardiopulmonary response to various modes of exercise in healthy subjects since, to understand pathology, one has to know healthy responses. With respect to the original collection of references, this book contains those that have been previously published in peer-reviewed journals. This is partially due to their novelty and partially to the fact that the referees of many journals are relatively more cautious with papers which are substantially innovative.

Book's Contents:

Chapter 1 discusses the knowledge about a broad range of exercise responses that can occur across time, intensities, and modes of exercise. Modes of exercise include dynamic aerobic, dynamic anaerobic, and isometric. Understanding exercise physiology can help to improve work capacity in health and disease. The chapter contains an introduction to general aspects and principles concerning exercise physiology. The main emphasis is on principles of altering in homeostasis during exercise and the compensatory mechanisms for returning as close as possible to homeostasis.

Chapter 2 focus on the respiratory system which acts by gasses exchange, and therefore functional capacity of the pulmonary under different exercise conditions and tests varies to influence physical performance, thus, may exclude existence of cardiovascular diseases. Additionally, cardiac output is affected by the phase of respiration with intrathoracic pressure changes influencing diastolic heart filling and therefore cardiac output.

Chapter 3 presents the cardiac output responses to exercise at sea level, altitude, and warm and cold ambient. It discusses the cardiac output dependency mainly on the type of exercise performed, metabolic demand, and fitness level.

Chapter 4 contains a review of the autoregulation mechanism which is characterized by its vasodilatation effect on the small arteries and arterioles, in spite of the domination of the sympathetic nervous system. Autoregulation is a manifestation of local blood flow regulation that assists to redistribute cardiac output so that the working muscles receive the most of it during exercise.

Chapter 5 is devoted to left ventricular function with and without coronary artery narrowing or ischemic heart disease. Normal left ventricular function is the contraction of the ventricle in order to eject maximal blood into the aorta. However, once left ventricular dysfunction occurs, a series of compensatory mechanisms are triggered which lead to a host of structural and neurohormonal adaptations.

Chapters 6 and 7 deal with cardiac risk factors and the role of exercise to minimize their impact upon the development of cardiac diseases. Cardiac risk factors are characteristics or traits that reliably predict an individual's chances of developing atherosclerosis or coronary artery disease. The greater the number or severity of cardiac risk factors that be relevant, the higher the chances are for cardiovascular disease. By identifying these cardiac risk factors and taking active step such as exercise, it may reduce their number or severity.

Chapter 8 examines several application problems with aging. Decline in physical performance is an important risk factor in developing cardiovascular diseases. It is estimated that 82% of people who die of coronary heart disease are 65 years and older. Aging is also associated with changes in the mechanical and structural properties of the vascular wall, which leads to the loss of arterial elasticity and reduced arterial compliance and may subsequently lead to coronary artery disease. The chapter discusses in details the physiological changes brought about following exercise training to the elderly population.

Chapter 9 is entirely devoted to the role of exercise in physical inactivity, its role in sudden cardiac death, and its cardioprotective benefits in coronary artery disease and healthy individuals.

Chapter 10 focuses on cardiac rehabilitation seen as a medically supervised program that helps improve the health and well-being of people who have heart problems. Cardiac rehabilitation programs include exercise training, education on heart healthy living, and counseling to reduce stress and help return to an active life. Focal point of this chapter is physiological and medical aspects.

Acknowledgements

In presenting this book, I would like to express my thanks to my colleagues who read parts of the written material and gave me constructive criticism, useful suggestions, and new cardiac problems to solve. They include Professor Ehud Goldhammer, a fine cardiologist; Professor David Ben-Sira, a statistician and biomechanist; and Mrs Roneet Sheer for her very useful professional work of the figures. Sincere thanks to my former professors who inspired me throughout my professional and personal life: the late Professor Peter G. Hanson and Professor William G. Reddan. I am thankful and blessed to have Limor, Ohad and Moran my children who gave my wife and me seven grandchildren. Last but not least to my wife Amira Sagiv, for her love, being a constant resource of patience and understanding.

Contents

1 Exercise Physiology 1
Introduction 1
Physical Activity 1
Exercise Physiology 2
Aerobic Exercise 3
Anaerobic Exercise 4
Isometric Exercise 6
Energy Expenditure 6
Metabolism 8
Metabolism of the Myocardium 12
Interplay Between Aerobic and Anaerobic Pathways 13
Lactic Acid Threshold 14
Gender Differences in Oxygen Extraction 16
Metabolic Demands in Diverse Populations 17
The Cardiovascular System 17
Coronary Artery Disease 19
Mitochondrial Changes in Skeletal Muscle 19
The Fick Equation 20
Efforts at Altitude 21
Exercise and Genetics 22
Physiological Measurements and Metabolic Calculations 23
Unit Measurements 23
Laboratory Equipments 24
Energy Cost 24
The Stress Test 25
Calculating Stepwise Work and Power 25
Calculating Metabolic Cost of Stepping 26
Calculating Bicycle's Work and Power 26
Calculating Metabolic Cost of Bicycle Ergometry 26
Calculating Treadmill's Work and Power 27
Metabolic Cost Treadmill Walking 28
Metabolic Cost of Treadmill Running 28
References 29

2 Pulmonary Function 33
Introduction 33
About the Gases 33

Minute Ventilation ... 35
Oxygen-Diffusing Capacity in the Lung ... 37
Transporting Oxygen and Carbon Dioxide by the Blood ... 38
Peak Oxygen Uptake (VO_{2peak}) ... 39
Oxygen Uptake (VO_2) ... 40
VO_2max Determination ... 41
Factors Affecting Oxygen Uptake ... 42
Genetics Role in Oxygen Uptake Variability ... 43
The Angiotensin-Converting Enzyme Genotype ... 44
Gender Effect on VO_2 ... 44
VO_2 in the Hot and Cold Ambient ... 45
VO_2max at Altitude ... 46
Peripheral Versus Central Theories ... 46
VO_2max in Cardiovascular Disease Patients ... 48
VO_2max Following Training ... 48
Oxygen-Carrying and Release Capacity of the Blood ... 49
Anemia ... 52
Role of the Pulmonary System in VO_2 ... 52
Gender Effect on Pulmonary Function ... 53
Pulmonary Function at Altitude ... 53
The Training Effect on the Pulmonary System ... 55
References ... 55

3 Cardiac Output ... 59
Cardiac Output in Normal Subjects ... 59
The Interplay Between Heart Rate and Stroke Volume ... 61
Supine Exercise ... 63
Control of Heart Rate ... 65
Factors Affecting Stroke Volume ... 67
Oxygen Extraction and Cardiac Output ... 69
Core Temperature Effect on Cardiac Output ... 70
Cardiac Output During Isometric Exercise ... 71
Cardiac Output During Anaerobic Exercise ... 74
Cardiac Output During Isodynamic Exercise ... 75
Cardiac Output in Coronary Artery Disease Patients ... 76
Isometric Exercise in Coronary Artery Disease Patients ... 77
Aerobic Training Effect on Cardiac Output ... 78
Isometric Training and Cardiac Output Adaptations ... 79
Aerobic Exercise Training in Coronary Artery Disease ... 81
References ... 82

4 Cardiac Output Redistribution ... 85
The Autoregulation Mechanism ... 85
Blood Flow During Exercise ... 86
Metabolic Theory of Blood Flow Regulation ... 87
Myogenic Theory of Blood Flow Regulation ... 89
Nitric Oxide and Kinins Influence on Blood Flow ... 89
Rennin-Angiotensin System ... 90
Myocardial Blood Flow ... 91

Cardiac Output Redistribution ... 96
Respiratory Muscle Work ... 98
Cardiac Output in Warm Environments ... 99
Cardiac Output Redistribution in Cold Environment ... 102
Cardiac Output at Altitude ... 102
References ... 104

5 Left Ventricular Function ... 109
Left Ventricular Function Measurements ... 109
Left Ventricular Function During Aerobic Exercise ... 110
Left Ventricular Function During Anaerobic Exercise ... 111
Left Ventricular Function During Isometric Exercise ... 111
Left Ventricular Systolic Function ... 113
Left Ventricular End-Systolic Pressure–Volume Ratio (*P*/*V*) ... 114
Left Ventricular Ejection Fraction ... 115
Left Ventricular Function in Coronary Artery Disease ... 117
Doppler Indices During Systole ... 117
Left Ventricular Diastolic Function ... 118
Left Ventricular Diastolic Indices ... 119
The Ratio of Peak Early Diastole/Presystole Maximal Velocity ... 120
Atrial Filling Fraction ... 121
Exercise Mode and Left Ventricular Hypertrophy ... 122
Genome and Left Ventricular Mass ... 123
Exercise and "Athlete's Heart" ... 125
Concentric Hypertrophy ... 127
Pathological Left Ventricular Hypertrophy ... 127
Left Ventricular Adaptations ... 128
References ... 130

6 Blood Pressure and Hypertension ... 135
Introduction ... 135
Exercise Effects on Atherosclerosis ... 136
Blood Pressure During Aerobic Exercise ... 138
Post-exercise Hypotension ... 139
Mean Arterial Blood Pressure ... 140
Hypertension and Arterial Baroreceptors ... 141
Blood Pressure Adaptations to Resistive Training ... 143
Anaerobic Bout ... 145
Total Peripheral Resistance ... 146
Arterials and Aortic Stiffening ... 147
Physical Activity in Hypertension ... 148
References ... 150

7 Metabolic Cardiovascular Risk Factors ... 155
Lipoproteins ... 155
Aerobic Exercise Effect on Lipoprotein ... 155
Strength Training Effect on Lipoprotein ... 157
High-Density Lipoprotein ... 157
Exercise and High-Density Lipoprotein Cholesterol Synthesis ... 158

Obesity . . . 159
Exercise in Obesity . . . 160
Resistive Exercise Training Effect on Obesity . . . 162
Diabetes . . . 162
Exercise's Effects on Diabetes . . . 163
References . . . 167

8 Cardiopulmonary Function in Elderly . . . 171
Aging Considerations . . . 171
Age Effect on Oxygen Uptake . . . 173
Aging Effect on Pulmonary Function . . . 174
Muscle Mass and Cardiopulmonary Function . . . 174
Influence of Physical Activity on Exercise Performance . . . 175
Aerobic Exercise Capacity . . . 176
Cardiac Changes and Cardiac Output . . . 176
Heart Rate Response . . . 178
Stroke Volume Response . . . 178
Stroke Volume Response to Training . . . 179
Left Ventricular Function During Aerobic Exercise . . . 179
Left Ventricular Function During Anaerobic Exercise . . . 181
Left Ventricular Function During Isometric Exercise . . . 182
Cardiovascular and Physical Performance . . . 182
Aging of the Arteries . . . 184
Training Effect on Cardiovascular Function . . . 185
Exercise Training for Elderly with CAD . . . 188
Exercise Benefits for Hypertensive Elderly . . . 188
Pulmonary Exercise's Benefits . . . 189
Metabolic Improvements . . . 190
References . . . 191

9 Exercise and Sudden Death . . . 195
Physical Inactivity and Cardiovascular Disease . . . 195
Are Exercise and Sudden Death Causally Related? . . . 196
Effect of Exercise on Risk of Sudden Death . . . 197
Levels of Physical Fitness . . . 198
Causes of Sudden Cardiac Death . . . 199
Pathophysiology . . . 201
Commotio Cordis . . . 202
Long QT Syndrome . . . 203
Catecholaminergic Polymorphic Ventricular Tachycardia . . . 203
Brugada Syndrome . . . 204
Hypertrophic Cardiomyopathy . . . 205
Coronary Artery Anomalies . . . 207
Mechanism of Ventricular Tachycardia . . . 207
Mechanism of Ventricular Fibrillation . . . 209
Arrhythmogenic Right Ventricular Dysplasia . . . 209
References . . . 211

10 Cardiac Rehabilitation 215
Program's Aims 215
All Causes Mortality 217
Physiology and Pathophysiology 218
Factors Determining Myocardial Oxygen Demand 219
Cardiovascular Benefits of Exercise 221
Impact of Exercise on Functional Capacity 221
Cardiac Biomarkers 223
How Much Exercise Is Enough? 229
What Is Moderate Intensity? 230
Exercise Stress Test in Coronary Artery Disease 231
Exercise Prescription in Coronary Heart Disease 233
Cardiac Power Output, Cardiac Reserve, and Circulatory Power 234
Cardiopulmonary and Ventilator Markers 235
The Minute Ventilation to Carbon Dioxide Ratio (VE/VCO2) 235
Pulmonary Ventilation-Perfusion Mismatch: During Exercise 237
Estimating Stroke Volume 238
References 239

Index 245

Exercise Physiology

1

Introduction

The knowledge about the broad range of exercise responses that can occur across time, intensities, and modes of exercise can help to improve work capacity and physical performance of humans in health and disease. Exercise alters physiological function in the organism, regardless of whether the effect is beneficial or harmful. Muscle contraction has both mechanical that produces movement and metabolic properties producing energy. *Isotonic dynamic exercise* shortens the muscle fibers. *Static isometric exercise* is an effort without fibers shortening. However, most physical activities involve both dynamic and static contractions and *aerobic* and *anaerobic* metabolism. Thus, activities tend to be classified on the basis of their dominant mechanical and/or metabolic characteristics.

Physical activity can give some estimation of the body's different systems range and abilities. It is however important to realize that the body's performance depends on the mode of exercise and more important if oxygen is available (aerobic) such prolong running, or without enough oxygen (anaerobic) such as 100-m dash or isometric bout. Therefore, the physiological responses of exercise demand coordination between functions of the heart, lungs, and skeletal muscles. This has to meet the increased metabolic demands in order to deliver oxygen to the working muscles and to eliminate carbon dioxide to the atmosphere. Since the responses of the heart and lungs to the metabolic demands are precise, it enables to predict the cardiopulmonary responses during aerobic exercise.

Cardiovascular adaptations to exercise have been systematically defined and differ according to type of conditioning: endurance training sometimes also described as dynamic, isotonic, or aerobic such as long-distance running and swimming; and strength training also referred to as static, isometric, power, or anaerobic such as wrestling, weightlifting, or throwing heavy objects. Long-term cardiovascular adaptation to dynamic training produces increased maximal oxygen uptake due to increased cardiac output and *arteriovenous oxygen difference* $(a\text{-}v)O_2$. Long-term cardiovascular adaptation to isometric training produces increase in strength and muscle mass.

Performing vigorous physical activity entails multiorgan system engagement, with the cardiovascular system playing a critical role. In order to provide enough oxygen to activate muscles during repeated physical activity of high intensity, the heart undergoes profound morphological, functional, and electrophysiological alterations, which have been identified as "athlete's heart syndrome" and are generally regarded as a benign increase in cardiac mass, with specific circulatory and cardiac morphological alterations, representing a physiological adaptation to systematic training [1].

Physical Activity

Aerobic physical activity is associated with hemodynamic changes which alter the loading conditions of the heart. In dynamic exercise, the emphasis is on movement with no or minimal development

M.S. Sagiv, *Exercise Cardiopulmonary Function in Cardiac Patients*,
DOI 10.1007/978-1-4471-2888-5_1, © Springer-Verlag London 2012

of force. The main hemodynamic features are increases in *heart rate* and *stroke volume*, the two components of *cardiac output*. Systemic vascular resistance drops, but the net result is a slight-to-moderate rise in blood pressure. The load on the heart is predominantly that of *volume overload*. During *static exercise*, force is developed with no or minimal movement. The hemodynamic consequences involve a slight elevation of cardiac output, caused by the increase of heart rate, and a more pronounced rise of *blood pressure*, resulting in a *pressure overload* on the heart. From a theoretical point of view, the hemodynamic alterations and the ventricular loading conditions during exercise could, in the long run, lead to *left ventricular hypertrophy*. Volume overload such as during aerobic exercise would lead to enlargement of the left ventricular internal diameter and a proportional increase of wall thickness; this type of adaptation is termed *eccentric left ventricular hypertrophy*. The *pressure overload* developed during isometric bout would induce thickening of the ventricular wall with unchanged internal dimension, or *concentric left ventricular hypertrophy*. It was suggested that these cardiac adaptations serve to normalize wall stress [2].

Exercise Physiology

Exercise physiology can be defined as "the identification of physiological mechanisms underlying physical activity, the comprehensive delivery of treatment services concerned with the analysis, improvement, and maintenance of health and fitness, rehabilitation of heart disease and other chronic diseases and/or disabilities, and the professional guidance and counsel of athletes and others interested in athletics, sports training, and human adaptability to acute and chronic exercise." The knowledge of exercise physiology can help out patients to get in a better shape for all around good health, or to treat patients with a medical condition through exercise. Exercise physiology is a field of study devoted to examining the body's response to physical activity. In a nutshell, its primary focus is "exercise as medicine." Topics of interest for someone working in the field of exercise physiology may include human energy expenditure, human energy transfer, and environmental effects on physiology. Exercise physiologists also devote a great deal of study to how physical activity influences the body's cardiovascular system, endocrine system, and musculoskeletal system.

Developing new and healthy habits for patients to enable them to manage their medical condition in the best way possible is a large part of their job. They can also work side by side with physiotherapists, occupational therapists, and podiatrists. The field of exercise physiology can be split into two primary areas of specialization: fitness and rehabilitation. Exercise physiologists who focus on fitness may work with professional athletes to improve their performance or counsel private clients who are trying to lose weight and get in shape. Exercise physiology professionals who specialize in rehabilitation often help people who are recovering from injuries or dealing with chronic conditions such as cardiovascular diseases by developing a customized exercise program that can be used as part of a comprehensive treatment strategy.

Physical rehabilitation is a common form of this restoring process. Often utilized after major surgery, an accident, or any event that robs the individual of mobility or function, this form of rehab pairs the patient with trained personnel who help him to recover as much of his former physical prowess as possible. Knowledge on the musculoskeletal, cardiopulmonary, and endocrine systems enables to prescribe a course of exercises for either fitness or rehabilitation. It may help in behavioral modification programs. Understanding exercise physiology can assist medical conditions such as obesity, diabetes, cancer, osteoporosis, depression, asthma, and cardiovascular diseases, as well as many other conditions. Therefore, an *exercise physiologist* is an allied health professional who prescribes exercise programs, also for cardiac and pulmonary patients referred by a physician, and educates people about the benefits of exercise. The exercise physiologist evaluates and assesses cardiovascular and metabolic effects, as well as the mechanisms, of exercise. Exercise physiologist studies acute and chronic physiological adaptation to physical activity and helps active people and athletes to improve and maintain their health and fitness level or performance.

Exercise physiology is the study of the acute responses and chronic adaptations to increased metabolic demand during a wide range of physical exercise conditions. It is related to various organ system responses under higher metabolic demand and psychological state. In its broadest sense, exercise physiology is the study of the exercise's effects on living organisms. In addition, it helps to study the effect that exercise has on pathology, and the mechanisms by which exercise can reduce or reverse disease progression. An exercise physiologist's area of study may include but is not limited to biochemistry, bioenergetics, cardiopulmonary function, hematology, biomechanics, skeletal muscle physiology, neuroendocrine function, and central and peripheral nervous system function. Furthermore, exercise physiologists range from basic scientists, to clinical researchers, to clinicians, to sports trainers.

The field of exercise physiology relies on anatomy, physiology, organic chemistry, biochemistry, cell biology, molecular biology, and psychology. In order to help the reader to have a more focused approach to the study of the human body responses to increased metabolic demand, this book will look into the influence of aerobic, anaerobic, and resistive exercises have on the *cardiopulmonary system.*

In terms of increase physical performance, it has traditionally been the beneficial effects that have been of specific interest. Because of the extensive use of physical efforts in health and disease, it will be necessary for members of the medical community, physical therapists, occupational therapists, and health promoters to have at least the basic knowledge of the different modes of exercise and the mechanisms of their action. For the purpose of this text, the effects of physical efforts on the function of the cardiopulmonary will be the primary concern. Most discussions of exercise physiology deal primarily with the beneficial effects of specific kind of physical efforts on human cardiopulmonary system, and the manner in which these physical efforts exert their effect.

With the increase of the overall size of the organism, cells had to be organized into organs and physiological systems. The exchange of substrates between the different water compartments, that is, exchange of substrates between the extracellular fluid, intracellular fluid, and blood, can increase very dramatically during exercise. With increased *metabolic demands* during exercise, these exchanges across the different water compartments create complicated and problematic situation to balance between production and removal of heat, carbon dioxide, lactic acid, and metabolites.

Aerobic Exercise

Aerobic exercise is a physical activity of relatively low intensity and long duration, which depends primarily on the aerobic energy system. The American College of Sports Medicine defines aerobic exercise as "any activity that uses large muscle groups, can be maintained continuously, and is rhythmic in nature." Aerobic exercise means with air or oxygen; it is rhythmically in nature, lasting for at least 15–20 min or longer while maintaining 60–80% of heart rate reserve. Aerobic activities include walking, biking, jogging, swimming, aerobic classes, and cross-country skiing. Anaerobic activity is short in duration and high in intensity. Anaerobic activities include racquetball, downhill skiing, weightlifting, sprinting, softball, soccer, and football.

Aerobic exercise is a constant moderate intensity work that uses up oxygen at a rate in which the cardiorespiratory system can replenish oxygen in the working muscles. Many types of exercise are aerobic and, by definition, are performed at moderate levels of intensity for extended periods of time. Aerobic exercise requires oxygen to be present for the generation of energy from fuels such as glucose, glycogen, and fat. Aerobic exercise results in no buildup of lactic acid as a result of metabolism. This process is more efficient than *anaerobic metabolism.* The *slow twitch fiber* (red fibers) muscles are more efficient at using oxygen to generate more fuel, that is, adenosine

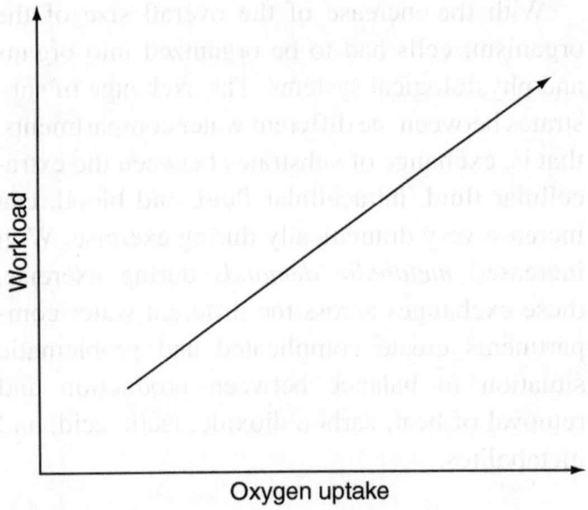

Fig. 1.1 Oxygen uptake is linearly related to the workload, and as exercise intensity increases, oxygen uptake increases proportionally

triphosphate (*ATP*) for continuous, extended muscle contractions over a long time. They fire more slowly than *fast twitch fiber* (white fiber) and can go for a long time before they fatigue. Therefore, slow twitch fibers helps athletes to run marathons and bicycle for hours.

Aerobic capacity describes the functional capacity of the cardiopulmonary system (the heart, lungs, and blood vessels). Aerobic capacity is defined as the maximum amount of oxygen the body can use during a specified period, usually during intense exercise, that is, there is a linear relationship between workload and oxygen uptake (Fig. 1.1). High-level aerobic capacity or *endurance* is a product of three physiological factors: a high *maximal oxygen uptake* (VO_{2max}), a high lactic acid threshold or *anaerobic threshold* (*AT*), and the efficient use of the three energy systems. Consequently, as athletes strive to push endurance to its limits, there has been a great body of research performed into what limits VO_{2max} and how it can be improved. Individuals who are unfit persons have a lower AT than trained individuals who are aerobically trained. The well-trained athlete may be able to approach 80% of the VO_{2max} aerobically without significant *lactic acid* production. Thus, muscle must be able to use oxygen efficiently to keep lactic acid during exercise to a minimum level.

To measure maximal aerobic capacity, an exercise physiologist or physician will perform a VO_{2max} test in which a subject will undergo progressively more strenuous exercise on a treadmill, from an easy walk through to exhaustion. The same test may be performed on bicycle also. Aerobic exercise and fitness can be contrasted with *anaerobic exercise*, of which *strength training* and short-distance running are the most prominent examples. The two types of exercise differ by the duration and intensity of muscular contractions involved as well as by how energy is generated within the muscle [3].

Aerobic exercise is a type of exercise that overloads the heart and lungs and causes them to work harder than at rest. Aerobic exercise conditions the heart and lungs by increasing the oxygen available to the body and by enabling the heart to use oxygen more efficiently. Exercise alone cannot prevent or cure heart disease. It is only one factor in a total program of risk reduction; examples of other factors are reduction of high blood pressure, cessation of cigarette smoking, reduction of high cholesterol level, and reduction of risk of cardiovascular disease. In addition to cardiovascular benefits, other benefits of aerobic exercise include:

- Control of body fat. (Aerobic exercise in conjunction with strength training and a proper diet will reduce body fat.)
- Increased resistance to fatigue and extra energy.
- Toned muscles and increased lean body mass.
- Decreased tension and aid in sleeping.
- Increased general stamina.
- Psychological benefits – exercise improves mood and reduces depression and anxiety.

Other benefits of aerobic exercise include an increased red blood cell count, which would transport oxygen much more efficiently throughout the body.

Anaerobic Exercise

Anaerobic exercise is intense enough to trigger *anaerobic metabolism* and therefore has a greater inherent risk of injury. Overall, anaerobic exercise burns fewer calories than does aerobic exercise and may be somewhat less beneficial for cardiovascular fitness. However, it is better at building strength and muscle mass and still benefits the heart and lungs. Anaerobic exercise helps keep muscles fit and strong (especially with aging, when muscles of the elderly tend to atrophy due to physical inactivity), and it can increase bone strength. This is especially important for women who are at risk for osteoporosis as they age. In addition, speed and general power for daily activities is increased.

In the long run, increased muscle mass helps an individual become leaner and manage his weight because muscle uses large amounts of calories. Anaerobic exercise such as weightlifting does not require large amounts of oxygen because the activity itself is very brief and intense. Because of this, instead of using oxygen, the muscles use glycogen.

Anaerobic exercise is used by athletes in non-endurance sports to promote strength, speed, and power and by body builders to build muscle mass. Anaerobic exercise include heavy weightlifting, all types of sprints (running, biking, etc.), jumping rope, hill climbing, interval training, isometrics, or any rapid burst of hard exercise. All-out exercise produces *lactic acid* and is usually of short duration. *Blood pH* can change from a slightly alkaline 7.4 at rest to as low as acidic 6.5 during all-out sprinting activity. This is primarily due to an increased reliance on anaerobic energy systems and the hydrogen ions (H+) accumulation [4]. With the onset of vigorous exercise, there is a temporary shortage of oxygen being delivered to the working muscles. *Lactic acid* is a by-product of producing energy anaerobically. When lactic acid accumulates at high levels in the blood, it causes muscular fatigue. This is why anaerobic exercises cannot last very long.

Anaerobic *energy expenditure* is difficult to accurately quantify, although several reasonable methods to estimate the anaerobic component to exercise are available [5]. Muscle energy systems trained using anaerobic exercise develop differently compared to aerobic exercise, leading to greater performance in short-duration, high-intensity activities, which last from mere seconds up to about 2 min. Any activity after about 2 min will have a large *aerobic metabolic* component. Intense exercise lasting upward of about 4 min such as mile race may still have a considerable anaerobic energy expenditure component.

Anaerobic metabolism, or anaerobic energy expenditure, is a natural part of whole-body metabolic energy expenditure [6]. Fast twitch skeletal muscle as compared to slow twitch muscle operates using anaerobic metabolic systems, such that any recruitment of fast twitch muscle fibers will lead to increased anaerobic energy expenditure. *Anaerobic metabolism* expenditure is part of whole-body metabolic energy expenditure. Because fast twitch fibers use anaerobic metabolism to create fuel (ATP), they are much better at generating short bursts of strength or speed than slow twitch fibers. However, they fatigue more quickly. *Fast twitch fibers* generally produce the same amount of force per contraction as slow muscles, but they are able to fire more rapidly. Having faster twitch fibers can be an asset to sprinters since they need to quickly generate high level of force.

Energy needed to perform anaerobic bout and high-intensity bursts of activity is derived from anaerobic sources within the cytosol of muscle cells, as opposed to aerobic respiration which utilizes oxygen, is sustainable, and occurs in the mitochondria. The quick energy sources consist of the chemical compound stored in muscle *phosphocreatine* (*PC*), fast *glycolysis*, and adenylate kinase. All of these systems resynthesize ATP, which is the universal energy source in all cells. The most rapid source, but the most readily depleted of the above sources, is the PC system which utilizes the enzyme creatine kinase. This enzyme catalyzes a reaction that combines PC and *adenosine diphosphate* (*ADP*) which is a reduced ATP by one phosphate into ATP and *creatine* (*C*). This resource is short lasting because oxygen is required for the resynthesis of PC via mitochondrial creatine kinase. Therefore, under anaerobic conditions, this substrate is finite and only lasts between approximately 10 and 30 s of high-intensity work. Fast glycolysis, however, can function for approximately 2 min prior to fatigue, and predominately uses intracellular glycogen as a substrate. *Glycogen* is broken down rapidly via glycogen phosphorylase into individual glucose units during intense exercise. Glucose is then oxidized to pyruvate and, under anaerobic condition, is reduced to *lactic acid*. This reaction oxidizes NADH to free enzyme nicotinamide adenine dinucleotide (NAD), thereby releasing a hydrogen ion, promoting acidosis. For this reason, fast glycolysis cannot be sustained for long periods of time. Lastly, adenylate kinase catalyzes a reaction by which 2 *ADP* are combined to form *ATP* and *adenosine monophosphate* (*AMP*). This reaction takes place during low-energy situations such as extreme exercise or conditions of hypoxia, but is not a significant source of energy. The creation of AMP resulting from this reaction stimulates AMP-activated protein kinase (AMP kinase) which is the energy sensor of the cell. After sensing low-energy conditions, AMP kinase stimulates various other intracellular enzymes geared toward increasing energy supply and decreasing all anabolic, or energy requiring, cell functions.

Anaerobic energy expenditure is difficult to accurately quantify, although several reasonable methods to estimate the anaerobic component to exercise are available [7–9]. In most conditions, anaerobic exercise occurs simultaneously with aerobic exercises because the less-efficient anaerobic metabolism must supplement the aerobic system due to energy demands that exceed the cardiopulmonary system's capacity.

Isometric Exercise

Isometric exercise is a type of strength training in which the joint angle and muscle length do not change during contraction. Isometric exercises are opposed by a force equal to the force output of the muscle, and there is no net movement. Isometric exercise is one method of muscular exercise. In contrast, isotonic exercise occurs when a contracting muscle shortens against a constant load, as when lifting a weight. Isometric comes from the Greek word "iso-," equal + "metron," measure = maintaining the same measure, dimension, or length. This mainly strengthens the muscle at the specific joint angle at which the isometric exercise occurs, with some increases in strength at joint angles up to 20° in either direction, depending on the joint trained [10]. In comparison, isotonic exercises strengthen the muscle throughout the entire range of motion of the exercise used. Isometric or *static exercise* is an activity in which muscles undergo no change in length with contraction. As a result, no physical work is done despite an increase in the metabolic rate. Intramuscular pressure is increased, thereby resulting in compression of the blood vessels and a mechanical occlusion of blood flow. It is observed that a 20–30% of maximal voluntary contraction can be maintained for 3–5 min duration [11].

Isometric muscle activity occurs in day-to-day tasks and has applications in physical training, sports, and recreational activities. It has been assumed that this type of activity is potentially dangerous for patients with *coronary heart disease* due to seemingly inappropriate *blood pressure* response [11]. Despite only moderate increases in metabolism, large increases in blood pressure occur in contractions of only 20–30% maximal voluntary contraction. This has the effect of placing a large *pressure load* on *the left ventricle* to increase metabolic demands on a heart already compromised by disease.

Energy Expenditure

In biology, *energy balance* is the biological homeostasis of energy in living systems. It is measured as follows (Eq. 1.1):

$$\text{Energy intake} = \text{internal heat produced} + \text{external work} + \text{storage} \quad (1.1)$$

It is also an aspect of bioenergetics, concerning energy flow through living systems.

It generally uses the energy unit kilogram calorie (kcal), which equals the energy needed to increase the temperature of liter of water by 1°C. This is about 4.184 kJ. Normal energy requirement, and therefore normal energy intake, depends mainly on age, sex, and physical activity level. Exercise represents one of the highest levels of extreme stresses to which the body can be

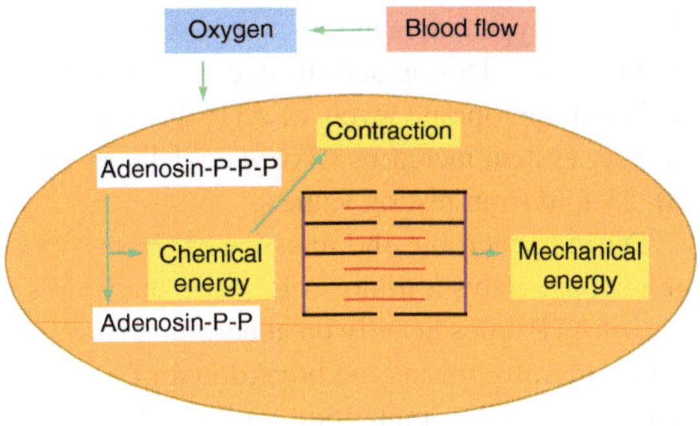

Fig. 1.2 ATP serves at least two functions in skeletal muscle systems: First, ATP disconnects actin from myosin, and second, ATP is hydrolyzed by the myosin molecule to produce the energy required for muscle contraction

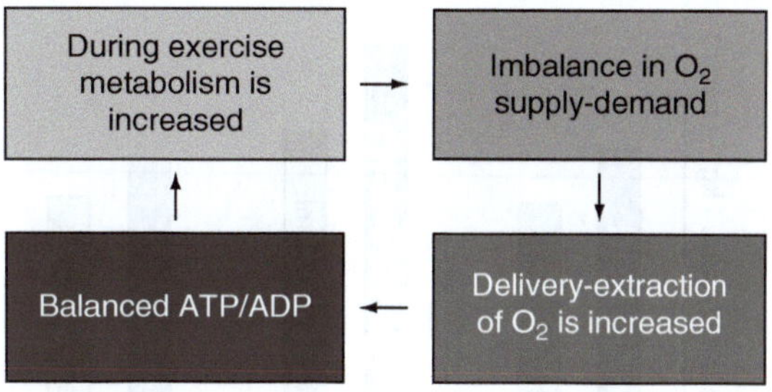

Fig. 1.3 Describes the changes in oxygen delivery-extraction during exercise. With increase in energy demand, an imbalance between oxygen supply and demand ensues. This in turn will increase oxygen delivery and extraction to keep balance between ATP and ADP

exposed. For example, in a person who has an extremely high fever approaching the level of lethality, the body metabolism increases to approximately 100% above normal; by comparison, the metabolism of the body during a marathon race increases to 2,000% above normal [12]. Humans are designed for motion basically by the muscles.

In comparison to other organs in the body, muscles are characterized by the ability to increase significantly its metabolic rate and their *oxygen uptake* (VO_2) in the range of 20–25-fold from resting values [13].

This VO_2 augmentation is in response to the increase in the need for ATP during exercise mainly for muscle contraction and the transport of various substances between cells. Thus, during exercise, there is a transformation of energy mediated by ATP which is a high-energy molecule from the chemical form into the mechanical one (Fig. 1.2).

Carbohydrates and *fatty acids* are the most important fuels for generating ATP in animal cells. In humans and animals, the metabolic processes at the muscle's cells depends on oxygen. During *aerobic exercise*, electrons from the chemical bonds of the fuel source combine with oxygen and hydrogen ions (H^+) to form water and carbon dioxide (CO_2). Cells couple this reaction to the production of ATP.

Humans have a high capacity to expend energy for many hours during sustained exercise. For example, one individual cycling at a speed of 26.4 km · h^{-1} across 8,204 km on 50 consecutive days may expend a total of 273,850 kcal with an average power output of 182.5 W [14]. Skeletal muscle burns 900.5 mmol of glucose each minute in repetitively extending the knee, generating ≈24 W of mechanical energy and, since muscle energy conversion is only 22–26% efficient, ≈76 W of heat energy. Resting skeletal muscle has a basal metabolic rate (resting energy consumption) of 0.63 W · kg^{-1} [15], making a 23-fold difference between the energy consumption of inactive muscle compared to active muscle. For short muscular exertion, energy expenditure can be far greater: an adult human male when jumping up from a squat mechanically generates 314 W · kg^{-1}. This energy expenditure is very large compared to the resting metabolism basal metabolic rate of the adult human body. This varies somewhat with size, gender, and age but is typically between 45 and 85 W. Total *energy expenditure* is very much higher and depends upon the average level of physical work and exercise mode during a day. Thus, exercise, particularly if sustained for very long periods, dominates the energy metabolism of the body. In order to keep the cell's physical and chemical balance, an exchange of molecules between intracellular fluid, extracellular fluid, and blood must be maintained at high rate. During *strenuous exercise*, the ability to keep the cell's ATP levels will depend mostly on supporting organs such as lung, heart, and oxygen extraction at the tissue level (Fig. 1.3).

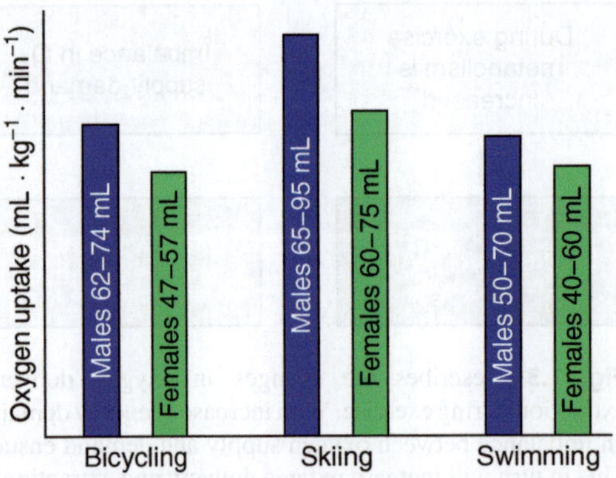

Fig. 1.4 Maximal oxygen uptake values for males and females during different sport activities

Exercise can give an estimation of the functional and work capacity of the body's different systems. In the broad sense, the ability to perform physical activity is defined by the following factors: (a) the ability to supply oxygen to the body, (b) the capacity of the metabolic system to utilize the oxygen to produce energy, (c) from the neuromuscular function including muscle strength, (d) coordination between nervous system and muscles or technique, (e) joint range of movement, and (f) psychological factor such as motivation and tactics. In different exercise conditions, one of these factors will dominant in the overall physical function. However, one has to keep in mind the mode of exercise performed, that is, with the presence of oxygen, *aerobic exercise*, or without enough oxygen, *anaerobic exercise* or *resistive effort* such as weightlifting. For example, during golf, where technique is essential, the energy cost is very low due to the nature of the activity.

To perform high jump, muscular strength and technique are crucial, while during long-distance running, oxygen supply and energy production rate will define performance (Fig. 1.4).

Therefore, the physiological changes needed during exercise must be well coordinated. Consequently, during exercise, significant increases in *cardiopulmonary system* and muscular functional capacity are noted to facilitate the increased metabolic demands, oxygen uptake, and carbon dioxide elimination. These physiological changes during aerobic exercise are so precise that it enables to evaluate the cardiopulmonary performance. At rest, oxygen demand is low, averaging 250 $mLO_2 \cdot min^{-1}$. During aerobic exercise, in order to maintain appropriate levels of ATP, the cardiopulmonary system increases its oxygen delivery up to 20–25-fold from resting values.

During anaerobic and resistive exercises, oxygen supply plays a minor role while the production of ATP relies heavily on anaerobic glycolysis which literally means the breakdown of glucose, that is, anaerobic metabolic pathway [16]. It is worth to point out that the heart and not skeletal muscle would be affected first by *anaerobic metabolism* since the heart is an aerobic organ with a very restricted anaerobic capacity [17].

Metabolism

Aerobic exercise is anything that involves or improves body's VO_2. Aerobic exercises increase metabolism because working muscles require additional calories to perform their tasks. Walking for 30 min a day will enhance metabolism slightly as this requires more calories than physical inactivity.

Aerobic exercises also slightly increase body's metabolism for a few hours after exercising. This increase in metabolism equals to almost 15% more calories than normal in the 48 h following effort. Thus, if an individual consumes 2,000 kcal/day by having three aerobic training sessions per week which adds 500 kcal a session then this individual could potentially burn an extra 3,600 kcal/week: 1,500 kcal from the three aerobic exercise sessions and an additional 300 kcal/day from the 15% post-workout increase. *Resistance training* also adds additional calories on top of the daily requirements during the workout by increasing muscle mass involved in the bout. Muscle tissue requires more calories to maintain its function than fat tissue. The difference is not huge; a kilo of muscle mass requires 13.25 kcal/day to maintain its function, while a kilo of fat tissue requires 4.4 kcal/day. Therefore, by performing regular resistance training and building muscle mass, it increases basal metabolic rate (BMR) and the overall amount of kcal utilized on a day-to-day basis. Both types of exercise are useful for increasing metabolism. Regular

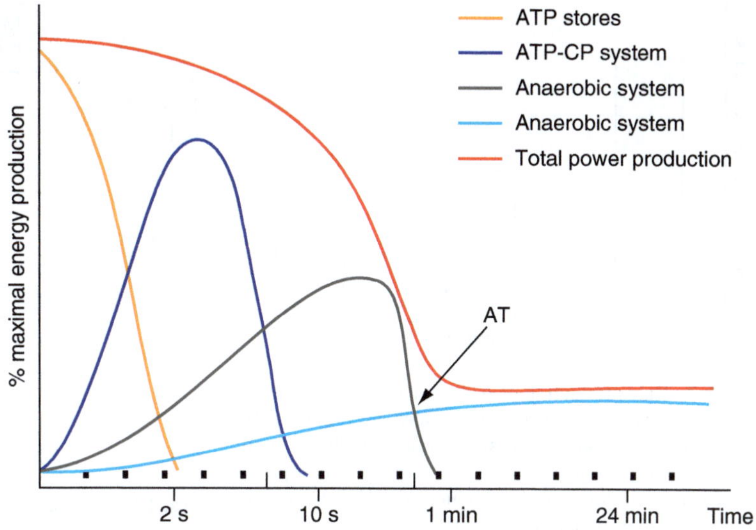

Fig. 1.5 Relative contribution of each energy pathway along time. At the anaerobic threshold (AT), the total energy required comes equally, from the anaerobic energy pathway 50% and 50% by the aerobic energy pathway

aerobic exercise increases the amount of calories used through physical activity while regular resistance training will increase lean muscle mass and therefore increase the number of calories used at rest. In combination, the two types of exercise can increase metabolism rate significantly.

During exercise, it is hard to discuss the *metabolic pathways* in absolute terms; the aerobic and anaerobic energy pathways do not work independently of one another. Though, the different metabolic pathways are independent as physiological systems, with tide relationships regarding energy supply and ATP production especially (Fig. 1.5). In most sport activities, the different metabolic pathways are well combined and coordinated to supply the amount energy needed. Thus, there are no anaerobic or aerobic efforts per se.

Because skeletal muscle is powered by one and only one compound, that is, ATP [18], and since the body stores only a small quantity of this ATP molecule within the cells and if for any reason, the energy system fails to supply chemical energy to regenerate ATP, then the amount of energy stored in ATP molecules can supply energy for 1 or 2 s.

However, this is not the usual case. The energy system in the body is very sensitive to the changes in ATP levels and regenerates them immediately to the needed levels at rest and during exercise [19]. Therefore, the body must replace or resynthesize ATP on an ongoing basis. Nevertheless, during exercise, the regeneration of ATP is immediate (Fig. 1.6). Whenever levels of ADP are higher than that of ATP, or when the ratio ATP/ADP is reduced, catabolism of glucose and fat starts in order to have energy to form ATP from ADP and *Pi* (inorganic phosphate). Every time that levels of ATP are higher than that of ADP, or when the ratio ATP/ADP is increased, anabolism of glucose and fat starts. The overall reaction of catabolism and anabolism is metabolism.

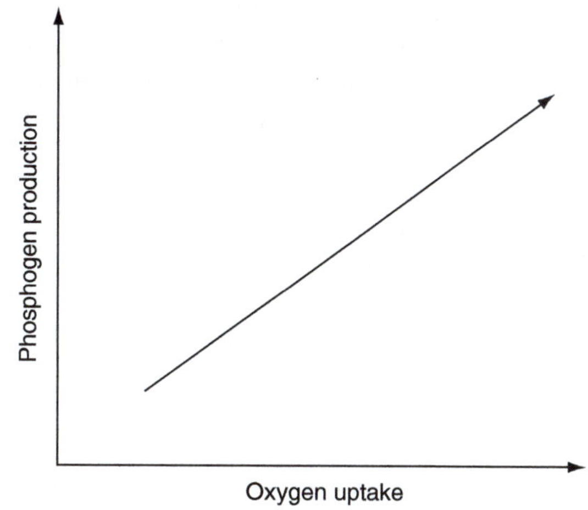

Fig. 1.6 There is a linear relationship between phosphogen production, CP, ADP, and ATP, and oxygen uptake during aerobic exercise

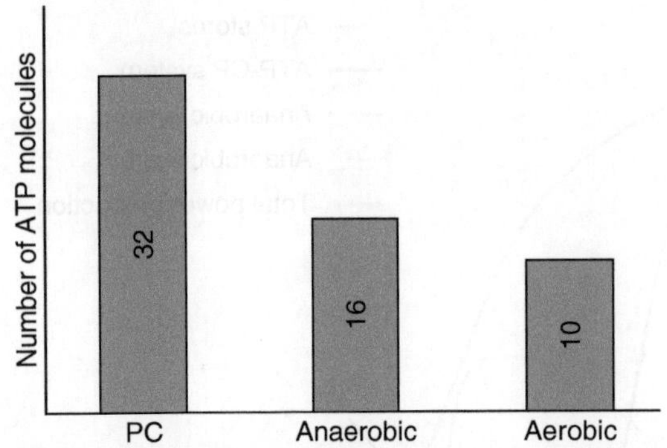

Fig. 1.7 Rate production of ATP molecules by the different metabolic pathways. Carbohydrates are broken down much faster than other fuels such as fats and thus provide quicker ATP for intense activity. The graph is comparing between the various energy production pathways and the amount of energy that they produce

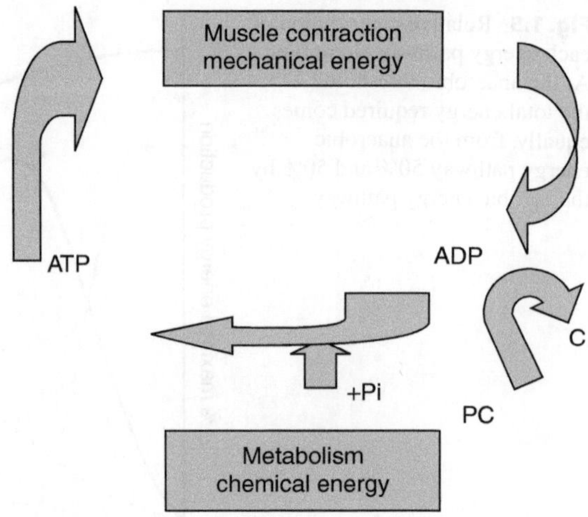

Fig. 1.8 ATP supply–demand balance of the muscle: the interplay between aerobic, anaerobic, and phosphogens for the production and utilization of ATP

The energy stored in any molecule with phosphates (phosphogen molecules) can be liberated each time that the phosphate is split from the molecule by means of enzymes or water. Such molecules are ATP, ADP, and PC (Eqs. 1.2, 1.3, and 1.4). Figure 1.7 shows that the ATP-PC system can generate energy at a rate of around 32 kcal · min^{-1} [20]:

$$\text{ATP} \rightarrow \text{ADP} + \text{ENERGY} \tag{1.2}$$

$$\text{ADP} + \text{PC} \rightarrow \text{ATP} + \text{C} \tag{1.3}$$

$$\text{ADP} + \text{ADP} \rightarrow \text{ATP} + \text{AMP} \tag{1.4}$$

PC is readily available to the cells and rapidly produces ATP. However, it exists in limited quantities. Splitting phosphate from ATP ends with muscle contraction (mechanical energy) while adding phosphate to ADP (chemical energy) is achieved from fuel catabolism (Fig. 1.8).

There are two types of anaerobic energy systems: (1) the high-energy phosphates, ATP and CP, and (2) *anaerobic glycolysis*. The high-energy phosphates are stored in very limited quantities within muscle cells. Anaerobic glycolysis exclusively uses glucose and glycogen as a fuel in the absence of oxygen or, more specifically, when ATP is needed at rates that exceed those provided by *aerobic metabolism*; the consequence of rapid glucose breakdown is the formation of lactic acid at biological pH levels. Physical activities that last up to about 30 s rely primarily on the former, ATP-PC *phosphagen* system. Beyond this time, both aerobic and anaerobic glycolytic metabolic systems begin to predominate. The by-product of anaerobic glycolysis, *lactic acid*, was traditionally thought to be detrimental to muscle function. However, this appears likely only when lactic acid levels are very high. In reality, many changes occur within and around muscle cells during intense exercise that can lead to fatigue, with elevated lactic acid levels being only one (fatigue that is muscular failure is a complex subject). Elevated muscle and blood lactic acid concentrations are a natural consequence of physical exertion, regardless of what form it takes: easy, moderate, hard, or severe. The effectiveness of anaerobic activity can be improved through training.

The capacity to generate power by each of the three energy systems can vary with training. The ATP-PC and glycolytic pathways may change by only 10–20% with training. The oxidative system seems to be far more trainable, although genetics play a limiting role here.

Carbohydrates (sugars and starches) are the most efficient source of energy, with the primary role to provide energy to cells in the body, particularly the brain, which is the only carbohydrate-dependent organ in the body. During strenuous *aerobic exercise* when oxygen supply is restricted, the catabolism of carbohydrates starts since the breakdown efficacy of carbohydrates in the utilization of oxygen yields 100%, while the breakdown efficacy of fat in the utilization of oxygen yields 90%. Thus, from the physiological stand point when oxygen supply is short, such as during strenuous exercise, the main source for energy will be the breakdown of carbohydrates. Anaerobic glycolysis can generate energy for a short time only, half as quickly at about 16 kcal · min^{-1} compared to the ATP-PC system, while the aerobic system has the lowest rate of about 10 kcal · min^{-1}. The energy stored in any molecule with phosphates (phosphogen molecules) can be liberated each time that the phosphate is split from the molecule by means of enzymes or water. Such molecules are ATP, ADP, and PC (Eqs. 1.2, 1.3, and 1.4). Figure 1.7 shows that the ATP-PC system can generate energy at a rate of around 32 kcal · min^{-1} [20].

In contrary, during light aerobic exercise when enough oxygen is available, the main source for energy is fat. In addition to fat and carbohydrates, proteins can be also source for energy. However, that will happen under extreme conditions: long fast or prolonged exercise lasting above 4 h [4]. It can be converted in the Cori cycle either into glucose or into other intermediates as alanine (Fig. 1.9), both used by the Krebs cycle such as acetyl coenzyme A. Protein might compose a more significant contribution during very prolonged activity, perhaps as much as 18% of total energy requirements [20]. A great deal can be understood about animal metabolism by comparing the VO_2 utilized by an organism to the volume of VCO_2 produced. The ratio VCO_2/VO_2 enables the assessment of important physiological indices, such as oxidation rate of energy substrate and energy expenditure [21], and the combination of the energy source being utilized: fat, carbohydrates, and protein.

The amount of oxygen needed to produce energy from the breakdown of glucose molecule is different from that of fat and protein. This is for the reason that the content of carbon and oxygen in carbohydrate, fat, and protein differ significantly.

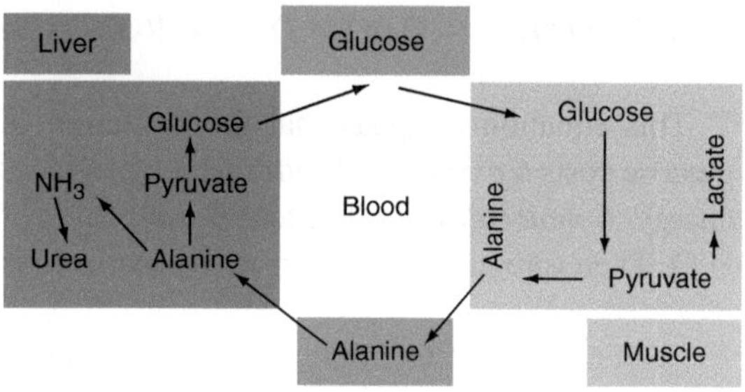

Fig. 1.9 Alanine released from the active muscle resynthesize glucose in the liver. This gluconeogenic process increases the limited carbohydrates reserve in the muscles and blood. The alanine cycle is less productive than the Cori cycle, which uses lactate, since a by-product of energy production from alanine is production of urea. Removal of the urea is energy-dependent, requiring four "high-energy" phosphate bonds; thus, the net ATP produced is less than that found in the Cori cycle

Glycolysis is the pathway by which glycogen and glucose are converted to two pyruvate molecules. In the presence of oxygen, pyruvate enters the Krebs cycle via acetyl COA.

Each turn of the Krebs cycle produces H^+ carriers that enter the electron transport chain and ultimately donate H^+ to oxygen to form water, allowing the electron transport chain to proceed to ATP. However, when oxygen is not present, the electron transport chain cannot proceed which prevents flux through the Krebs cycle and results in a buildup of pyruvate. If this was allowed to continue then glycolysis would stop, and no further ATP would be resynthesized. Fortunately, pyruvate can accept the H^+ carrier, forming *lactic acid* via lactate dehydrogenase. The conversion of *glycogen* to lactic acid yields only 3 mol ATP per molecule of glycogen, but this can occur in the absence of oxygen, and the maximum rate of glycolysis can be reached within a few seconds from the onset of exercise. In contrast, complete breakdown of glycogen via glycolysis, the Krebs cycle, and the electron transport chain yields 39 ATP per molecule of glycogen. When utilizing *glucose*, the efficiency is 100% since the respiratory exchange ratio is 1 as seen in the next equations (Eqs. 1.5 and 1.6):

$$C_6H_{12}O_6 + 6O_2 \rightarrow 6CO_2 + 6H_2O + \text{ENERGY} \quad (1.5)$$

This equation suggests that the oxidation of glucose costs *6 oxygen molecules* which produces energy, *6 molecules* of CO_2, and 6 molecules of H_2O. Therefore, the *respiratory exchange ratio* is

$$6CO_2 / 6O_2 = 1 \quad (1.6)$$

Fatty acids are more energy dense than glycogen, and there are very large stores of fat in adipose tissue. In fact, if all of the energy stored as fat were stored as glycogen, body mass would increase by ~50 kg. *Fatty acids* are catabolized via β-oxidation and then entry to the Krebs cycle and the electron transport chain. If it is fully oxidized, a typical fat (Palmitate) yields 129 molecules of ATP. Given that stores of *fat* in the body are so vast, they would allow exercise at a maximal intensity (i.e., sprinting) to continue for more than 1 h. However, the rate of ATP resynthesis from fat is too slow to be of great importance during high-intensity activity. Therefore, although fat is the preferred substrate and dominates the energy contribution to resting metabolism, *carbohydrate* stores are available when energy requirements increase, for example, at the onset of exercise. As exercise continues, however, fat metabolism may become more important, particularly if muscle glycogen stores become depleted.

Traditionally, *protein* is not considered to contribute to energy provision except under conditions of starvation or in ultra-endurance events. This is unsurprising on the basis that most of the protein in the body is functional in nature, for example, contractile proteins in skeletal muscle.

The respiratory exchange ratio with the oxidation of *fat* will be approximately 0.7 as suggested by the following equation (Eqs. 1.7 and 1.8):

$$C_{15}H_{31}COOH \rightarrow 16CO_2 + 16H_2O + \text{ENERGY} \quad (1.7)$$

This equation suggests that the oxidation of fat costs *23 oxygen molecules* which produce energy, *16 molecules of CO_2*, and 16 molecules of H_2O. Therefore, the respiratory exchange ratio is 0.7:

$$16CO_2/23O_2 = 0.7 \quad (1.8)$$

Calculating the respiratory exchange ratio of *protein* reveals mean ratio of 0.82.

Both the aerobic and anaerobic energy pathways make a contribution to produce ATP molecules; however, one will usually predominate [13]. For that reason, it is more appropriate to consider the metabolic pathways as a continuous combination of energy supply sources. Figure 1.10 shows how much (percentage) each of the metabolic pathways aerobic and anaerobic contributes to meet the energy demands during different duration of physical activity.

Metabolism of the Myocardium

The *myocardium* is adapted to be highly resistant to fatigue: It has a large number of mitochondria, enabling continuous aerobic respiration via oxidative phosphorylation, numerous myoglobins, and a good blood supply, which provides nutrients and oxygen. The myocardium is so tuned to aerobic metabolism that it is unable to pump sufficiently in ischemic conditions. At basal metabolic rates, about 1% of energy is derived from anaerobic metabolism. This can increase to 10% under moderately hypoxic conditions, but under more severe hypoxic conditions, not enough energy can be liberated by lactic acid production to sustain ventricular contractions [22]. Under basal aerobic conditions, the majority of energy comes from *free fatty acids* and *triglycerides*, and the rest comes from carbohydrates. However, these proportions vary widely according to nutritional state. For example, during starvation, *lactic acid* can be recycled by the heart. This is very energy efficient, because one *NAD^+* is reduced to NADH and H^+ (equal to 3 ATP molecules) when lactic acid is oxidized to pyruvate, which can then be consumed aerobically in the Krebs cycle, liberating much more energy. In the condition of diabetes, more fat and less carbohydrate are used due to the reduced induction of *GLUT4* glucose transporters to the cell surfaces. Therefore, contraction itself plays a part in bringing GLUT4 transporters to the surface [23]. This is true of skeletal muscle as well, but relevant in particular to cardiac muscle due to its continuous contractions.

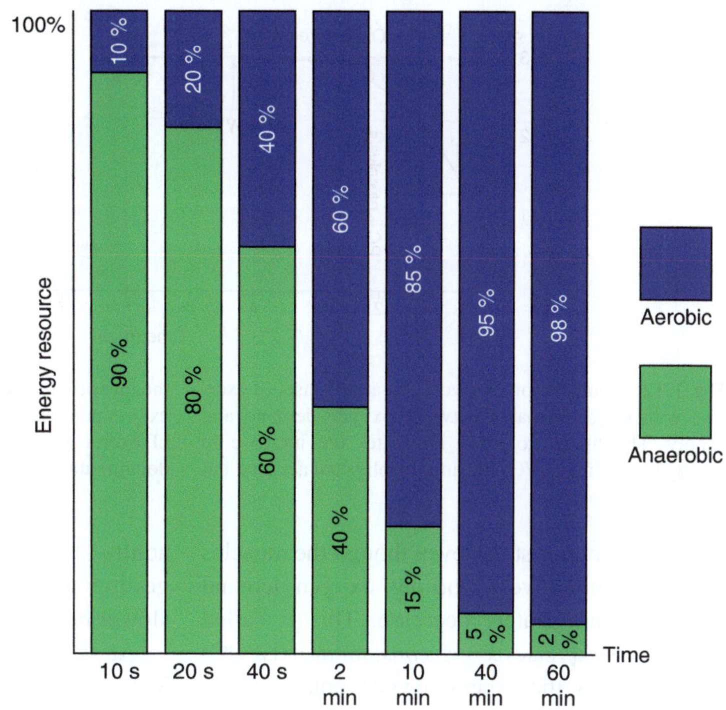

Fig. 1.10 Percentage contributed by each metabolic pathway during different length of physical activity

Interplay Between Aerobic and Anaerobic Pathways

Figure 1.11 shows some examples of sports events and how each of the metabolic pathways contributes to meet the physical stress imposed [19]. The factor that coordinates between the aerobic and anaerobic pathways is oxygen availability. In the occasion that the cardiopulmonary keeps up with the body's *oxygen demand*, the aerobic metabolic pathway will dominate and vice versa. The contribution of each pathway depends on the mode, duration, and intensity of the exercise.

Although *heart rate* increases rapidly with the onset of activity, providing exercise intensity remains constant, heart rate will level off. This is known as *steady-state* heart rate where the demands of the active tissues can be adequately met by the *cardiopulmonary system*. However, there is an exception to this.

With the onset of constant aerobic exercises for few minutes, the anaerobic energy systems (ATP-CP and glycolysis) supply the basic needed *ATP* for this effort. The energy provided during this deficit phase of exercise is employed until the cardiopulmonary system delivers more oxygen by increasing heart rate, stroke volume, and minute ventilation. At this phase, a *steady state* is reached, indicating that mitochondrial respiration is the dominant energy system being utilized (Fig. 1.12).

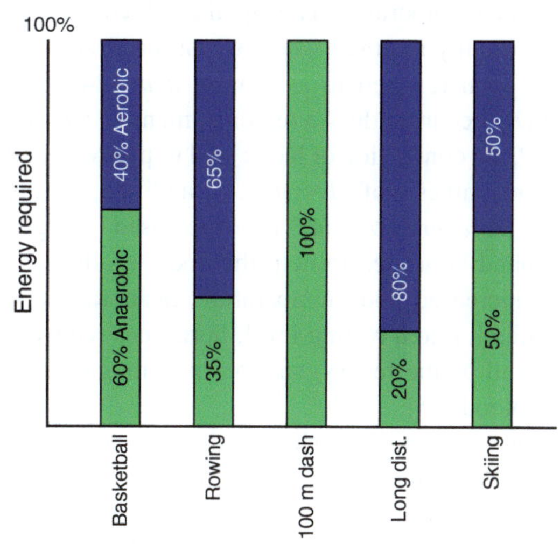

Fig. 1.11 Contribution of each metabolic pathway during various sports activities. The shorter the activity, the more is the reliance on the anaerobic pathway

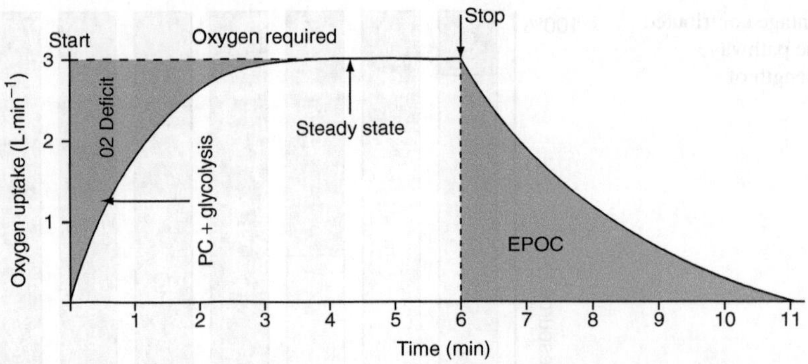

Fig. 1.12 Contribution of glycolysis at the onset of exercise with large mismatch between oxygen demand and supply. The figure not only illustrates the increase in energy expenditure (VO_2) during the physical activity, but the increase in energy expenditure in recovery. The EPOC, excess post-exercise VO_2, depends more on the intensity of exercise than the duration of exercise and has been documented to last up to 24 h after exercise

When exercise stops, even though the muscles are no longer actively working, oxygen demand does not immediately decrease. This is called *excess post-exercise oxygen consumption* (EPOC) which defines the excess oxygen uptake above the resting level in recovery. Instead, VO_2 remains elevated temporarily. This uptake, which exceeds that usually required when at rest, has traditionally been referred to as *oxygen debt* [24]. The *EPOC* occurred due to replenishment of *CP* and *ATP*, the conversion of lactic acid to pyruvate and the resynthesis of glycogen. In addition, during this *recovery period*, the increased oxygen demand is needed to help the body in adjusting the increased body temperature, heart rate, and ventilation to a resting level, hormones recovery as well as the re-oxygenation of hemoglobin in the blood [25].

In young adults, whether the slower oxygen kinetics are due to a slower delivery of oxygen to working muscle or a delayed activation or slowing of the metabolic processes of oxidative phosphorylation remains unclear [26]. However, Mizuno et al. [27] reported in healthy young adults that perfusion was well matched to metabolism in five areas of the quadriceps muscles during rest and recovery from exhaustive exercise. Contribution levels of glycolysis during the onset of exercise depends upon whether the load brings about a large mismatch between VO_2 and delivery; thus, the Krebs cycle cannot produce aerobically enough ATP molecules required. In older adults, slower heart rate kinetics is observed, suggesting that oxygen delivery adaptation to the slower heart rate may be limited [28].

At *the steady-state* phase and up to 50% of VO_{2max}, ATP is achieved mainly via the aerobic metabolic pathway, and thus, water and CO_2 are the end products of carbohydrates and fat. Also, at the steady-state phase glycolysis still provides ATP in small quantities and lactic acid from carbohydrates breakdown. At this stage, part of the lactic acid is transformed in the *Cori cycle* to glucose, and part of it is utilized by the myocardium to produce ATP. Above approximately 50% of VO_{2max} and until VO_{2max} is reached, more and more the anaerobic pathway becomes dominant since the cardiopulmonary cannot supply the oxygen required.

Lactic Acid Threshold

Accurately measuring the *lactic acid threshold* involves taking blood samples from the pinprick, finger, earlobe, or thumb during an incremental test where the exercise intensity is progressively increased. Measuring the threshold can also be performed noninvasively using gas-exchange (respiratory quotient) methods, which requires a metabolic cart to measure air inspired and expired. Although the lactic acid threshold is defined as the point when lactic acid starts to accumulate, some testers approximate this by using the point at which lactic acid reaches a concentration of

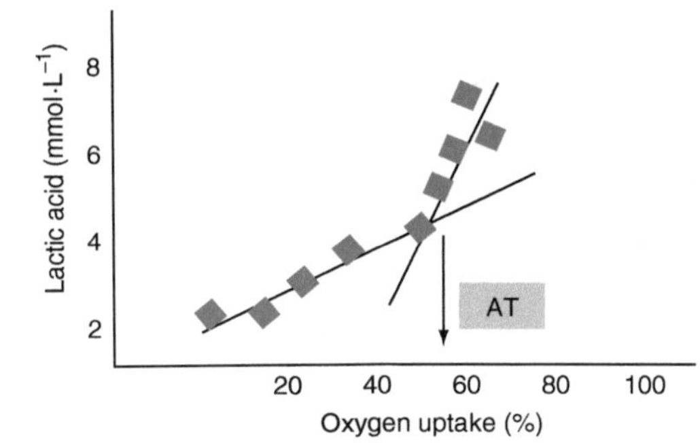

Fig. 1.13 Description of blood lactic acid response to exercise as a function of oxygen uptake percentage. The anaerobic threshold (AT) indicates the onset of significant anaerobic metabolism and the increase in the production of lactic acid, which occurs in sedentary individuals at approximately 45–55% of maximal oxygen uptake

4 mmol · L^{-1} (at rest, blood lactic acid is about 1.0–1.5 mmol · L^{-1}). The lactic acid threshold is the exercise intensity at which lactic acid starts to accumulate in the blood stream. This happens when lactic acid is produced faster than it can be removed (metabolized). This point is sometimes referred to as the *lactic acid threshold*, AT, or the onset of blood lactate accumulation (OBLA). At this stage, the body accommodates by increasing glycolysis. However, glycolysis becomes limited by the fact that it cannot shuttle the NADH+H+ (from Step 6 of glycolysis) through the mitochondrial membrane.

Figure 1.13 describes the AT and OBLA; as exercise intensity increases, a point is reached where the body begins to accumulate more lactic acid in the blood stream. The reason for the acidification of the blood at strenuous exercise intensities is twofold: The muscle releases H^+ ions, as they are co-transported out of the muscle into the blood via the monocarboxylate transporter due to the high rates of ATP hydrolysis, and also bicarbonate stores in the blood begin to be used up. This happens when lactic acid is produced faster than it can be eliminated. During this demanding exercise, mitochondrial respiration is unable to keep up with the pace of the oxygen demand.

When exercising below the AT intensity, any lactic acid produced by the muscles is removed by the body without it building up. The AT is a useful measure for deciding exercise intensity for training and racing in endurance sports, such as long-distance running, cycling, rowing, swimming, and cross-country skiing, but varies between individuals and can be increased with training. Interval training takes advantage of the body being able to temporarily exceed the AT and then recover by reducing blood lactic acid while operating below the threshold and while still doing physical activity. Fartlek training and interval training are similar, the main difference being the structure of the exercise. Interval training can take the form of many different types of exercise and should closely replicate the movements found in the sport.

Therefore, pyruvate reacts in the cytoplasm with NADH+H+ to form lactic acid, which begins to accumulate in the blood. The intensity at the lactic acid threshold represents the maximal intensity at which steady-state exercise can be maintained.

Training the lactic acid threshold is similar to training for strength. The body adapts to stress overload placed upon it by becoming more efficient. To stress the body to cause an increase in efficiency, the individual needs to increase the lactic acid above that which individual can tolerate. This is done in training by exercising at a high intensity for several short periods and recovering between hard bouts, allowing excess *lactic acid* to clear the muscle. A proper mix of hard efforts with short recovery, and some medium hard efforts with longer recovery, will raise both the lactic acid threshold and the VO_{2max}. Aerobic training is known to increase the size and number of mitochondria in active muscle and increase ability to VO_2 proportionately, that is, mitochondrial density in the muscle is proportional to VO_{2max} (Fig. 1.14). In addition, while training the aerobic energy system, the individual will also be training the phosphagen and glycolytic system [21].

Other ways for the elimination of lactic acid during aerobic exercise are: (a) its utilization by the myocardium which is rich with mitochondria and is an aerobic organ, and (b) through the *Cori cycle* that converts lactic acid to glucose in the liver (Fig. 1.15).

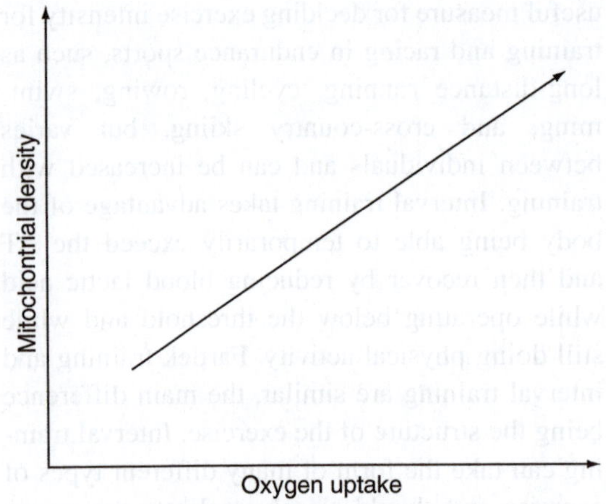

Fig. 1.14 Exercise training can improve exercise capacity (VO_2) by increasing mitochondrial density since oxygen uptake is proportional to the number of mitochondria in active muscles

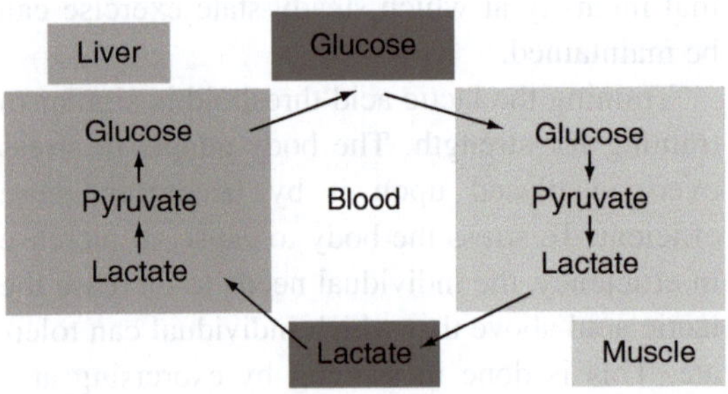

Fig. 1.15 Lactic acid released from the active muscle resynthesizes glucose in the liver. This gluconeogenic process increases the limited carbohydrate reserve in the muscles and blood. The Cori cycle involve the utilization of lactic acid, produced by glycolysis in non-hepatic tissues, such as muscle as a carbon source for hepatic gluconeogenesis. In this way, the liver can convert the anaerobic by-product of glycolysis, lactic acid, back into more glucose for reuse by non-hepatic tissues

Gender Differences in Oxygen Extraction

In general, the exercise-related measurements established for women follow the same general principles as those established for men, except for the quantitative differences caused by differences in body size, body composition, and levels of testosterone. In women, the values of muscle strength, pulmonary ventilation, and cardiac output (all variables related with muscle mass) are generally 60–75% of the exercise physiology values recorded in men. When measured in terms of strength per square centimeter, the female muscle can achieve the same force of contraction as that of a male.

During strenuous exercise that genders a significant lactic acidosis, oxygen uptake continues to rise until exercise is terminated, or exhaustion ensues [29]. In healthy subjects, it has been found that during aerobic exercise, VO_2 of male exceeds that of female due to gender-related variance in heart size [30, 31]. Mean values for VO_2 in children, adolescents, and adults are consistently greater in males than females (Fig. 1.16), whether VO_2 is expressed in absolute terms or relative to body mass [32]. Factors linked mainly to oxygen-carrying capacity and cardiac size have been shown to contribute significantly to this gender-related difference [33].

The mechanism that facilitates oxygen extraction by males is due to the different skeletal muscle fiber recruitment patterns [33]. Males have larger skeletal muscle fibers than females but similar fiber composition, influencing metabolism and the adaptive response to exercise [34]. The mechanism that enables the females to increase their oxygen extraction during exercise is the lower velocity of contraction by skeletal muscles [26]. From in vitro studies, it has been observed that at low contraction velocities, the

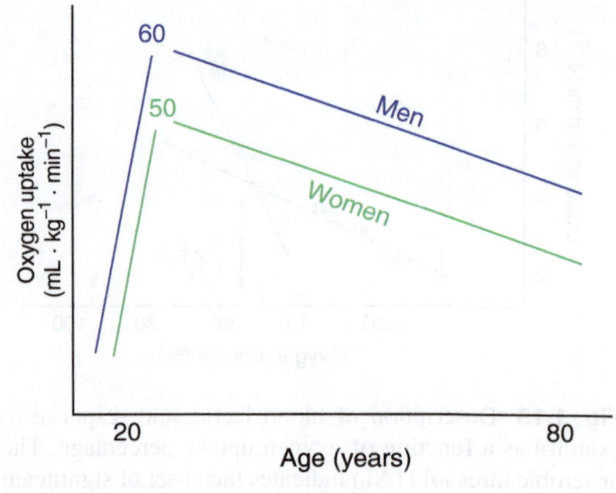

Fig. 1.16 Maximum oxygen uptake increases to age of 20–25 years and decreases thereafter. Maximal oxygen uptake in children, adolescents, and adults are consistently greater in males than females

efficiency of slow twitch fibers is higher than of fast twitch fibers, and the reverse is observed at high speeds [26, 35]. *Cardiopulmonary* responses (delivery) and metabolic (oxygen extraction) responses during incremental exercise differ between men, women, adolescents, and elderly despite a relatively similar fitness [18].

During the period of adolescence, many structural, hormonal, biochemical, and physiological changes take place that interfere with the oxygen delivery and extraction relationship [36]. As a consequence, at peak aerobic test that creates a significant lactic acidosis [37], *left ventricular contractility* and function in healthy adolescent subjects may be altered. The intracellular accumulation of Na+ and Ca2+ plays a key role in ischemia-induced myocardial injury that may be manifested as left ventricular mechanical dysfunction, dysrhythmias, or infarction. ATP hydrolysis produces H+, and the resulting intracellular acidosis directly impairs left ventricular contractility. However, it is the accumulation of intracellular H+ and the activation of N+ –dependent pH regulatory mechanisms. Intracellular Na+ accumulation causes Ca2+ overload and further left ventricular mechanical dysfunction [38, 39].

Metabolic Demands in Diverse Populations

Since metabolic demands during incremental exercise are increased over time, diverse populations may have different rate of reaction for energy supply between oxygen delivery and extraction [31]. With the onset of exercise blood plasma volume decreases due to the increase in blood pressure and changes in intramuscular osmotic pressures, forcing water from the vascular compartment to the interstitial space. However, this reduced plasma volume in turn increases the concentration of hemoglobin. Although no extra red blood cells have been produced, the greater concentration of hemoglobin per unit of blood significantly increases the blood's oxygen-carrying capacity. Even though oxygen delivery to the working muscle may be reduced and since metabolic demand during incremental exercise is increased over time to maximum, these populations may maintain the energy supply due to the balance between oxygen delivery and extraction.

At rest conditions, the oxygen content of blood varies from about 20 $mLO_2 \cdot dL^{-1}$ of arterial blood to 16–17 $mLO_2 \cdot dL^{-1}$ of venous blood [7]. As exercise intensity increases, the $(a\text{-}v)O_2$ also increases, and at maximal exertion, the difference between arterial and venous blood oxygen content can be three times that at a resting level.

The Cardiovascular System

The cardiovascular system (Fig. 1.17) provides for the transport and exchange of gases, ions and electrolytes, hormones, nutrients, fluids, antigens, cells, and other biological elements moved by the blood among the different organs of the body. The force that moves the blood through a complicated network of blood vessels is generated by the heart. The myocardium is innervated by the autonomic nervous system, both sympathetic and parasympathetic nerve fibers. *During exercise*, precise regulatory mechanisms are required to allow the cardiopulmonary system to adjust to the metabolic demands of the skeletal muscles and myocardium. The extent to which other regulatory reflexes, such as vestibular-autonomic reflexes, are able to impact upon the cardiovascular and respiratory systems during exercise is largely unknown.

The heart controls the movement of oxygenated and non-oxygenated blood throughout the body, including the heart itself. The circulatory system is a closed-loop and flexible system, flow through the circulatory system is the result of pressure differences between the two ends of the system, the left ventricle with 90 mmHg and the right atrium which is approximately 0 mmHg.

The heart is able to increase its functional capacity in response to the wide range of demands made by the body especially during exercise, and to supply blood to the organs, thus meeting the body's metabolic needs. The limits of adaptation by the heart to constantly changing bodily

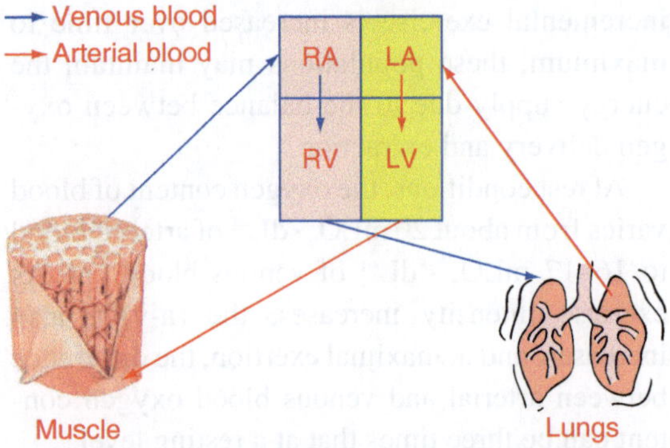

Fig. 1.17 The cardiopulmonary system consists of the heart, pulmonary, and skeletal muscles; it is a closed-circuit vessels. The red vessels are rich with oxygen (*red arrows*), while the *blue ones* are deoxygenated and with carbon dioxide. *RA* right atrial, *LA* left atrial, *RV* right ventricular, *LV* left ventricular

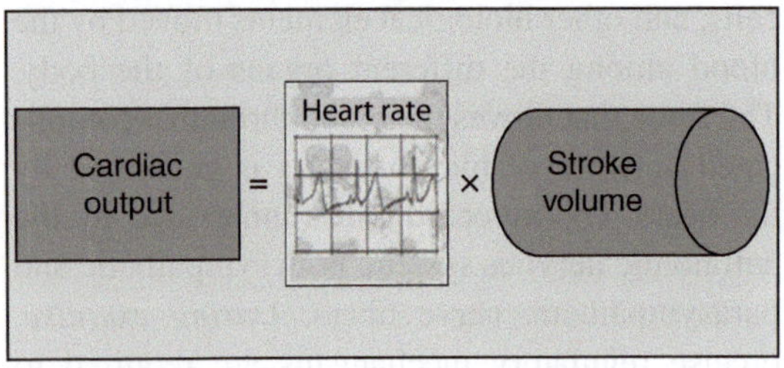

Fig. 1.18 Cardiac output is the sum of heart rate multiplied by stroke volume

demands range from very low, such as during sleep, up to maximal demand during maximal aerobic exercise.

Metabolic demands force the heart to increase blood supply, that is, *cardiac output* to the body by increasing its beats per minute (heart rate) and by increasing the force of cardiac contraction which in turn increases the amount of blood ejected by the ventricles each beat (stroke volume). Cardiac output is the amount of blood ejected by one of the ventricles in 1 min (Fig. 1.18). Thus, increasing either *heart rate* or *stroke volume* increases cardiac output.

Effects attributable to *angiotensin II* may involve the regulation of body fluid balance via increased aldosterone secretion. This in turn results in retention of Na+ and water, leading to increased venous return, larger end diastolic volume, and subsequently to increased stroke volume due to the Starling's law. There is also evidence that the angiotensin-converting enzyme (*ACE*) D allele is associated with ventricular hypertrophy [40] and left ventricular mass of athletes [41].

The vascular system is a special, unusual, and complicated *hydraulic system*. It has a number of features that are unique when compared to other hydraulic systems:

- It is *a* system that expends *during exercise*.
- The system is filled by fluid along with positive pressure, independent of cardiac contraction activity.
- The ventricles are largely filled (up to 80%) passively without any energy cost. The other 20% is done actively by the atriums. *During exercise*, these 20% are decreased.
- Due to this passive filling, the heart is regulated mainly by peripheral factors and the skeletal muscles especially during exercise.
- Blood flow to the aorta and pulmonary arteries are non-consecutive, while because of the aorta function, blood is pumped to the body and returns to the heart consecutively.
- *Exercise* is the most *potent trigger* for increasing *cardiac output* to its maximal level.
- Arterial blood pressure is regulated independently of cardiac and local blood flow regulation.

Exercise places an increased demand on the cardiovascular system. Oxygen demand by the muscles increases sharply. Metabolic processes speed up, and more waste is created. More nutrients are used, and body temperature rises. In order to perform as efficiently as possible, the cardiovascular system must regulate these changes and meet the body's increasing demands [9].

The *cardiopulmonary system* acts as an integral unit. It is composed of two main parts: a muscular pump (the heart), which generates force to propel blood throughout the system, and the circulatory system made up of a systemic circuit comprised of multiple (parallel) pathways, each with its own local control or autoregulation mechanism, plus pulmonary circulation.

Coronary Artery Disease

Coronary heart disease, also called *coronary artery disease*, is a condition in which plaque builds up inside the coronary arteries. These arteries supply oxygen-rich blood to the myocardium. Plaque is made up of fat, cholesterol, calcium, and other substances found in the blood. When plaque builds up in the arteries, the condition is called *atherosclerosis*. The buildup of plaque occurs over many years. If the flow of oxygen-rich blood to the heart muscle is reduced or blocked, angina or a heart attack may occur. Over time, coronary artery disease can weaken the myocardium and lead to heart failure and arrhythmias. Heart failure is a condition in which the heart cannot pump enough blood to meet the body's needs. Arrhythmias are problems with the rate or rhythm of the heartbeat. This has negative consequences on the heart performance especially during exercise, that is, reduced *cardiac output*, increased *heart rate*, and *left ventricular* dysfunction. Therefore, it has been suggested to exercise coronary artery disease patients to gain benefits following exercise training as seen in normal subjects.

Physical inactivity is recognized as a risk factor for coronary artery disease. Regular aerobic physical activity increases exercise capacity and plays a role in primary and secondary prevention of cardiovascular disease [42]. Exercise training increases cardiovascular functional capacity and decreases *myocardial oxygen demand* at any level of physical activity in apparently healthy persons as well as in most subjects with cardiovascular disease. Regular physical activity is required to maintain these training effects. The potential risk of physical activity can be reduced by medical evaluation, risk stratification, and supervision [43].

Exercise training is a useful therapeutic intervention for most normal, untrained adults and for many coronary artery disease patients with established cardiovascular disease. Participation in the rehabilitation program requires a rational selection and evaluation of patients combined with an understanding of exercise physiology and anticipated responses to training. *Physical activity* can improve heart's and body's fitness level and hence health. Physical activity is the cornerstone of a good cardiac rehabilitation program. A structured or prescribed aerobic program, regularly followed, has been shown to reduce the incidence of coronary disease, increase the quality of living, and probably reduce the incidence of further heart attacks in the postcoronary patient. The following are the benefits of exercising regularly in patients with *coronary artery disease*: reduces or eliminates the risk of future heart diseases, improves heart *left ventricular contractility* and function, reduces blood pressure, reduces lipids and cholesterol levels in the blood leading to weight loss, improves diabetic patient's cardiopulmonary function, improves management of stress, improves physical fitness and energy levels, and thus, increases ability to perform higher workloads.

Mitochondrial Changes in Skeletal Muscle

In order to decrease the heart work, the skeletal muscles has to increase the $(a\text{-}v)O_2$, meaning by improving the muscle's ability to extract more oxygen from the blood delivered. On the other hand, the high prevalence of skeletal muscle atrophy and its relation to exercise intolerance and abnormal muscle metabolism in patients with heart failure suggest that patients with chronic heart failure frequently develop significant skeletal muscle atrophy and metabolic abnormalities. Atrophy contributes modestly to both the reduced exercise capacity and altered muscle metabolism [18].

Skeletal muscle adapts to endurance exercise such as long-distance running, with an increase in the capacity for aerobic metabolism. Muscle and energy system metabolism is the sum of all the chemical reactions that occur within the muscle. Each bout of contractile activity results in a coordinated alteration in the expression of a variety of nuclear deoxyribonucleic acid (DNA) and mitochondrial DNA (mtDNA) gene products, leading to phenotypic adaptations. This is reflected in an increased capacity of whole homogenates and of the mitochondrial fraction of muscle to oxidize pyruvate and long chain fatty acids. This is the result of an increase in muscle mitochondrial volume and changes in organelle composition, referred to as mitochondrial biogenesis. The functional consequence of this biogenesis is an improved increase in *mitochondria* size and number in the muscle cells [44]. These changes in mitochondrial volume and size bring to an increase in the levels of a number of mitochondrial enzymes. These include the enzymes involved in fatty acid oxidation, the enzymes of the citric acid cycle (Krebs cycle), and the components of the respiratory chain that link the oxidation of succinate and NADH to oxygen. An alteration in mitochondrial composition also occurs, with some mitochondrial enzymes increasing twofold. As a result of these and other exercise-induced biochemical adaptations, skeletal muscle tends to become more like heart muscle in its enzyme pattern, that is, more aerobically. This will increase oxygen demand and may partly explain the observed elevation in whole body VO_2 during aerobic exercise [45].

Other factor affecting oxygen extraction by the muscle is the increase of capillary density in the muscle after exercise training, which is probably due to the angiogenic response to training in human skeletal muscle [46]. The third factor is the increased levels of *myoglobin* of the muscle following physical training [47]. Myoglobin is a compound that helps in the storage and transport of oxygen within the muscle cell.

These three factors facilitate the transfer of oxygen from the red blood cells in capillary to the muscle's cell. At rest, alveolar oxygen partial pressure equals to 100 mmHg, while venous blood oxygen partial pressure is 40 mmHg; thus, the pressure gradient is 60 mmHg. In addition, at rest, cardiac output is low, and therefore blood flow is slow. This pressure gradient and the slow blood flow are sufficient to oxygenate 97–98% of the red blood cells leaving the lung. The slow blood flow allows enough time to unload oxygen from the capillary's red blood cells to the muscle cell. Though, *during exercise*, the increase in *cardiac output* and thus blood flow speed are so significant that it interferes with the oxygen unloading to the muscle, that is, there is not enough time and gradient pressure to unload the oxygen. But the increase in mitochondrial size and number, capillaries' number, and myoglobin compensate for this oxygen-unloading interference to the muscle since the oxygen molecule is engulfed by these three factors. The end result is increased $(a\text{-}v)O_2$, and thus, based on the Fick equation, it will reduce heart rate.

The Fick Equation

The *Fick equation* is a mathematical estimation of an athlete's theoretical maximal oxygen uptake. Understanding the individual components that comprise VO_{2max} can help to determine the specific types of workouts to focus on to increase this important training variable. Although the scope of this book is the cardiopulmonary function, it is inevitable to discuss in brief the role of the skeletal muscles with regard to the cardiac function. The Fick equation states that VO_{2max} equals the amount of blood pumped per heart beat at maximum heart rate times the amount of oxygen the working muscles are able to extract from the blood passing through them. The maximal heart rate times the volume of blood pumped per beat is referred to as maximal cardiac output.

During exercise, the $(a\text{-}v)O_2$ by working muscles can decrease or increase heart rate. This extraction can be measured by subtracting venous oxygen content from arterial oxygen content. Fick equation shows that VO_2 is the product of cardiac output and $(a\text{-}v)O_2$ (Eq. 1.9):

$$VO_2 = Q(a - v)O_2, \qquad (1.9)$$

where VO_2 = oxygen uptake, Q = cardiac output, and $(a\text{-}v)O_2$ = arteriovenous oxygen content difference.

And since cardiac output is the product of heart rate and stroke volume, the above equation (Eq. 1.9) can be rearranged (Eq. 1.10) as follows:

$$VO_2 = (SV \cdot HR)(a - v)O_2, \qquad (1.10)$$

where VO_2 = oxygen uptake, HR = heart rate, SV = stroke volume, and $(a\text{-}v)O_2$ = arteriovenous oxygen content difference.

Therefore, any increase in $(a\text{-}v)O_2$ extracted by the muscles will end in a reduction of heart rate. The muscles can further increase its $(a\text{-}v)O_2$ by a dynamic aerobic exercise training program that produces anatomical and biochemical changes in the muscles. This is why, for a given workload, heart rate will be lower in trained individual compared to untrained individuals.

Efforts at Altitude

Under stress condition such as altitude compared to conditions at sea level, there are changes in the cardiopulmonary function due to *hypoxia*. In height above 3,000 m, people are disconnected from the atmospheric environment known to them. At this point, subject starts to feel the environment stress due to the decline in oxygen, that is, hypoxia. The body's function is influenced by the response of the *cardiopulmonary system* in order to deliver more oxygen in hypoxic conditions. As elevation increases, oxygen has a progressively lower partial pressure with the same 20.93% oxygen fraction in the atmospheric air [19]. At altitude of 4,000 m, barometric pressure is 480 mmHg, and oxygen partial pressure is 100 mmHg as compared to 159 mmHg at sea level (Fig. 1.19). The implication of Fig. 1.19 is that for the same air volume, the number of molecules is reduced progressively with increase in height (gas law, Avogadro's law). The higher the subject climbs, the less air there is above him in the column, so the lower the air pressure and the less dense the gas. Less air means less oxygen which forces the cardiopulmonary system to deliver oxygen under abnormal conditions.

In 1968, the Olympic Games in Mexico City with oxygen partial pressure of approximately 125 mmHg drew considerable attention to their specific effect on athletic performance. It was found that the reduced barometric pressure has a negative influence on any physical activity lasting above 2 min due to *hypoxia*. It makes sense then that any reduction in the pressure of oxygen entering the pulmonary will reduce the pressure difference or gradient. The result is less oxygen being driven from the pulmonary into the blood. Therefore, at high altitude, in spite of the lower barometric pressure and oxygen molecules, weightlifting and anaerobic physical activity such as long and high jumps and sprints for 100, 200, 400, and 800 m are not influenced, and the results are even improved.

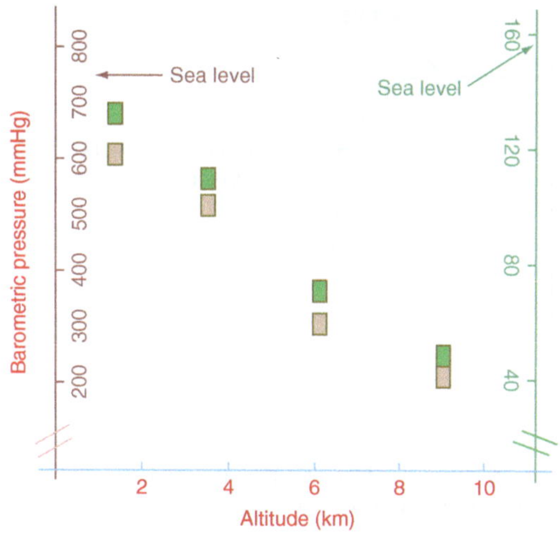

Fig. 1.19 Barometric (*brown*) and oxygen partial pressures (*green*) at different altitudes

Athletes that compete above 1,500 m aerobic exercise have more difficulties and limited performance [19]. This is accompanied by *hyperventilation*, increase in *hemoglobin* and *cardiac output* by means of significant increase in *heart rate*. Following few weeks of acclimatization, hyperventilation is attenuated, and cardiac output decreases to sea level values, while hemoglobin keeps increasing.

At elevations above 2,400 m, breathing irregularities appear for short period due to the inability of the pulmonary system to eliminate CO_2. At elevations above 6,300 m, all people experience apnea and breathing irregularities. Apnea further reduces oxygen content in the blood. Above 2,400 m, 24% of all people experience apnea while sleeping, which in turn reduces the sleep quality, reaching early fatigue during the daylight and

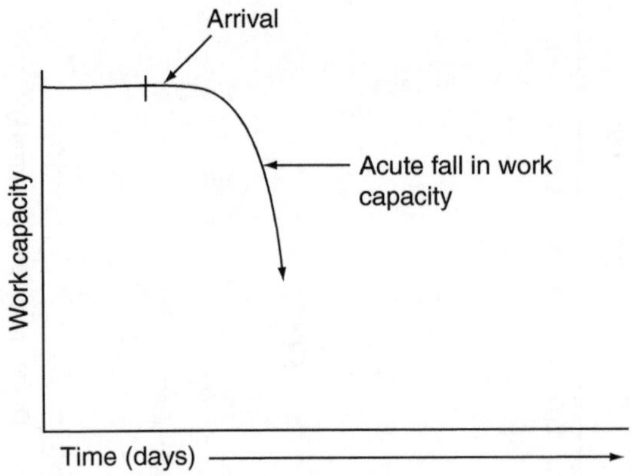

Fig. 1.20 Acute reduction in work capacity with the exposure to a low oxygen partial pressure

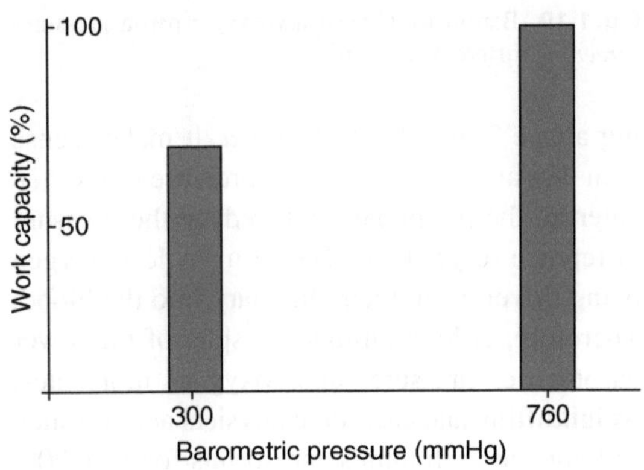

Fig. 1.21 Work capacity at different barometric pressures

an acute reduction in work capacity (Fig. 1.20). Acclimatization improves significantly in the quality of sleep and work capacity; however, in altitudes above 4,500 m, acclimatization does not improve sleep. With diminished oxygen partial pressure, VO_{2max} decrease, but aerobic exercise demands the same amount of oxygen as at sea level.

This imbalance between muscular oxygen demand and *cardiopulmonary* supply, and hence *hypoxia*, brings about a reduction in work capacity. The muscle in turn will produce ATP by means of *anaerobic metabolism.* With hypoxic condition, the chemoreceptors signal the *sympathetic nervous system* to increase cardiopulmonary output, even though hypoxia still exists although in reduced levels (Fig. 1.21).

Exercise and Genetics

The basic mechanism by which exercise activates genes involves a stimulus signal to the DNA, then transcription via messenger ribonucleic acid (mRNA), and finally translation into protein [48, 49]. However, if the genetic predisposition is set for a lower-level range, changes due to *physical activity* can be trained up to a certain extent. Physical exercise has positive effects on a variety of biological systems. Evidence from animal models has indicated a role for exercise in angiogenesis, neurogenesis, learning, and cognition [50, 51]. Exercise training may also affect the immune response by increasing levels of pro-inflammatory cytokines (e.g., TNF-α, IL-6, IL-1) and stress proteins (heat shock protein 72) and by altering circulating populations of peripheral blood mononuclear cells. Furthermore, regular exercise protects against cardiovascular and neurological diseases, decreases mortality and morbidity, and improves disease outcome.

The interaction of *genes* and *exercise* in modifying health status occurs at multiple levels. At the molecular level, the direct mechanism by which exercise alters gene expression involves activation of signal transduction pathways resulting in enhanced transcription of mRNA and subsequently increased translation into protein [52, 53]. In recent years, genetic research driven by genomic scans in humans (linkage studies, association studies) and studies in animal models has evaluated the impact of heritable factors on physical performance, health-related fitness phenotypes, and individuals' responses to regular exercise. It is now well appreciated that traits related to physical functioning such as endurance phenotypes, trainability, muscle mass and strength, cardiopulmonary function, hemodynamic response, and body composition have a strong genetic component. This section will examine the evidence that has accumulated for a strong genetic influence on human cardiac hypertrophy, with an emphasis on two modes of exercise, namely endurance and resistive, which are particularly important for performance in a variety of sports.

Regular exercise has a great impact on cardiovascular risk factors and chronic diseases such as obesity, hypertension, diabetes, cardiovascular disease, and stroke. The knowledge of the importance of genes to health outcome is still growing. Specific genes have been linked to cardiovascular disease, atherosclerosis, Alzheimer, and other disorders. Genetic epidemiological studies have evaluated the role of genes in hypertension, obesity, asthma, chronic obstructive pulmonary disease, and cancer. Studies on human cohorts suggest strong involvement of genetic factors in determining the degree of age-associated osteoporosis and sarcopenia, bringing about a loss of muscle strength function [54, 55]. Finally, putative genes may also play a role in longevity.

The complex interplay of different physiological responses to *exercise* with *genetic polymorphism* can be found in the origins of left ventricular mass in health and disease. Trained athletes usually develop adaptive *left ventricular hypertrophy*, and *ACE gene polymorphisms* may regulate myocardial growth. However, little is known about the impact of the ACE/DD genotype and D allele dose on cardiac changes in adult endurance athletes, with the ACE/DD genotype associated with the extent of exercise-induced left ventricular hypertrophy in *endurance athletes*, regardless of other known biological factors [56–58]. The mechanisms that regulate the development of human physiological cardiac hypertrophy for young and elderly, healthy or ill, remain poorly understood. The renin-angiotensin system, which is modulated by genetic polymorphism, plays an important role in the regulation of vascular tone and myocardial hypertrophy [57].

Physiological Measurements and Metabolic Calculations

Measurements of *functional capacity*, *energy cost*, and *mechanical power output* have significant application in variety of exercises, for example, knowledge on the energy expenditure needed to perform *physical activity*, such as running, walking, and biking, is important for exercise prescription in health and disease. This knowledge of the energy cost is also practical in medicine, exercise physiology, coaching, physical education, physical fitness, and physiotherapy.

The selection of an appropriate protocol for assessing work capacity is of critical importance. The *Bruce Test* commonly utilizes treadmill exercise stress test. It was developed as a clinical test to evaluate patients with suspected *coronary heart disease*, though it can also be used to estimate cardiovascular fitness. *The purpose* of The Bruce Test is to evaluate cardiac function and fitness. It is performed on a treadmill and starts with a speed of 2.74 km · h^{-1} (1.7 mph) and at an incline of 10%. Thereafter, at each 3-min intervals (2–3 min), the treadmill's speed and grade are increased. The *Balke* and *Naughton* protocols, which involve only modest increases in treadmill elevation at a constant speed, are preferable for this purpose. In athletes and healthy individuals, functional capacity can also be accurately determined with the use of protocols in which small increments in work rate occur at intervals of 30–60 s. Regardless of the specific protocol chosen, the protocol should be tailored to the individual to yield a fatigue-limited exercise duration of ≈10 min. Shorter durations may produce a nonlinear relationship between VO_2 and work rate, whereas durations >12 min may cause subjects to terminate exercise because of muscle fatigue or orthopedic factors.

Unit Measurements

Most of the measurements in life sciences are expressed by the *metric system*. This system uses *decimal units*. For example, *kilo* means thousand, *centi* is hundred, and *milli* is a fraction of thousand. In physiology, units are expressed by the *System International* (*SI*), which is an update of the metric system. The base units are the meter, kilogram, second, ampere, kelvin, candela, and mole, respectively, representing length, mass, time, electric current, temperature, luminous intensity, and amount of substance. By multiplying a base unit by itself or by combining two or more basic units by multiplication or division, many units can be formed, known as SI-derived units.

Examples of derived units are the square meter, cubic meter, mole per cubic meter, pascal (Pa), and joule (J). Exceptions in the biomedical sciences include blood pressure (mmHg), oxygen pressure (mmHg) and enzyme activity (IU), H+ concentration (pH), temperature (°C), and volume (L). The measurements expressed as SI most commonly are used in life sciences in general and exercise physiology specifically.

Laboratory Equipments

When it is not possible to measure VO_2, physical performance can be measured by means of *ergometer* (in Greek, ergon = work and metry = measure). Equations related to mechanical work rate are helpful in estimating the metabolic equivalent of the physical effort done. These metabolic measurements are appropriate for clinical and general population use. The ergometer gives a good control to the estimated increase metabolic demand during different exercise modes and intensities. Each metabolic equation includes the resting metabolic cost, the horizontal component, and the vertical one. Laboratory ergometry equipment such as stairs, bicycle, and treadmill are necessary items to increase metabolic demand and to bring about physiological changes during exercise. Work and power are measured during exercise stress tests, physical performance test, training, and physical rehabilitation.

Energy Cost

Metabolic cost is a corner stone in the evaluation of physical performance. When it is impossible to measure *VO_2* by metabolic cart, it is possible to estimate the *metabolic cost* by using regression equations. These equations were validated in laboratories and are connected between mechanical measurements and metabolic cost. The equations are utilized at the laboratories and clinical purposes when using standard equipment. The equations can be practical to evaluate metabolic cost during aerobic exercises such as walking, running, biking, swimming, and stepwise performed outdoors. However, one has to keep in mind that measurements of VO_2 by open-circuit spirometry at a given workload can be repeated with great accuracy. However, with the use of the equations, there is the possibility of inter-variation between subjects tested. Therefore, a repeated measurement might be inaccurate by 7%, and sometimes even higher than that.

Regression equations are practical only during submaximal exercises at steady state. At peak exercise, these equations my over estimate VO_2.

In spite that the accuracy of the equations is not influenced by heat or cold, it is possible that changes in mechanical efficiency will reduce significantly the accuracy of the predicted VO_2.

When using the regression equations intelligently and right, it is possible to have a good tool in spite the above two notifications. One good measurement that helps to have a reasonable evaluation of VO_2 is the MET. The *metabolic equivalent of task* (*MET*), or simply *metabolic equivalent*, is a physiological concept expressing the energy cost of physical activities [59] as multiples of resting metabolic rate and is defined as the ratio of metabolic rate (and therefore the rate of energy consumption) during a specific physical activity to a reference rate of metabolic rate at rest, set by convention to $3.5\ mLO_2 \cdot kg^{-1} \cdot min^{-1}$ or equivalently $1\ kcal \cdot kg^{-1} \cdot h^{-1}$ or $4.184\ kJ \cdot kg^{-1} \cdot h^{-1}$. By convention, 1 MET is considered as the resting metabolic rate obtained during quiet sitting [60]. See Eqs. 1.11 and 1.12:

$$VO_{2rest} = 3.5\ mL{\cdot}kg^{-1}{\cdot}min^{-1} \quad (1.11)$$

Or in a man weighing 70 kg, 1 MET for the *whole body* will be:

$$\begin{aligned} VO_2 &= 3.5\ mL{\cdot}kg^{-1}{\cdot}min^{-1}{\cdot}70\ kg \\ &= 245\ mLO_2{\cdot}min^{-1} \end{aligned} \quad (1.12)$$

The Stress Test

The stress response is induced by exercise or drug stimulation. *Exercise stress tests* compare the coronary circulation while the patient is at rest with the same patient's circulation observed during maximum physical exertion, showing any abnormal blood flow to the myocardium tissue. The results can be interpreted as a reflection on the general physical condition of the test patient. This test can be used to diagnose ischemic heart disease, and for patient prognosis after a myocardial infarction. The cardiac stress test is done with heart stimulation, either by exercise on a treadmill or pedaling a stationary exercise bicycle ergometer, with the patient connected to an electrocardiography [61]. The level of mechanical stress is progressively increased by adjusting the difficulty steepness of the slope and speed. The test administrator or attending physician examines the symptoms and blood pressure response. With use of electrocardiography, the test is most commonly called a cardiac stress test, but is known by other names, such as exercise testing, stress-testing treadmills, exercise-tolerance test, stress test, or exercise electrocardiography test.

The American College of Cardiology/American Heart Association [61] has published guidelines that state that patients with suspected coronary disease and an intermediate pretest probability are appropriate candidates for *exercise electrocardiography test*, while those with low or high pretest probability are not. However, the value of exercise testing in detecting myocardial ischemia resulting from coronary atheroma remains controversial as a diagnostic test for *coronary artery disease*. It has been suggested that methodological problems may explain the wide range of sensitivity and specificity found for exercise electrocardiography testing [62], suggesting that exercise electrocardiography alone may not be a sufficient screening test. Determining the true value of exercise testing requires methodological improvements in patient selection, data collection, and data analysis. Though, the exercise electrocardiography had a good diagnostic value in normal subjects [63].

Calculating Stepwise Work and Power

During stepwise test (Fig. 1.22), the tested individual is asked to perform a series of steps or flights of steps for passing from one level to another. Work done on a stepwise is calculated by multiplying the individual's weight by the distance achieved during the test. As an example for such calculations for a man weighing 70 kg, working on a stepwise with 0.5 m height up and down 30 times for 10 min. Therefore (Eqs. 1.13, 1.14, 1.15, 1.16, and 1.17)

$$\text{Distance} = 30\ \text{times} \cdot 0.5\ \text{m height} \cdot 10\ \text{min} = \mathbf{150\ m} \tag{1.13}$$

$$\text{Work} = 70\ \text{kg weight} \cdot 150\ \text{m distance} = \mathbf{10{,}500\ kgm} \tag{1.14}$$

$$\text{Power} = 10{,}500\ \text{kgm work} / 10\ \text{min} = \mathbf{1{,}050\ kgm{\cdot}min^{-1}} \tag{1.15}$$

$$\text{SI units} = 1{,}050\ \text{kgm}{\cdot}\text{min}^{-1} / 6.12\ \text{kgm} = \mathbf{171.6\ W} \tag{1.16}$$

Or

$$\text{SI units} = 1{,}050\ \text{kgm}{\cdot}\text{min}^{-1} / 0.101\ \text{kgm} = \mathbf{10{,}396.04\ J}. \tag{1.17}$$

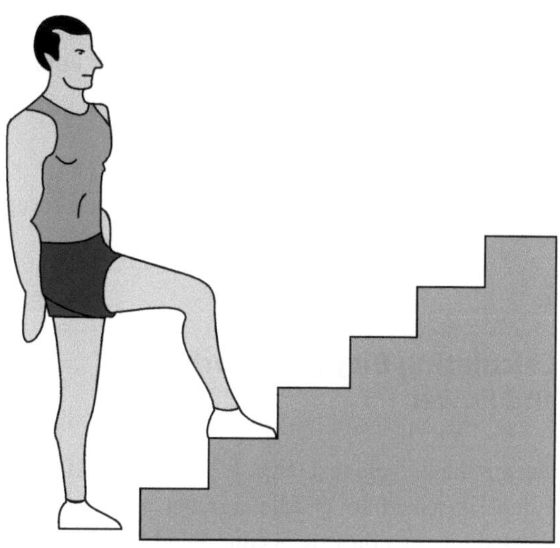

Fig. 1.22 stepwise test; up and down

Calculating Metabolic Cost of Stepping

Calculating oxygen uptake is based on four components: horizontal, slopped, climbing up, and down (Eq. 1.18):

$$VO_2 = \left[\begin{matrix}(\text{steps } \#\cdot 1.8\cdot \text{height in m}\cdot 1.33)\\ +(\text{steps } \#/10)\end{matrix}\right] + 3.5, \quad (1.18)$$

where 1.8 = oxygen cost ($mLO_2 \cdot kg^{-1} \cdot min^{-1}$) of moving vertically during stepping, 1.33 = correction factor for negative (down) component of stepping ($mLO_2 \cdot kg^{-1} \cdot min^{-1}$) of moving vertically during stepping, steps #/10 = correction factor for positive (up) component of stepping (10 is a constant #), and 3.5 = VO_2 at rest ($mLO_2 \cdot kg^{-1} \cdot min^{-1}$).

In essence, VO_2 is the best indicator of exercise intensity because it is tied closely to energy expenditure.

As an example, what will be the VO_2 cost of a person weighing 70 kg that goes up and down 40 $\cdot\ min^{-1}$ at a height of 0.5 m for 10 min?

Anwswer: $VO_2 = [(40 \cdot 1.8 \cdot 0.5 \cdot 1.33) + (40/10)] + 3.5$ $= \mathbf{55.38\ mLO_2 \cdot kg^{-1} \cdot min^{-1}}$.

Question: How many METs are 55.38 $mLO_2 \cdot kg^{-1} \cdot min^{-1}$?

Answer: 55.38/3.5 = **15.8 METs**.

Question: What was the total VO_2 (whole body) for the 10 min?

Answer: 55.38 $mLO_2 \cdot kg^{-1} \cdot min^{-1} \cdot$ 70 kg $\cdot$ 10 min $= \mathbf{38{,}766\ mLO_2 \cdot min^{-1}}$.

Question: How many litters of oxygen equals 38,766 $mLO_2 \cdot min^{-1}$?

Answer: 38,766/1,000 = **38.766 LO_2**.

Question: How many kcal equals 38.766 LO_2?

Answer: Each LO_2 equals 5 kcal; therefore, 38.766 LO_2 = **193.83 kcal**.

Calculating Bicycle's Work and Power

During the bicycle test (Fig. 1.23), the tested individual is asked to peddle against a resistance. Work done on a bicycle is calculated by multiplying paddling revolution per minute (rpm) with the resistance in kg. An example for such calculations is a man weighing 70 kg, paddling on a bicycle at a rate of 60 rpm, resistance of 1.5 kg for 10 min (Eqs. 1.19, 1.20, 1.21, 1.22, and 1.23).

Therefore,

$$\text{Distance} = 60\ \text{rpm}\cdot 6\ \text{m pre revolution} \cdot 10\ \text{min} = \mathbf{3{,}600\ m} \quad (1.19)$$

$$\text{Work} = 1.5\ \text{kg resistance} \cdot 3{,}600\ \text{m distance} = \mathbf{5{,}400\ kgm} \quad (1.20)$$

$$\text{Power} = 5{,}400\ \text{kgm work}/10\ \text{min} = \mathbf{540\ kgm\cdot min^{-1}} \quad (1.21)$$

$$\text{SI units} = 540\ \text{kgm}\cdot\text{min}^{-1}/6.12\ \text{kgm} = \mathbf{88.24\ W} \quad (1.22)$$

Or

$$\text{SI units} = 540\ \text{kgm}\cdot\text{min}^{-1}/0.101\ \text{kgm} = \mathbf{5{,}346.53\ J.} \quad (1.23)$$

Calculating Metabolic Cost of Bicycle Ergometry

Calculating oxygen uptake is based on whole body energy cost (Eq. 1.24):

$$VO_2 = (\text{rpm}\cdot 6\ \text{m}\cdot 2\ \text{mLO}_2\cdot\text{resistance}) + (\text{body weight}\cdot 3.5\ \text{mLO}_2\cdot\text{kg}^{-1}\cdot\text{min}^{-1}), \quad (1.24)$$

where rpm = paddling per minute, 6 m = for each revolution of the wheel moves 6 m, 2 mLO_2 = oxygen cost for each revolution, resistance = the friction on the wheel (kg), and whole *body resting* VO_2 = body weight (kg) $\cdot$ 3.5 $mLO_2 \cdot kg^{-1} \cdot min^{-1}$.

Note: Calculations on the bicycle ergometry are for whole-body $mLO_2 \cdot min^{-1}$ and not $mLO_2 \cdot kg^{-1} \cdot min^{-1}$.

As an example, what will be the oxygen uptake cost of a person weighing 70 kg that paddles 60 rpm with resistance of 5 kg and exercise for 10 min?

Answer: $VO_2 = (60 \cdot 6 \cdot 2 \cdot 5) + (70 \cdot 3.5) = \mathbf{3{,}845\ mLO_2 \cdot min^{-1}}$.

Question: How many METs are 3,845 $mLO_2 \cdot min^{-1}$?

Answer: 3,845 $mLO_2 \cdot min^{-1}$/245 = **11 METs**.

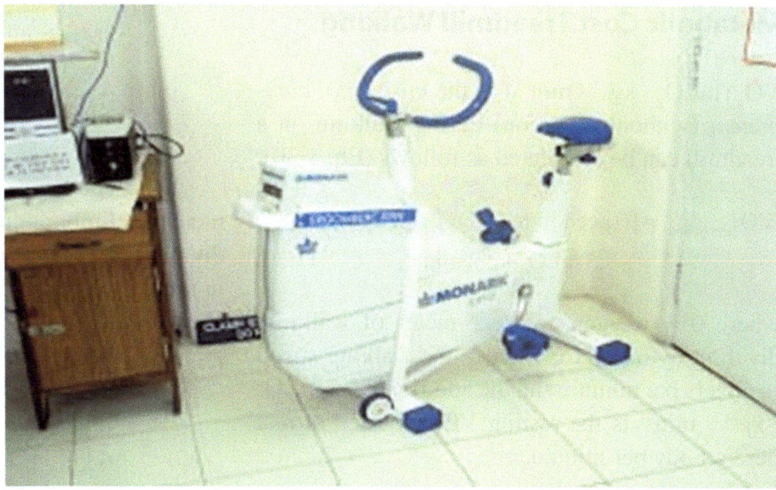

Fig. 1.23 Mechanical bicycle ergometry

Question: What was the total VO_2 (whole body) for the 10 min?

Answer: 3,845 $mLO_2 \cdot min^{-1} \cdot 10$ min = **38,450 mLO2 · min**$^{-1}$.

Question: How many litters of oxygen equals 38,450 mL · min^{-1}?

Answer: 38,450/1,000 = **38.45** LO_2.

Question: How many kcal equals 38.450 LO_2?

Answer: Each LO_2 equals 5 kcal; therefore, 38.450 LO_2 = **192.25 kcal**.

Calculating Treadmill's Work and Power

During treadmill test (Fig. 1.24), the tested individual is asked to walk/run on a motor drive belt. Work done on a treadmill is calculated by multiplying working time by the horizontal and vertical components.

An example for such calculations is a man weighing 70 kg, running on a treadmill at a speed of 200 m · min^{-1} for 10 min (Eqs. 1.25, 1.26, 1.27, 1.28, and 1.29):

$$\text{Distance} = 200\ \text{m}\cdot\text{min}^{-1}\cdot 10\ \text{min} = \mathbf{2{,}000\ m} \quad (1.25)$$

$$\begin{aligned}\text{Work} &= 70\ \text{kg weight}\cdot 2{,}000\ \text{m distance}\\ &= \mathbf{140{,}000\ kgm}\end{aligned} \quad (1.26)$$

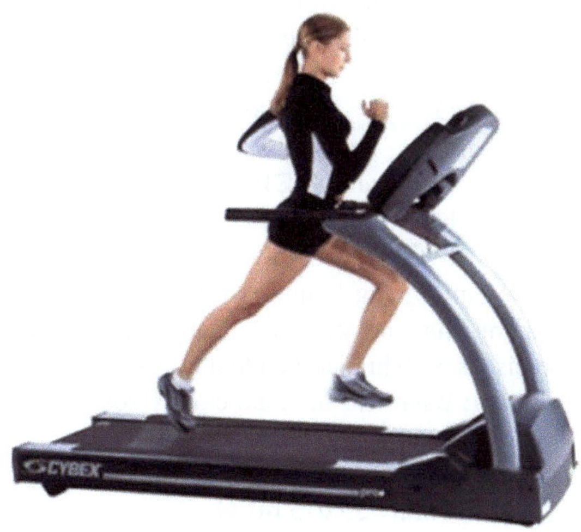

Fig. 1.24 Motor drive treadmill ergometer

$$\begin{aligned}\text{Power} &= 70\ \text{kg weight}\cdot 2{,}000\ \text{m distance}\\ &= 140{,}000\ \text{kgm}/0.10\ \text{kgm}\\ &= \mathbf{14{,}000\ kgm\cdot min^{-1}}\end{aligned} \quad (1.27)$$

$$\begin{aligned}\text{SI units} &= 14{,}000\ \text{kgm}\cdot\text{min}^{-1}/6.12\ \text{kgm}\\ &= \mathbf{228{,}758\ W}.\end{aligned} \quad (1.28)$$

Or

$$\begin{aligned}\text{SI units} &= 14{,}000\ \text{kgm}\cdot\text{min}^{-1}/0.101\ \text{kgm}\\ &= \mathbf{13{,}861.39\ J}.\end{aligned} \quad (1.29)$$

Metabolic Cost Treadmill Walking

VO_2 ($mLO_2 \cdot kg^{-1} \cdot min^{-1}$) of the *horizontal component* (without elevation) during walking on a treadmill can be calculated as follows (Eq. 1.30):

$$VO_{2horizontal} = [(\text{speed in m} \cdot 0.1O_2)/(60\ \text{min})] + 3.5\ mLO_2 \cdot kg^{-1} \cdot min^{-1}, \quad (1.30)$$

where 0.1 = oxygen cost per meter of walking, dividing by 60 min is to have the walking speed in meters per minute, and the additional 3.5 $mLO_2 \cdot kg^{-1} \cdot min^{-1}$ is the resting VO_2 required at rest per kg body per minute.
For example:

Question: What will be the energy cost of a man weighing 70 kg that walks on a treadmill without elevation at a speed of 6 $km \cdot h^{-1}$ (6,000 $m \cdot h^{-1}$) for 35 min?
Answer: $VO_{2\ horizontal}$ = (6,000 · 0.1) + 3.5 = **13.5 $mLO_2 \cdot kg^{-1} \cdot min^{-1}$**.
Question: How many METs equals 13.5 $mLO_2 \cdot kg^{-1} \cdot min^{-1}$?
Answer: METs = 13.5 $mLO_2 \cdot kg^{-1} \cdot min^{-1}$/3.5 $mLO_2 \cdot kg^{-1} \cdot min^{-1}$ = **3.86**
Meaning that the subject's energy cost during exercise is 3.86 higher than that at rest.
Question: What was the total energy cost for the 35 min of exercise?
Answer: VO_2 = 13.5 $mLO_2 \cdot kg^{-1} \cdot min^{-1}$ · 70 kg · 35 min = **33,075 mLO_2**.
Question: How many litters of oxygen equals 33,075 mLO_2?
Answer: 33,075/1,000 = **33.075 LO_2**.
Question: How many kcal are in 33.075 LO_2?
Answer: If 1 L of oxygen equals 5 kcal, then 33.075 LO_2 equals **165,375 kcal**.

During walking on a sloped treadmill, VO_2 will be higher compared to that without elevation. VO_2 will be the sum of the *vertical* and *horizontal components*. The horizontal component is calculated as shown in Eq. 1.30:

$$VO_{2\ horizontal} = \left[(\text{speed in m} \cdot 0.1O_2)/(60\ \text{min})\right] + 3.5\ mLO_2 \cdot kg^{-1} \cdot min^{-1}. \quad (1.30)$$

The vertical component is calculated as follows (Eq. 1.31):

$$VO_{2\ vertical} mLO_2 \cdot kg^{-1} \cdot min^{-1} = (\text{speed in m} \cdot 1.8O_2 \cdot \text{grade}\ \%) / (60\ \text{min} \cdot 100\%), \quad (1.31)$$

where speed = $m \cdot h^{-1}$, 1.8 = oxygen cost per meter of climbing uphill, grade = % of inclination dividing by 60 min is to have the walking speed in meters per minute, and 100%.
For example:

Question: What will be the energy cost of a man weighing 70 kg that walks on a treadmill with 12% elevation at a speed of 6 $km \cdot h^{-1}$ (6,000 $m \cdot h^{-1}$) for 35 min?
Answer: Calculated as before, $VO_{2\ horizontal}$ = (6,000 · 0.1) + 3.5 = **13.5 $mLO_2 \cdot kg^{-1} \cdot min^{-1}$**:
$VO_{2\ vertical}$ = (6,000 · 1.8 · 12)/(60 · 100) = 21.6 $mLO_2 \cdot kg^{-1} \cdot min^{-1}$.
Question: What was the overall metabolic cost?
Answer: VO_2 horizontal + VO_2 vertical = 13.5 + 21.6 = **35.1 $mLO_2 \cdot kg^{-1} \cdot min^{-1}$**.
Question: How many METs equals 35.1 $mLO_2 \cdot kg^{-1} \cdot min^{-1}$?
Answer: METs = 35.1 $mLO_2 \cdot kg^{-1} \cdot min^{-1}$/3.5 $mLO_2 \cdot kg^{-1} \cdot min^{-1}$ = **10 METs**.
Question: What was the total energy cost for the 35 min of exercise?
Answer: VO_2 = 35.1 $mLO_2 \cdot kg^{-1} \cdot min^{-1}$ · 70 kg · 35 min = **85,995 mLO_2**.
Question: How many litters of oxygen equals 85,995 $mLO_2 \cdot min^{-1}$?
Answer: 85,995/1,000 = **85.995 LO_2**.
Question: How many kcal are in 85.995 LO_2?
Answer: If 1 L of oxygen equals 5 kcal, then 33.075 LO_2 equals **430 kcal**.

Metabolic Cost of Treadmill Running

During running on a sloped treadmill, VO_2 will be higher compare to that without elevation. VO_2 will be the sum of the *vertical* and *horizontal components*. The VO_2 ($mLO_2 \cdot kg^{-1} \cdot min^{-1}$) of the *horizontal component* (without elevation) during running on a treadmill can be calculated as follows (Eq. 1.32):

$$VO_{2\ horizontal} = \left[(\text{speed in m} \cdot 0.2O_2)/(60\ \text{min})\right] + 3.5\ mLO_2 \cdot kg^{-1} \cdot min^{-1}, \quad (1.32)$$

where 0.2 = oxygen cost per meter of running since at a point both legs are in the air, dividing by 60 min is to have the running speed in meters per minute, and the additional 3.5 $mLO_2 \cdot kg^{-1} \cdot min^{-1}$ is the resting VO_2 required at rest per kg per minute.

The vertical component is calculated as follows (Eq. 1.33):

$$VO_{2\,vertical} mLO_2 \cdot kg^{-1} \cdot min^{-1} = (\text{speed in m} \cdot 1.8O_2 \cdot \text{grade } \%) / (60 \text{ min} \cdot 100\%), \quad (1.33)$$

where speed = $m \cdot h^{-1}$, 1.8 = oxygen cost per meter of climbing uphill, grade = % of inclination dividing by 60 min is to have the walking speed in meters per minute, and 100%.

For example:

Question: What will be the energy cost of a man weighing 70 kg that runs on a treadmill with 3% elevation at a speed of 12 km $\cdot h^{-1}$ (12,000 $m \cdot h^{-1}$) for 50 min?

Answer: $VO_{2\ horizontal}$ = (12,000 · 0.2) + 3.5 = **43.5 $mLO_2 \cdot kg^{-1} \cdot min^{-1}$**:

$VO_{2\ vertical}$ = (12,000 $m \cdot h^{-1} \cdot 1.8\ O_2 \cdot 3\%$)/(60 min · 100%) = **10.8 $mLO_2 \cdot kg^{-1} \cdot min^{-1}$**.

Question: What was the total VO_2 for 1 min?

Answer: 43.5 + 10.8 = **54.3 $mLO_2 \cdot kg^{-1} \cdot min^{-1}$**.

Question: How many METs it equals?

Answer: METs = 54.3 $mLO_2 \cdot kg^{-1} \cdot min^{-1}$/3.5 $mLO_2 \cdot kg^{-1} \cdot min^{-1}$ = **15.5 METs**.

Question: What was the total energy cost for the 50 min of exercise?

Answer: VO_2 = 54.3 $mLO_2 \cdot kg^{-1} \cdot min^{-1} \cdot$ 70 kg · 50 min = **190,050 mLO_2**.

Question: How many liters of oxygen equals 190,050 $mLO_2 \cdot min^{-1}$?

Answer: 190,050/1,000 = **190.050 LO_2**.

Question: How many kcal are in 190.050 LO_2?

Answer: If 1 L of oxygen equals 5 kcal, then 190.050 LO_2 equals **950.25 kcal**.

References

1. Maron BJ, Pelliccia A. The heart of trained athletes: cardiac remodeling and the risks of sports, including sudden death. Circulation. 2006;114:1633–44.
2. Fagard RH. The ALLHAT trial: strengths and limitations. J Hypertens. 2003;21:229–32.
3. Ben Sira D, Amir R, Amir O, Yamin C, Eynon N, Meckel Y, Sagiv M, Sagiv M. Effect of different sprint training regimes on the oxygen delivery-extraction in elite sprinters. J Sports Med Phys Fitness. 2010; 50:121–5.
4. McArdle WD, Katch FI, Katch VL. Essentials of exercise physiology. 2nd ed. Philadelphia: Lippincott Williams & Wilkins; 2000.
5. Scott CB. A primer for the exercise and nutrition sciences: thermodynamics, bioenergetics, metabolism. Totowa: Humana Press; 2008. 166pp.
6. Scott CB, Kemp RB. Direct and indirect calorimetry of lactate oxidation: implications for whole-body energy expenditure. J Sports Sci. 2005;23:15–9.
7. Ashok C. Test your physical fitness. Gyan Publishing House; New Delhi, India. 2008. p. 30.
8. Renna BF, Kubo H, MacDonnell SM, Crabbe DL, Reger PO, Houser SR, Libonati JR. Enhanced acidotic myocardial Ca^{2+} responsiveness with training in hypertension. Med Sci Sports Exerc. 2006;38:847–55.
9. Wilmore JH, Costill DL, Kenney WL. Physiology of sport and exercise. 4th ed. Champaign: Human Kinetics; 2008.
10. Mademli L, Arampatzis A, Morey-Klapsing G, Brüggemann GP. Effect of ankle joint position and electrode placement on the estimation of the antagonistic moment during maximal plantarflexion. J Electromyogr Kinesiol. 2004;14:591–7.
11. Sagiv M, Hanson P, Besozzi M, Nagle F. Left ventricular responses to upright isometric handgrip and deadlift in men with coronary artery disease. Am J Cardiol. 1985;55:1298–302.
12. Guyton AC, Hall JE. Textbook of medical physiology. 9th ed. Philadelphia: Saunders; 1996.
13. Wilson TM, Tanaka H. Metaanalysis of the age-associated decline in maximal aerobic capacity in men: relation to training status. Am J Physiol Heart Circ Physiol. 2000;278:H829–34.
14. Gianetti G, Burton L, Donovan R, Allen G, Pescatello LS. Physiologic and psychological responses of an athlete cycling 100+ miles daily for 50 consecutive days. Curr Sports Med Rep. 2008;7:343–7.
15. Elia M. Energy expenditure in the whole body. Energy metabolism. Tissue determinants and cellular corollaries. New York: Raven Press; 1992. p. 61–79.
16. Astrand PO, Rodahl K, Dahl HA, Stromme SB. Textbook of work physiology. 4th ed. Champaign: Human Kinetics; 2003.
17. Noakes TD. Physiological models to understand exercise fatigue and the adaptations that predict or enhance athletic performance. Scand J Med Sci Sports. 2000;10:123–45.
18. Kang J, Hoffman JR, Chaloupka EC, Ratamess NA, Weiser PC. Gender differences in the progression of metabolic responses during incremental exercise. J Sports Med Phys Fitness. 2006;46:71–8.
19. Wilmore JH, Costill DL. Physiology of sport and exercise. 3rd ed. Champaign: Human Kinetics; 2005.
20. Baechle TR, Earle RW. Essentials of strength training and conditioning. 2nd ed. Champaign: Human Kinetics; 2000.

21. Hargens TA, Griffin DC, Kaminsky LA, Whaley MH. The influence of aerobic exercise training on the double product break point in low-to-moderate risk adults. Eur J Appl Physiol. 2011;111:313–8.
22. Barrett KE, Barman SM, Boitano SH. Ganong's review of medical physiology. 23rd edn. LANGE Basic Science; New York, 2009.
23. Bu G, Adams H, Berbari EJ, Rubart M. Uniform action potential repolarization within the sarcolemma of in situ ventricular cardiomyocytes. Biophys J. 2009;96: 2532–46.
24. Noordhof DA, de Koning JJ, Foster C. The maximal accumulated oxygen deficit method: a valid and reliable measure of anaerobic capacity? Sports Med. 2010;40:285–302.
25. Scott JM, Esch BT, Haykowsky MJ, et al. Sex differences in left ventricular function and beta-receptor responsiveness following prolonged strenuous exercise. J Appl Physiol. 2007;102:681–7.
26. Fox J, Garber P, Hoffman M, et al. Morphological characteristics of skeletal muscles in relation to gender. Aging Clin Exp Res. 2003;15:264–9.
27. Mizuno M, Kimura Y, Iwakawa T, et al. Regional differences in blood flow and oxygen uptake in resting muscle and their relationship during recovery from exhaustive exercise. J Appl Physiol. 2003;95: 2204–10.
28. Scheuermann BW, Bell C, Paterson DH, Barstow TJ, Kowalchuk JM. Oxygen uptake kinetics for moderate exercise are speeded in older humans by prior heavy exercise. J Appl Physiol. 2002;92:609–16.
29. Endo MY, Kobayakawa M, Kinugasa R, et al. Thigh muscle activation distribution and pulmonary VO_2 kinetics during moderate, heavy, and very heavy intensity cycling exercise in humans. Am J Physiol Regul Integr Comp Physiol. 2007;293:R812–20.
30. Ben-Sira D, Sagiv M. The effect of gender on left ventricular systolic function at Peak Wingate Anaerobic Test. Eur J Appl Physiol. 1997;75:549–53.
31. Sagiv M, Metrany R, Fisher N, Fishman ZE, Kellerman JJ. Comparison of hemodynamic and left ventricular responses to increased after-load in healthy males and females. Int J Sports Med. 1991;12:41–5.
32. Schaufelberger M, Drexler H, Schieffer E, et al. Angiotensin-converting enzyme gene expression in skeletal muscle in patients with chronic heart failure. J Card Fail. 1998;4:185–91.
33. Batterham A, George K, Mullineaux D. Allometric scaling of left ventricular mass by body dimensions in males and females. Med Sci Sports Exerc. 1997;29: 181–6.
34. Tossavainen M, Nummela A, Paavolainen L, Mero A, Rusko H. Comparison of two maximal anaerobic cycling tests. Int J Sports Med. 1996;17 Suppl 2:S120–4.
35. Gurd BJ, Peters SJ, Heigenhauser GJ, LeBlanc PJ, Doherty TJ, Paterson DH, Kowalchuk JM. Prior heavy exercise elevates pyruvate dehydrogenase activity and muscle oxygenation and speeds O2 uptake kinetics during moderate exercise in older adults. Am J Physiol Regul Integr Comp Physiol. 2009;297:R877–84.
36. Jansen RK, Nassas G. Growth of segment principal movements of interia between four and twenty years. Med Sci Sports Exerc. 1988;20:594–604.
37. Toft I, Ilindal S, Bonaa KH, Jenssen T. Quantitative measurement of muscle fiber composition in a normal population. Muscle Nerve. 2003;28:101–8.
38. Clanachan AS. Contribution of protons to post-ischemic Na(+) and Ca(2+) overload and left ventricular mechanical dysfunction. J Cardiovasc Electrophysiol. 2006;17 Suppl 1:S141–8.
39. Rowland T, Goff D, Martel L, Ferrone L. Influence of cardiac functional capacity on gender differences in maximal oxygen uptake in children. Chest. 2000;117:629–35.
40. Schunkert H, Hense HW, Holmer SR, et al. Association between a deletion polymorphism of the angiotensin-converting-enzyme gene and left ventricular hypertrophy. N Engl J Med. 1994;330:1634–8.
41. Fatini C, Guazzelli R, Manetti P, et al. RAS genes influence exercise-induced left ventricular hypertrophy: an elite athletes study. Med Sci Sports Exerc. 2000;32:1868–72.
42. Chandrashekhar Y, Anand IS. Exercise as a coronary protective factor. Am Heart J. 1991;122:1723–39.
43. Wenger NK, Froelicher ES, Smith LK, et al. Cardiac rehabilitation as secondary prevention. Clinical practice guideline no. 17. Rockville: US Department of Health and Human Services, Public Health Service, Agency for Health Care Policy and Research and the National Heart, Lung, and Blood Institute; ACHCPR Publication No. 96–0672; 1995.
44. Hood DA, Irrcher I, Ljubicic V, Joseph AM. Coordination of metabolic plasticity in skeletal muscle. J Exp Biol. 2006;209:2265–75.
45. Fernstrom M, Bakkman L, Tonkonogi M, et al. Reduced efficiency, but increased fat oxidation, in mitochondria from human skeletal muscle after 24-h ultraendurance exercise. J Appl Physiol. 2007;102: 1844–9.
46. Huber-Abel FA, Gerber M, Hoppeler H, Baum O. Exercise-induced angiogenesis correlates with the up-regulated expression of neuronal nitric oxide synthase (nNOS) in human skeletal muscle. Eur J Appl Physiol. 2012;112(1):155–62. Epub 2011 Apr 20.
47. Ookawara T, Suzuk K, Haga S, et al. Transcription regulation of gene expression in human skeletal muscle in response to endurance training. Res Commun Mol Pathol Pharmacol. 2002;111:41–54.
48. Britton SL, Koch LG. Animal genetic models for complex traits of physical capacity. Exerc Sport Sci Rev. 2001;1:7–14.
49. Macarthur DG, North KN. Genes and human elite athletic performance. Hum Genet. 2005;116:331–9.
50. Cotman CW, Berchtold NC. Exercise: a behavioural intervention to enhance brain health and plasticity. Trends Neurosci. 2002;25:295–301.
51. Ding Q, Vaynman S, Akhavan M, Ying Z, Gomez-Pinilla F. Insulin-like growth factor I interfaces with brain-derived neurotrophic factor-mediated synaptic plasticity to modulate aspects of exercise-induced cognitive function. Neuroscience. 2006;140:823–33.

52. Baar K, Blough E, Dineen B, Esser K. Transcriptional control in response to exercise. Exerc Sport Sci Rev. 1999;27:333–79.
53. Bolster DR, Kimball SR, Jefferson LS. Translational control mechanisms modulate skeletal muscle gene expression during hypertrophy. Exerc Sport Sci Rev. 2003;31:111–6.
54. Livshits G. Genetic epidemiology of skeletal system aging in apparently health human population. Mech Ageing Dev. 2005;126:269–79.
55. Pantsulaia I, Trofimov S, Kobyliansky E, Livshits G. Genetic regulation of the variation of circulating insulin-like growth factors and leptin in human pedigrees. Metabolism. 2005;54:975–81.
56. Hernández D, de la Rosa A, Barragán A, et al. The ACE/DD genotype is associated with the extent of exercise-induced left ventricular growth in endurance athletes. J Am Coll Cardiol. 2003;42:527–32.
57. Kasikcioglu E, Kayserilioglu A, Ciloglu F, et al. Angiotensin-converting enzyme gene polymorphism, left ventricular remodeling, and exercise capacity in strength-trained athletes. Heart Vessels. 2004; 19: 287–93.
58. Tanriverdi H, Evrengul H, Kaftan A, et al. Effects of angiotensin-converting enzyme polymorphism on aortic elastic parameters in athletes. Cardiology. 2005; 104:113–9.
59. Byrne NM, Hills AP, Hunter GR, Weinsier RL, Schutz Y. Metabolic equivalent: one size does not fit all. J Appl Physiol. 2005;99:1112–9.
60. Rezzi S, Martin FP, Shanmuganayagam D, Colman RJ, Nicholson JK, Weindruch R. Metabolic shifts due to long-term caloric restriction revealed in nonhuman primates. Exp Gerontol. 2009;44:356–62.
61. Gibbons R, Balady G, Timothybricker J, et al. ACC/AHA 2002 guideline update for exercise testing: summary article. A report of the American College of Cardiology/American Heart Association Task Force on Practice Guidelines. J Am Coll Cardiol. 2002; 40:1531–40.
62. Morise AP. Are the American College of Cardiology/American Heart Association guidelines for exercise testing for suspected coronary artery disease correct? Chest. 2000;118:535–41.
63. Cortigiani L, Bigi R, Rigo F, Landi P, Baldini U, Mariani PR, Picano E. Diagnostic value of exercise electrocardiography and dipyridamole stress echocardiography in hypertensive and normotensive chest pain patients with right bundle branch block. J Hypertens. 2003;21:2189–94.

2 Pulmonary Function

Introduction

The purpose of respiration is to provide oxygen to the tissues and to remove CO_2 from the tissues [1]. Humans are able to extract oxygen from the atmosphere and transport it to their cells where it is utilized for essential metabolic processes. The oxygen pathway from environment to mitochondria can be viewed as a cascade of resistances in chain, each one being overcome by a specific pressure gradient (Fig. 2.1). However, there are several elements in the oxygen transport pathway from mouth to mitochondria that have the individual potential to limit oxygen supply during exercise and therefore VO_{2max} [2]. Changes of VO_2 could be induced by altering the blood oxygen-carrying capacity, peripheral function, or both.

During heavy exercise, large volumes of oxygen are transported through the links of the cardiopulmonary transport system to mitochondrial cytochromes for synthesis of ATP in the electron transport chain. Exercise causes these elements to change. But the body is designed to maintain homeostasis by regulating diffusion of oxygen and carbon to and from the blood, by transporting oxygen and CO_2 by the blood, and by regulating ventilation and other aspects of respiration.

About the Gases

The respiratory system acts by gases exchange, and therefore, it is important to understand the factors that affect gases responses:

Gas volume changes under the conditions that it being measured, this, in spite of the fact that the number of molecules is even. Thus, when comparing gases volume measured under different conditions, it is necessary to take into account the following factors:

Temperature (*T*) – Volume of a gas is linearly related to temperature. Increase in temperature will force the gas molecules to move faster, the gas mixture expends, bringing about a larger volume (*Charles's law* $V=K \cdot T$). *Charles's law*: As the temperature of an amount of gas increases, so does its volume (Eq. 2.1):

$$V_1 / T_1 = V_2 / T_2, \tag{2.1}$$

where *T* is the absolute temperature of the gas (in Kelvin) and assuming the pressure and moles of gas is constant (in $m^3 \cdot K^{-1}$) is the constant produced.

At standard temperature and pressure, a mole of gas occupies 22.4 L. The actual value for CO_2 and N_2O is about 22.2 L.

Pressure (*P*) – Volume of a gas is inversely related to the pressure exerted on it. Increase in pressure force the molecules to get closer to each other; thus, the gas mixture decreases relatively to the pressure increment (*Boyle's law* $P \cdot V=K$). *Boyle's law*: In a container filled with gas, if the volume is decreased, the pressure will correspondingly increase and vice versa.

Water vapor – Gas volume is increased when the amount of water vapor is low when it is dry and larger when it has water vapor.

M.S. Sagiv, *Exercise Cardiopulmonary Function in Cardiac Patients*,
DOI 10.1007/978-1-4471-2888-5_2, © Springer-Verlag London 2012

Fig. 2.1 Oxygen transport from the atmosphere to the mitochondria and carbon dioxide from the cell to the atmosphere. The pathway for oxygen from the atmosphere to the muscle contains a series of steps that include mechanical work, pressure gradient, and chemical reactions

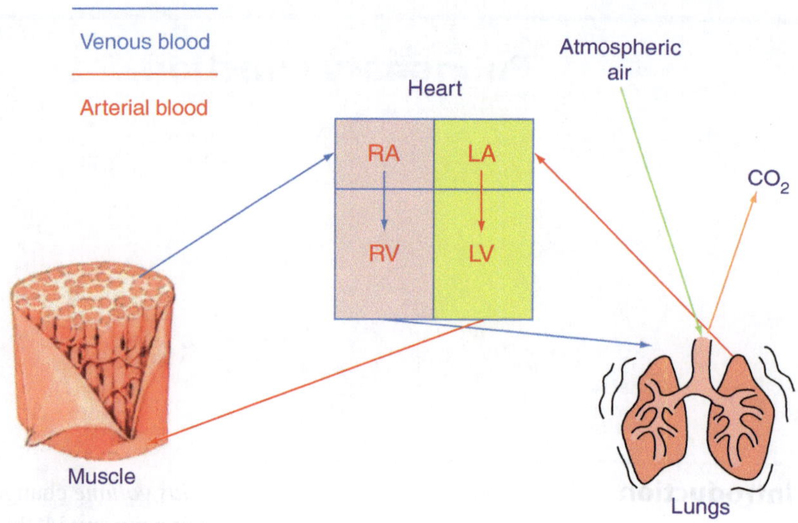

Gases can be expressed in four ways:

STPD = it means that the gas under standard conditions, in which ambient temperature is corrected to 0°C, barometric pressure of 760 mmHg at sea level and dry air. Expressing gas in *STPD* units enables to compare gas volumes measured under different temperatures, ambient pressure, and percentage of water in the air.

BTPS units are related to a gas volume expressed under conditions of, core body temperature, a given barometric pressure and saturated with water vapor of 47 mmHg.

ATPS units are related to a gas volume expressed under conditions of ambient temperature, a given barometric pressure, and saturated with water vapor of the ambient.

ATPD units are related to a gas volume expressed under conditions of ambient pressure and temperature and dry.

In general, gases move from an area of high pressure to areas of low pressure. If there are mixtures of gases in a container, each gas behaves as if it were on its own: it exerts a *partial pressure* that is independent of that exerted by other gases in the mixture (*Dalton's Law*). At sea level, the *atmospheric pressure* equals 760 mmHg (1 atm of pressure = 760 mmHg = 101 kPa = 15 L bs/sq in.). The air is composed out of 20.9% oxygen, 78% nitrogen, and small quantities of CO_2, argon, and helium. The pressure exerted by the main two gases individually, when added together, equals the total surrounding pressure or atmospheric pressure. The *oxygen partial pressure* of dry air at sea level is therefore (Eq. 2.2)

$$(20.9/100\%)\cdot 760\ \text{mmHg} = 159\ \text{mmHg}. \tag{2.2}$$

However at the trachea, the air has been warmed and humidified; since the vapor pressure in the trachea is 47 mmHg, the oxygen partial pressure (PO_2) in the trachea when breathing will be (Eq. 2.3)

$$PO_2 = \left[(760 - 47\ \text{mmHg})(21/100\%)\right] = 150\ \text{mmHg}. \tag{2.3}$$

When oxygen has reached the alveoli, the oxygen partial pressure has fallen to about 100 mmHg. This is because the oxygen partial pressure of the gas in the alveoli (PAO_2) is a balance between two processes: the removal of oxygen by the pulmonary capillaries and its continual supply by alveolar ventilation (breathing).

Oxygen moves down the pressure or concentration gradient from a relatively high level in air (760 mmHg), to the levels in the respiratory tract and then alveolar gas (100 mmHg) by means of diffusion, the arterial blood (95–97 mmHg), capillaries, and finally the cell. The oxygen partial pressure reaches the lowest level (4–20 mmHg)

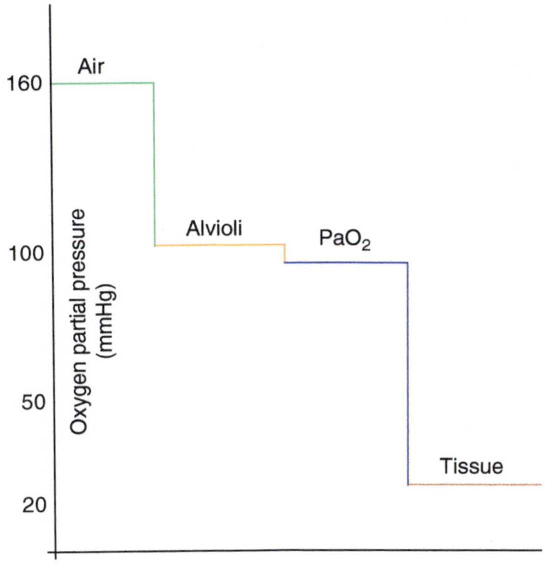

Fig. 2.2 The oxygen cascade

in the mitochondria (Fig. 2.2). This decrease in oxygen partial pressure from air to the mitochondrion is known as the *oxygen cascade*, and the size of any one step in the cascade may be increased under pathological circumstances and may result in hypoxia.

Minute Ventilation

Minute ventilation (V_E) is the volume of gas inhaled or exhaled from a person's lungs in 1 min. It is an important parameter in respiratory medicine due to its relationship with blood CO_2 levels. *Arterial partial pressure of* CO_2 *(*$PaCO_2$*)* levels generally vary inversely with V_E. For example, a person with increased V_E due to hyperventilation should demonstrate a lower Arterial blood CO_2 level. Hyperventilation is the term for having a V_E higher than physiologically appropriate. Hypoventilation describes a V_E less than physiologically appropriate. The healthy human body will alter V_E in an attempt to maintain physiologic homeostasis. A normal V_E in humans at rest is about 5–8 L · min^{-1}. V_E generally decreases when at rest, and increases with *exercise*. For example, during light aerobic activities, V_E may be around 12 L · min^{-1}. Paddling a bicycle increases V_E by a factor of 2–4 depending on the level of exercise involved. During moderate exercise V_E may be between 40 and 60 L · min^{-1} [3]. Note that although V_E implies that it is a volume, V_E is actually a flow, it represents a volume change over time. Measurements of V_E are expressed in liters and can be calculated by multiplying *tidal volume* (V_T) by *breathing frequency* (f) (Eq. 2.4):

$$V_E = V_T \cdot f \tag{2.4}$$

where V_T = the volume of air that the subject inhales with each breath and f = the number of breaths that the subject takes each minute.

At *rest*, in normal young males, weighting 70 kg V_E equals to 6–7.5 L · min^{-1} from 12 to 15 · min^{-1} breathes and a V_T of 0.5 L. At maximal intensity of exercise, VO_2, CO_2 formation, and total pulmonary and *alveolar ventilation* (V_A) increase by approximately 20-fold. At relatively low exercise intensities, V_T and f increase proportionally. However, at higher relative intensities, V_T reaches a plateau and further increases in V_E depend exclusively upon increasing f.

During maximal exercise, V_E in normal sedentary subjects may reach 120–150 L · min^{-1}. The increase in pulmonary ventilation is attributable to a combination of increases in V_T and f and closely matches the increase in VO_2 and CO_2 output. Hemoglobin continues to be fully saturated with oxygen throughout exercise in people with normal respiratory function.

The maximal voluntary ventilation is approximately 40% greater than the actual pulmonary V_E during maximal exercise. In sedentary individuals, V_T is 3.0–3.5 L while f is 40–55 · min^{-1}. Top *athletes* at *peak exercise* V_E may reach values of 200 L · min^{-1} breathing 60–70 · min^{-1} with tidal volume of 3.8–4.0 L (Figs. 2.3 and 2.4). Untrained relies on f since V_T is limited while well-trained and top athletes are able to increase both f and V_T. Therefore, the respiratory system itself is not usually the most limiting factor in the delivery of oxygen to the working muscles during maximal muscle aerobic metabolism.

Regulation of ventilation is complex and under the influence of several mechanisms. With the onset of exercise, V_E increases rapidly followed by gradual increase. The primary mechanism

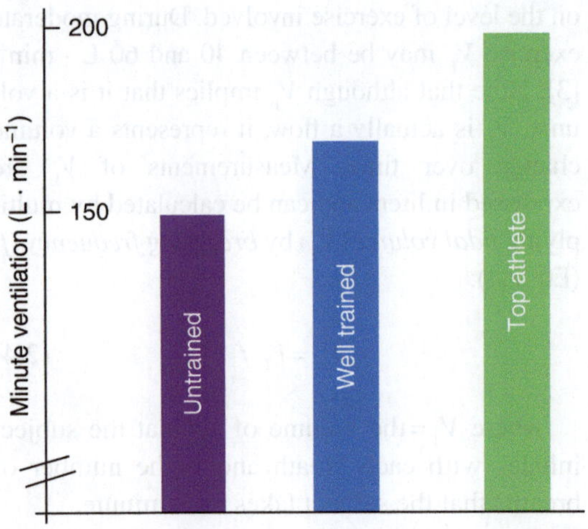

Fig. 2.3 Comparison between untrained, well-trained individuals, and top athletes in minute ventilation at maximal aerobic exercise

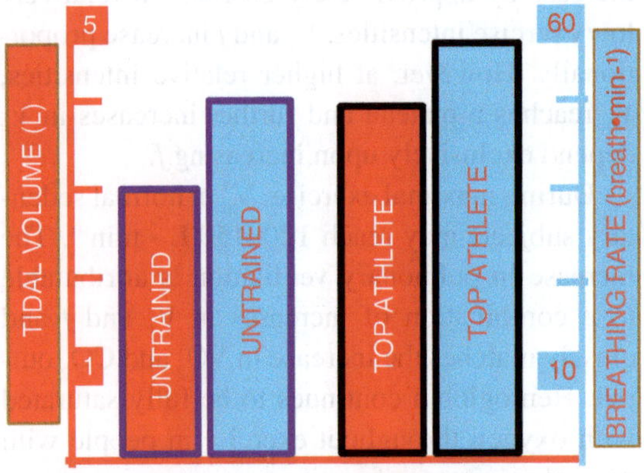

Fig. 2.4 The relationships between breathing rate (*blue*) and tidal volume (*red*) in untrained and top athlete. Untrained is restricted in tidal volume and therefore increases mainly breathing rate, while top athlete is able to increase both: rate of breathing and tidal volume

during exercise is a neural input that likely originates from the same area of the motor cortex in the brain and afferent impulses from the limbs, joints, and muscles. This would explain the rapid increase and decrease of V_E with the onset and cessation, respectively, of exercise.

The increased V_E far exceeds the increase in the amount of blood that can be circulated through the lungs during exercise, which is typically only five to eight times the resting value. Following the rapid increase in V_E a constant regulation of

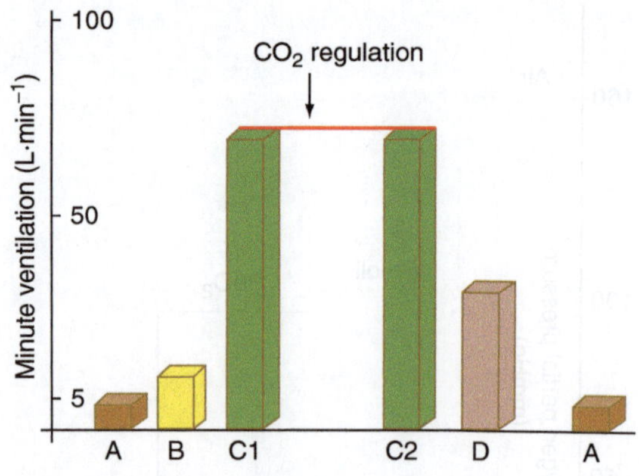

Fig. 2.5 Minute ventilation regulation: from *A to B*, neural input due to anticipation; from *B to C1* is a rapid increase due to afferent impulses from the limbs, joints, and muscles; *C1 to C2* is during exercise regulated mainly by the CO_2 chemoreceptors followed by a sharp decrease; from *C2 to D*, owed to the cessation of the afferent impulses from the limbs, joints and muscles; and from *D to A* is the time for rebuilding PC and ATP along with the reduction in blood lactic acid levels

V_E during exercise is accomplished mainly by the peripheral chemoreceptors, most likely by the CO_2 chemoreceptors. Figure 2.5 illustrates the different control mechanisms before, during, and after effort exercise. This means that the cardiovascular system is the limiting factor, and there will be no overload on the lungs that forces them to increase their capacity over time due to regular aerobic exercise.

Control of breathing in man is immensely complex. It takes place at three levels in the control of breathing: the anterior horn cell, the brainstem, and feedback regulation. Two sets of chemoreceptors regulate breathing: *central chemoreceptors* which are usually by far the most important. They respond mainly to changes in cerebrospinal fluid pH. As arterial partial pressure of CO_2 rises, so erebrospinal fluid CO_2 partial pressure will increase, this causing a drop in pH. Breathing is stimulated, reducing arterial partial pressure of CO_2, and so on. With prolonged respiratory acidosis or alkalosis, the response becomes dulled, possibly related to compensatory normalization of the cerebrospinal fluid pH by movement of $HCO3^-$ ions. Severe hypoxia may depress central chemoreceptors.

Less important in normal man than the central chemoreceptors, the *carotid bodies* become stimulated with *hypoxemia*, low arterial pH (whether due to CO_2 partial pressure or not), hypoperfusion, fever, and certain drugs such as acetylcholine and nicotine. These bodies, the metabolically most active tissue in the body, contain glomus cells which synapse with nerve endings of the glossopharyngeal nerve, and their stimulation results in stimulation of respiration. The peripheral response to CO_2 arterial partial pressure is about one-fifth of the central one. The relationship between oxygen arterial partial pressure and V_E at constant CO_2 arterial partial pressure is complex and nonlinear, but if it is plotted as saturation against V_E, a convenient almost linear curve down to a saturation of about 70% will be obtained.

The response to hypoxia is enhanced by hypercarbia, acidosis, and exercise. During maximal exercise, highly trained individuals often reach the mechanical limits of the lung and respiratory muscle for producing large V_A. This level of ventilation is achieved at a considerable metabolic cost but with a mechanically optimal pattern of breathing and respiratory muscle recruitment and without sacrifice of a significant alveolar hyperventilation [4]. It is important to realize that the potential of gas exchange between the lung and blood is the amount of gas reaching the alveolus. At rest, the V_A fraction is 70% of the V_T while 30% is the *anatomical dead space* (V_D) while at peak exercise, V_A increases up to 85–90% (10–15% is the physiological dead space). *Physiological dead space* can be calculated using Bohr's method (Eq. 2.5):

$$\text{Physiological dead space} = [CO_2]_A * (V_T - V_D) = [CO_2]_{\text{expired}} V_T \qquad (2.5)$$

where $(CO_2)_A$ = alveolar carbon dioxide concentration, V_T = tidal volume, V_D = dead space, and $(CO_2)_{\text{expired}}\ V_T$ = tidal volume and the expired concentration of CO_2.

In other words, the product of alveolar CO_2 concentration and the amount of inspired air reaching the alveoli equals the expired CO_2 concentration times the V_T. It is easy to measure the tidal volume and the expired concentration of CO_2, so all which needed to determine physiological dead space is the alveolar CO_2 concentration. In most cases, it can simply substitute in the CO_2 arterial partial pressure, as the two are generally very similar.

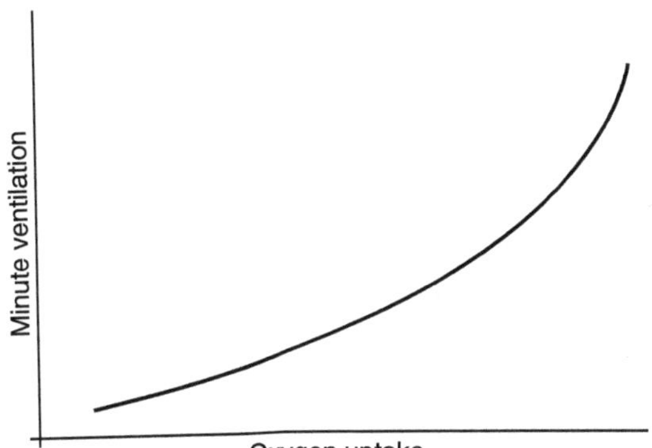

Fig. 2.6 The relationship between minute ventilation and oxygen uptake

Normally, V_A is unconsciously regulated to maintain constant arterial blood gas tensions particularly CO_2, despite variable levels of VO_2 and CO_2 production. In order to meet the increased metabolic demand during exercise, V_E is increased up to 60% of VO_{2max} somehow in a linear mode while above 60% of VO_{2max} the curve increases in an exponential way (Fig. 2.6). The exponential increase in V_E above 60% of VO_{2max} is due to increase in *lactic acid production* and H^+ ions in the blood. This nonlinear response suggests that V_E is regulated by the levels of CO_2. Thus, V_E is increased linearly with CO_2 levels (Fig. 2.7).

Oxygen-Diffusing Capacity in the Lung

Oxygen-diffusing capacity is a measure of the rate at which oxygen can diffuse from the alveoli into the blood. Lung diffusing capacity is known to vary with hemoglobin concentration and alveolar lung volume. An increase in diffusing capacity is observed in a state of *maximal exercise*.

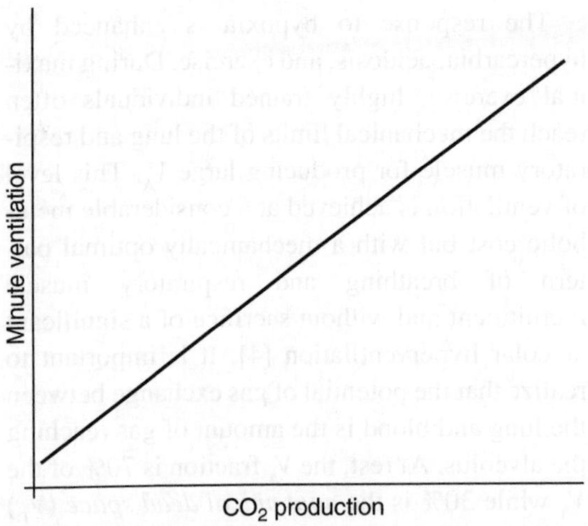

Fig. 2.7 The relationship between minute ventilation and carbon dioxide production (CO_2) from rest to maximal effort

Diffusing capacity can more than double as *cardiac output* increases from rest to peak exercise in normal subjects, the increase results from the fact that *blood flow* through many of the pulmonary capillaries is low in the resting state. With exercise, increased blood flow through the lungs causes all of the pulmonary capillaries that were unperfused to be perfused at their maximal level, providing a greater surface area through which oxygen can diffuse into the pulmonary capillary blood. Capillaries recruitment is critical for maintaining normal arterial oxygen saturation as VO_2 increases. Trained individuals who require greater amounts of oxygen per minute have been found to have higher diffusing capacities, but the exact reason why is not yet known. The effectiveness of the capillaries recruitment can be described by how the diffusing capacity/cardiac output ratio changes as exercise load increases; when the diffusing capacity/cardiac output ratio declines below a critical level, *arterial oxygen saturation* falls. Although one would expect the oxygen pressure of arterial blood to decrease during strenuous exercise and CO_2 pressure of venous blood to increase far above normal, this is not the case. Both of these values remain close to normal. In addition, recently, it has been demonstrated that genetic variation of the α-subunit of ENaC at amino acid 663 influences lung diffusion at peak exercise in healthy humans, suggesting differences in alveolar Na^+ and, therefore, fluid handling. These findings could be important in determining who may be susceptible to pulmonary edema in response to various clinical or environmental conditions [5].

Transporting Oxygen and Carbon Dioxide by the Blood

When oxygen reaches the cells, it is released. The excreted CO_2 from cells is transported approximately 60% via bicarbonate, 20% via hemoglobin, and 10% in plasma which contributes to the partial pressure of carbon dioxide in the body. The bicarbonate (H_2CO_3) reaction is CO_2 mixes with H_2O in the presence of the enzyme carbonic anhydrase to form H_2CO_3, which breaks up into the bicarbonate ion HCO3⁻ and free H^+. It is only transported in this way, and when it arrives to the lungs, the reaction occurs in reverse to reform CO_2, which is then excreted from the lungs through diffusion. CO_2 produced in the tissue cells diffuses into the blood plasma. The largest fraction of CO_2 diffuses into the red blood cells. The CO_2 in the red blood cells is transported as dissolved CO_2, combined with hemoglobin, or with the largest fraction as H_2CO_3. The formation of HCO_3^- *hydration* (Eq. 2.6) and *dissociation* (Eq. 2.7) takes place by the following reactions:

$$\text{Hydration of } CO_2\text{: } CO_2 + HOH \rightarrow H_2CO_3 \quad (2.6)$$

$$\text{Dissociation of } H_2CO_3\text{: } H_2CO_3 \rightarrow H^+ + HCO_3^- \quad (2.7)$$

Combining Eqs. 2.6 and 2.7 (Eq. 2.8),

$$CO_2 + H_2O \leftrightarrow H_2CO_3 \leftrightarrow H^+ + HCO_3^- \quad (2.8)$$

The H_2CO_3/HCO_3^- ratio acts as the primary buffer of the blood. The H^+ of H_2CO_3 is a slow process but occurs rapidly in the red blood cells because a high concentration of the enzyme carbonic anhydrase catalyzes the reaction. H_2CO_3 diffuses out of the red blood cells into the plasma in venous blood and in opposition to arterial blood. Chloride ion always diffuses in an opposite direction of HCO_3^- ion in order to maintain a charge balance. This is referred to as the "chloride shift."

Oxygen diffuses from the lungs and diffuses into the circulatory system where it is transported 98.5% via the hemoglobin molecule (red blood cells) and 1.5% in the plasma as solution, which contributes to the partial pressure of oxygen in the body. Four oxygen molecules can be carried at one time by hemoglobin which is found in red blood cells. The hemoglobin then transports the oxygen to cells that need it, and when they release the oxygen, the hemoglobin carries back CO_2 to the lungs where most of it is exhaled. The changes in concentration of CO_2 or HCO_3^- can influence slight acid/base balance in the blood even though it is buffered. At the same time, the concentration of H^+ ions will influence the concentrations of CO_2 and HCO_3^- ions.

The reactions for both oxygen and CO_2 are coupled together and work in cooperation with each other. The main reason for this effect is that both systems are influenced by H^+ ions and equilibrium principles. At the *lungs*, the diffusion of oxygen into the blood triggers the reactions. The oxygen reacts with and attaches to hemoglobin. This oxygenation reaction with hemoglobin produces excess H^+ ions which react with HCO_3^- ions to produce $H_2CO_3^-$. The carbonic acid decomposes to CO_2 which diffuses out of the blood.

Peak Oxygen Uptake (VO_{2peak})

Myocardial functional changes in *cardiovascular disease patients* include decline in maximum heart rate, stroke volume, and contractility, and an increase in peripheral vascular resistance. The changes in structure and function of the cardiopulmonary system result in *peak oxygen uptake* (VO_{2peak}) decline, which is the best single indicator of physical working capacity. During the past two decades, VO_{2peak} (Fig. 2.8) compared to VO_{2max} has been consistently confirmed as an independent predictor of *mortality* in patients with cardiovascular disease [6].

Because maximal exertion is not without risk in elderly and *cardiac patients*, VO_{2peak} is used

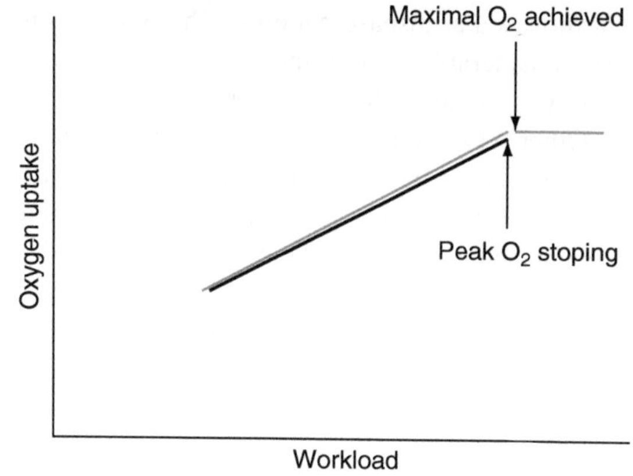

Fig. 2.8 Two different reference points determining peak oxygen uptake and maximal oxygen uptake. The determination of peak oxygen uptake is different from the maximal oxygen uptake that has a maximal oxygen uptake with increased workload, while VO_2peak is defined when the subject withdrawal voluntarily from the test

during maximal exercise testing. VO_{2peak} differs from VO_{2max} by not having a plateau in oxygen uptake with increased workload, namely VO_{2peak} is defined as the point that the subject withdraws voluntarily from the test. An early study suggested that a specific VO_{2peak} cut-point was able to distinguish patients with low and high probability of survival [7].

High-intensity aerobic interval exercise is superior to moderate exercise for increasing VO_{2peak} in stable *coronary artery disease patients*. As VO_{2peak} seems to reflect a continuum between health and cardiovascular disease and death, the present data may be useful in designing effective training programs for improved health in the future. Several limitations additionally have been attributed to VO_{2peak} as an indicator of the severity of cardiac performance. It can be affected by age, sex, motivation, body composition, and muscle deconditioning [8]. It has also been claimed that the exercise capacity for a given level of cardiac dysfunction may vary with the etiology of disease. Thus, these data suggest that VO_{2peak} is only an indirect indicator of the cardiac response to exercise. In addition, it may be unfavorably affected by alterations in skeletal muscle characteristics. Also, one has to keep in mind that muscle mass plays an important role in the definition of VO_{2peak}.

Cardiovascular disease patients exhibited in general considerably lower total skeletal muscle mass and VO_{2peak} than healthy controls.

Other VO_2 exercise-derived parameters have emerged as predictors of outcomes in cardiovascular disease patients [9]. They mainly include percent achieved of predicted VO_{2peak} and VO_2 kinetics during and after exercise [10]. Patients who are unable to reach 50% of predicted VO_{2peak} have increased *mortality*, but the prognostic value of VO_2 percent over VO_{2peak} alone has not been confirmed in a number of studies [11]. Yet it is still matter of debate whether VO_2 variables are superior to VO_{2peak} in the prognostic evaluation of cardiovascular disease [12].

In healthy subjects, the VO_{2peak} or VO_2 is limited by maximal capacity of oxygen delivery to active tissues and/or oxygen release from hemoglobin. Since metabolic demands during incremental exercise are increased over time, diverse populations may maintain the energy supply in an imbalance between oxygen delivery and extraction and hence different VO_2 rate of reaction. The mechanisms of *exercise intolerance* in *cardiovascular disease patients* in comparison with rest indices of cardiac performance, measures of pulmonary function, and peripheral vasodilator capacity were more closely associated with exercise VO_{2peak}. Furthermore, the associations were independent of each other and together accounted for 50% of the variance in VO_{2peak} [13]. This suggests that *pulmonary* and *peripheral vascular* adaptations may be important determinants of exercise intolerance in cardiovascular disease. In fact, it has been suggested that under elevated pressure loads as during isometric bouts, a failure in the performance of the *left ventricle* in susceptible subjects may compromise *contractility* and *stroke volume*, with the consequent lower *oxygen delivery* to the working muscles [11].

Oxygen Uptake (VO_2)

VO_{2max} is achieved under maximal aerobic metabolism. This rate in short-term studies is found to increase only 10% with the effect of training. However, that of a person who runs in marathons is 45% greater than that of an untrained person. This is believed to be partly genetically determined: stronger respiratory muscles, larger chest size in relation to body size and partly due to long-term training. The fastest rate at which the body can utilize oxygen during heavy exercise is defined as the maximum rate of VO_2, which is an index of maximal cardiovascular function [14]. Therefore, it might be hypothesized that VO_{2peak} or VO_{2max} is dependent on *oxygen delivery* and by the tissues ability to *extract oxygen* [15]. Pulmonary capacity, maximal cardiac output, and total hemoglobin content are considered central conditioning factors for VO_2, the total *hemoglobin* content, and *oxygen release capacity* of the blood defined by the $(a\text{-}v)O_2$.

VO_2 and aerobic capacity are all terms used interchangeably with VO_{2max}. One factor that can determine an individual's capacity to perform sustained exercise and is linked to aerobic endurance is VO_{2max}. It is the maximum capacity of an individual's body to transport and use oxygen during incremental exercise, which reflects the physical fitness of the individual. It is measured as milliliters of oxygen used in 1 min/kg of body weight ($mLO_2 \cdot kg^{-1} \cdot min^{-1}$). This measurement is generally considered the best indicator of an individual's cardiovascular fitness and aerobic endurance. Theoretically, the more oxygen the individual can use during high level exercise, the more energy he/she can produce. This is often the case with elite endurance athletes who typically have very high VO_{2max} values. VO_{2max} results vary greatly. The average for a sedentary individual is close to 35 $mLO_2 \cdot kg^{-1} \cdot min^{-1}$ while, elite endurance athletes often average 70 $mLO_2 \cdot kg^{-1} \cdot min^{-1}$. One of the highest recorded VO_{2max} results (94 $mLO_2 \cdot kg^{-1} \cdot min^{-1}$) was that of a cross-country skier.

VO_2 is of vital importance for both health and sport performance [16]. Although VO_{2max} is generally considered the best indicator of *cardiopulmonary function* and endurance, it is more useful as an indicator of a person's aerobic potential or upper limit than as a predictor of success in endurance events. While a high VO_{2max} may be a prerequisite for performance in endurance events at the highest level, other markers such as *lactic acid threshold* are more predictive of performance [17]. The speed at *lactic acid threshold* (LT) is more significant than the actual value itself. Yet, VO_{2max} varies greatly between individuals as does cardiac output and even between elite athletes that compete in the same sport. Therefore, VO_{2max} should not be confused with the LT or anaerobic threshold, which refers to the point during exhaustive, all-out exercise at which lactate builds up in the muscles during exercise. With proper training, individuals are often able to substantially increase their anaerobic threshold and exercise lasting longer at a higher intensity.

VO_2 increases very rapidly with a half-time of around 30 s after a sudden increase in exercise workload. This may occur either as a result of oxygen delivery to the tissues, by the increased *cardiac output*, or of an increase in the $(a\text{-}v)O_2$, or a combination of both factors. One of the fundamental beliefs in exercise physiology is that there is a lag between the onset of an increase in exercise workload and the arrival of the hypoxic blood from the exercising muscle at the lungs. This traditional belief, however, was questioned by Casaburi et al. [18], who found that pulmonary artery desaturation occurred in humans within 4 s after a transition between rest and 150 W cycle exercise, that is, earlier than the predicted circulation time of around 12–17 s [19].

VO_{2max} Determination

VO_{2max} can be determined through a number of physical evaluations. These tests can be *direct* or *indirect*. Direct testing requires sophisticated metabolic carts to measure the volume and gas concentrations of inspired and expired air. There are many protocols used on treadmills, cycle ergometers, and other exercise equipment to measure VO_{2max} directly. Accurately measuring VO_{2max} requires an all-out effort usually on a treadmill or bicycle, effort sufficient in duration to fully stress the aerobic energy system. It should be performed under a strict protocol in an exercise physiology laboratory. The subject is typically connected to a metabolic cart to measure VO_2, and the workload is increased incrementally over a fixed duration of time. These protocols for clinical and athletic testing involve a graded exercise test in which exercise intensity is progressively increased while measuring the volume and oxygen concentration of inhaled and exhaled air. This determines how much oxygen the individual is using.

The method for measuring oxygen uptake is called *open circuit spirometry* (Fig. 2.9). It measures simultaneously and on line oxygen and CO_2, multiply by V_E in order to have VO_2 and volume of CO_2 production. VO_{2max} is reached when VO_2 remains at steady state despite an increase in workload (Fig. 2.10).

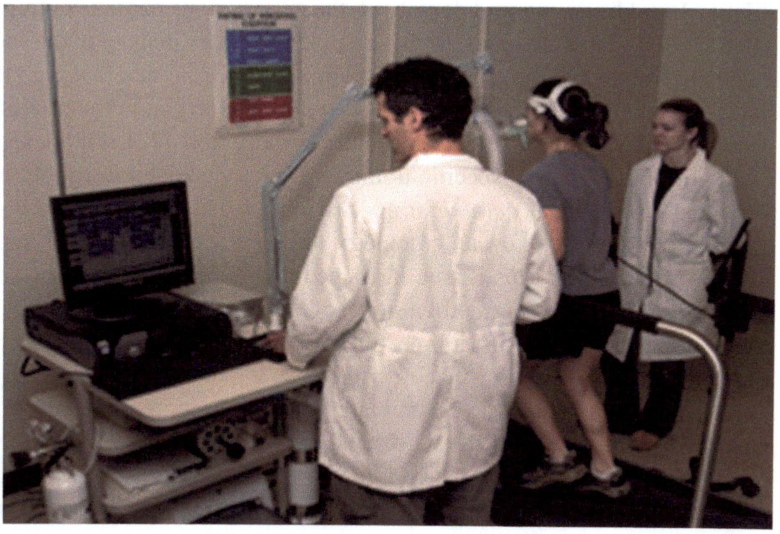

Fig. 2.9 Open circuit spirometry metabolic cart to define oxygen uptake in a direct method on line in real time (With permission from Skidmore College)

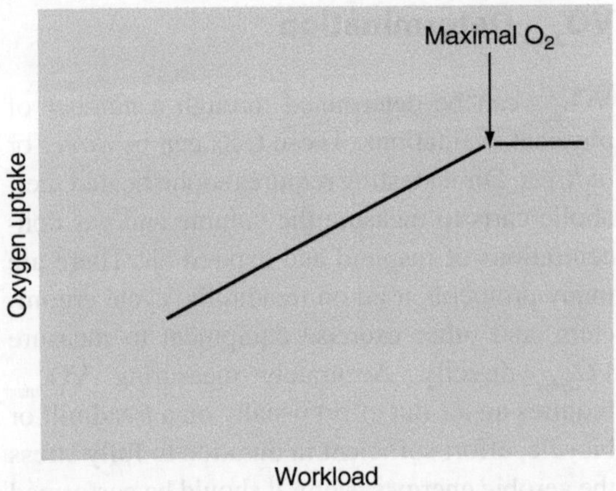

Fig. 2.10 The concept of maximal oxygen uptake. It is reached when VO_2 remains at steady state despite an increase in workload. Oxygen uptake plateaus even if the exercise intensity increases

An individual's VO_2 increases in a linear relationship with exercise intensity up to a point, in which oxygen uptake plateaus even if the exercise intensity increases [20]. This plateau marks the VO_{2max}. At this point, the individual moves from aerobic metabolism to anaerobic metabolism. From here, it is not long before muscle fatigue forces the individual to stop exercising. VO_{2max} varies greatly between individuals and even between elite athletes that compete in the same sport. The test usually takes between 6 and 8 min. Tests that last longer than that may force the individual to withdrawal from the test due to fatigue. In addition, normal length of the test, requires from an individual to be completely rested and motivated to endure the pain long enough to find the true VO_{2max}.

VO_{2max} defined at peak exercise depends on the mode of exercise and the specific training of the individual. Incremental *aerobic stress test* on a treadmill compared to cycle ergometry has a higher VO_{2max} values. This is true in trained and untrained subjects. However, professional cyclists participating in major competitions such as the Tour de France exceptions, that is, will have a higher VO_{2max} values on the cycle ergometry compared to the treadmill. Anyhow, in most cases, VO_{2max} values measured on a treadmill will be higher by 10% than that of the cycle ergometry.

Calculating VO_2 is somehow a simple process: in addition to the Fick equation discussed in the previous chapter, by subtracting volume of oxygen expired from volume of oxygen inspired, it is possible to express the volume of oxygen consumed (Eq. 2.9) Therefore,

$$VO_2 = V_E\left(F_IO_2 - F_EO_2\right), \quad (2.9)$$

where VO_2 = oxygen uptake, V_E = minute ventilation, F_EO_2 = fractional of oxygen expired (%), and F_IO_2 = fractional of oxygen inspired (%).

In an attempt to compare the cardiopulmonary system in different populations, VO_2 is usually expressed relative to bodyweight because VO_2 and total energy needs, among other factors, are also determined by body size. Another possibility is to normalize VO_2 to body surface area, which can be more accurate when comparing children and gender.

Factors Affecting Oxygen Uptake

Performance in VO_{2max} is related to several physiological variables, such as the anaerobic threshold, long-lasting aerobic exercise, running economy, and anaerobic capacity [21]. Factors affecting VO_2 are often divided into supply and demand factors [22].

Supply is the transport of oxygen from the lungs to the mitochondria including lung diffusion, cardiac output, blood volume, and capillary density of the skeletal muscle, while demand is the rate at which the mitochondria can reduce oxygen in the process of oxidative phosphorylation [22]. Of these, the supply factor is often considered to be the limiting one [22, 23]. However, it has also been argued that while trained subjects probably are supply limited, untrained subjects can indeed have a demand limitation [24].

Noakes [25] described a number of variables that may affect VO_{2max}: age, gender, fitness and training, changes in altitude, and action of the ventilatory muscle. Noakes [25] also asserts that VO_{2max} is a relatively poor predictor of performance in runners due to variations in running economy and fatigue resistance during prolonged exercise [25].

Although the past controversy is regarding VO_2 limiting factors, central vs. peripheral origin, it is now widely accepted that VO_{2max} is mainly determined by central factors, namely pulmonary ability to saturate *hemoglobin*, *cardiac output*, and hemoglobin capacity to *release oxygen* to the tissues [26]. However, the interplay of the cardiopulmonary (central limitation) and cellular (peripheral limitation) should be always examined according to age, sex, and health status in order to better understand the real contribution of those factors to limit VO_2. Indeed, in young and old males and females, the peripheral machinery is matched to the growth (puberty) and loss (aging) of muscle mass [12]. Moreover, it can be assumed that cardiac *stroke volume* capacity may adjust following the changes in muscle mass following physical activity or inactivity [27]. For instance, remarkable increases in endurance performance are related to relatively small changes in VO_{2max}. Consequently, there has been great interest in identifying the physiological factors that limit VO_2 and determining the role of this variable in endurance and anaerobic performances.

Today, it is universally accepted that there is a physiological upper limit to the body's ability to deliver and consume oxygen. In the scientific literature, an increase in VO_2 is the most common method of demonstrating cardiopulmonary and physical performance ability. In addition, VO_2 is frequently used in the development of an exercise prescription in health and cardiovascular diseases. Given these applications of VO_2, there has been large interest in defining the relative contribution of cardiopulmonary physiological factors that limit VO_2 in healthy subjects and *cardiac patients* of different ages, sex, and training status.

Genetics Role in Oxygen Uptake Variability

It is well known that different individuals have different DNA sequences. In general, DNA sequence differences occurring in more than 1% of the population and are termed polymorphisms. Polymorphisms may account for some of the differences in performance capacity between individuals, including VO_{2max}. *Genetics* plays a major role in the variability of VO_2 and cardiac output or in the responsiveness to training [28]. It is suggested that heredity can account for up to 25–50% of the variance seen between individuals [29]. *Mitochondrial DNA* is of particular interest, because it contains the genes for several enzymes involved in VO_2. Mitochondrial DNA contains genes for 13 proteins of the *electron transport chain* as well as 22 transfer RNAs and two ribosomal RNAs required for their intramitochondrial synthesis [30]. Variation in the DNA sequence of these genes could therefore contribute to the differences in endurance performance between individuals. Research shows that although VO_{2max} has a genetic component, it can also be increased through training. Research in this area has focused on mitochondrial DNA sequences, genes for creatine kinase, and genes for angiotensin-converting enzyme [31].

The two methods for increasing VO_{2max} include increases in both training volume and intensity. Research also indicates that the more sedentary an individual is, the further he/she can increase its VO_{2max} through training. In fact, novice exercisers have been able to increase VO_{2max} by 20% through proper training. Well-trained athletes have a harder time increasing their VO_{2max}, most likely because they are already so near to their genetic potential. Chromosomes 1p31 and 5q23 were used to identify *human genomic regions* that are linked to VO_{2max} in sedentary individuals or to the responsiveness of VO_{2max}. Results of a genomic scan based on 289 polymorphic markers covering all 22 pairs of autosomes performed on the Caucasian families of the HERITAGE Family Study indicated that in response to a 20-week standardized endurance training program, results showed linkages between VO_{2max} and markers on 4q, 8q, 11p, and 14q for VO_{2max} before training and with markers on 1p, 2p, 4q, 6p, and 11p for the change in VO_{2max}. These chromosomal regions harbor many genes that may qualify as candidate genes for these quantitative traits [32].

The Angiotensin-Converting Enzyme Genotype

Endurance athletic performance has been related to *angiotensin-converting enzyme* (ACE) genotype [33]. Several potential mechanisms may explain how angiotensin-converting enzyme genotype affects endurance performance. Angiotensin-converting enzyme is widely expressed in human tissues, including skeletal muscle [34] and may play a metabolic role *during exercise* [35]. The angiotensin-converting enzyme DD *genotype* level and activity is higher in identical pairs of genes for any given pair of hereditary characteristics (*homozygous*). The identical pairs have the same alleles at one or more gene loci on homologous chromosome segments [36].

In some studies, higher VO_{2max} levels, which indicate an improved oxidative capacity, were found to be related with angiotensin-converting enzyme D *allele* [37]. The increased *angiotensin-converting enzyme* activity associated with the DD genotype may lead to enhanced production of angiotensin II, which is the predominant biological product of *renin-angiotensin system* (*RAS*), mediating many of the local effects of angiotensin-converting enzyme on skeletal muscle. *Angiotensin II* increases blood pressure by stimulating the Gq protein in vascular smooth muscle cells which in turn activates contraction by an IP3-dependent mechanism which is a necessary factor in mediating vascular smooth muscle growth, and affects capillary density in skeletal muscle [35]. Moreover, angiotensin II has direct hypertrophic effect on skeletal muscle, and angiotensin II type I receptor AT1R-mediated angiotensin II is crucial for optimal overload-induced skeletal muscle hypertrophy [38]. Angiotensin II has been shown to regulate VO_2 and affect muscle energy expenditure as well [39]. Aside from genetic factors, four other components have a large influence on VO_{2max}: age, gender, ambient temperature, and altitude.

Gender Effect on VO_2

During strenuous exercise that genders a significant *lactic acidosis*, VO_2 continues to rise until exercise is terminated, or exhaustion ensues [40]. VO_2 values observed in sedentary *trained men* and *women* of the same ages vary primarily due to anatomical and physiological differences in *maximal stroke volume* between subjects, given that considerably less variation exists in maximal heart rate and systemic oxygen extraction. In addition, it has been found that during *aerobic exercise* VO_2 of male exceeds that of female due to gender-related variance in heart size [41]. The highest ever recorded VO_{2max} is 94 $mLO_2 \cdot kg^{-1} \cdot min^{-1}$ in men and 77 $mLO_2 \cdot kg^{-1} \cdot min^{-1}$ in women. Both were cross-country skiers [42]. Untrained *girls* and *women* typically have a VO_{2max} 20–25% lower than untrained *boys* and *men*. However, when comparing elite athletes, the gap tends to close to about 10%. Taking it step further, if VO_2 is adjusted to account for fat free mass in trained and untrained males and females, the differences disappear in some studies. Pardaens et al. [43] suggested that sex-specific essential fat stores account for the majority of metabolic differences in running between men and women. Comparing *gender responses* during a 1-h treadmill run, similar gender physiologic and perceptual responses were generally found [44]. In addition, it has been suggested that normal exercise capacity as determined by VO_{2peak} is related to the indexed *stroke volume* in males and left atrial pressure in females. These native normal differences between genders may explain the known vulnerability of women to *endurance exercise* compared to men [44].

Comparing the exercise cardiac function during endurance exercise of young *women* and *men* suggest that compared to women, men had a higher *blood volume* and *hemoglobin*. At maximal heart rate, *men* had a *higher cardiac output* (31.0 ± 0.6 vs. 24.1 ± 0.9 $L \cdot min^{-1}$) and stroke volume than *women*. When expressed relative to body mass (kg), there were no gender differences in maximal *stroke volume index* [44]. Factors linked mainly to oxygen-carrying capacity and cardiac size have been shown to contribute significantly to this gender-related difference [45].

VO_2 in the Hot and Cold Ambient

Core temperature is sensed by the hypothalamic thermoregulatory center. This center then sets off a number of circulatory adjustments in an effort to dissipate heat. Primarily, this involves increasing *cardiac output* and redistributing blood from the visceral organs to the *working muscles* and *skin*. Severe *heat stress* has been shown to markedly suppress VO_{2max} and work capacity without altering the initial rate of rise in whole-body VO_2 [46]. Thus, endurance performance is impaired in hot environment as compared to temperate environment, and the time to exhaustion is influenced by alterations of *heat stress* and increase in body temperature [47]. The mechanisms underlying the compensatory adjustments to heat stress early in exercise and the subsequent precipitated fatigue have never been investigated. However, it has been proposed that, during heat stress, skin blood flow may be up to 20-fold higher than at resting level. Sweat glands become more active for increasing evaporative heat loss. During *heavy exercise* in *normal environments*, fatigue is often preceded by a plateau or even a decline in VO_{2max}. However, no study to date has determined whether central hemodynamic and skeletal muscle circulation are indeed impaired before fatigue during exercise that requires maximal aerobic capacity. It has been proposed that in the *heat*, *pulmonary system* may limit VO_{2max} of elite athletes by way of CO_2 changing acid–base regulation. In the average person, CO_2 partial pressure falls toward VO_{2max}, suggesting that there are expiratory flow limitations. However, in elite athletes, CO_2 levels actually rise as VO_2 reaches its maximum secondary to their greater capacity to utilize oxygen, and potentially, CO_2 may limit VO_{2max} [2].

Several sports are contested outdoors during winter months, including ice hockey, road, or cross-country footraces, snowboarding, alpine or cross-country skiing, and ice-skating. Other sports and recreational activities sometimes occur when the air temperature is cold; these include American football, soccer, baseball, hiking, and rock climbing. Performance in these sports and activities may be negatively affected if core body temperature decreases. From a physiological point of view, cold is an ambient temperature that forces humans to behave accordingly in order to help the thermoregulatory system to achieve homeostasis. V_E increases slightly at rest and during light exercise in neutral environments compared to the cold environment. This is a response to the impulses coming from the heat receptors in the subcutaneous blood vessels. However, V_E increases as workload is increased in both environments to the same extent. It is possible that the V_E response in the cold environment is a result of adaptations of the peripheral receptors to the cold environment. Thus, healthy individuals need not to be concerned about the acute effects of cold air exercise on the lungs. During swimming in different water temperatures, VO_2 is higher in the coldest water.

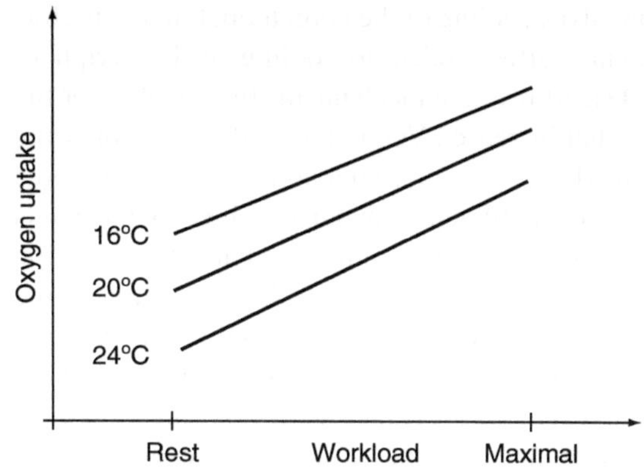

Fig. 2.11 Oxygen uptake at rest is higher in ambient temperature of 16°C with the lower in ambient temperature of 24°C. At maximal effort, these differences are reduced

In the cold at rest, heat production will increase VO_2 by fivefold compared to rest in normal ambient temperatures. This relatively increase in VO_2 will be found also during efforts in the cold. However, with increase in effort's load, the difference between the environments is reduced. Figure 2.11 illustrates the large differences in VO_2 at rest between the three different ambient temperatures. It also demonstrates that at maximal effort, these differences are reduced.

While humans maintain body *core temperature* within a strict homeostatic range, *skin* and peripheral muscle temperature may experience a wide temperature variation. Much of the literature investigating cooling on human performance involves cooling of the core, though many performance effects relate to cooling of the periphery [48]. At rest, the mechanisms responsible for the higher increased VO_2 in the cold are (a) shivering and (b) reduced muscular ability to generate force due to inefficient movements. External work is the same in different environments. However, the reduced ability of the muscle to generate force imposes to recruit more motor units, and by doing so, VO_2 is increased. In addition, the inefficient movements contradict the agonist and antagonist synchronization and (c) increase levels of catecholamine in the blood with reduced ambient temperatures especially in the water. This increase in the blood's catecholamine influences metabolism and thus VO_2.

In the cold environment, *during exercise*, *oxygen delivery* has the greatest impact on the reduction of VO_{2max} following the decrease in whole body temperature, occurring if exercise lasts long in cold air. The VO_{2max} decrement is due to (a) fall in cardiac output following decreases in maximal heart rate and unchanged stroke volume, (b) *oxygen extraction* by skeletal muscles decrease when blood temperature decreases below normal core temperature due to interference in oxygen release from the hemoglobin to muscle tissue, and (c) blood flow to skeletal muscle during exercise decreases; thus, energy is produced by *glycolysis* with increasing *lactic acid* levels. One solution is a pre-exercise warm-up that prepares muscles and the cardiovascular system, prevents injury, and promotes metabolic efficiency. The optimal preparation for exercise in the cold involves moderate exercise intensity and longer duration. Warming up with a short duration and high-intensity protocol is ineffective.

In the *cold ambient*, the muscles are impaired from most of their functional properties like power, force production, and velocity Therefore, *strength* and muscular power decrease [49]. There is general agreement that rate properties are slowed with almost any level of cooling thereby most substantially reducing muscle power. Specific decrements, subsequent to muscle cooling, occur in jumping and sprinting events. The decrement in maximal voluntary contraction ranges from 11% to 19% when the muscle temperature decreases below 27°C [48]. The slowed enzymatic processes and slowed nerve conduction that impair rate of force development also likely reduce local muscular endurance during strength contractions and impair manual dexterousness.

VO_{2max} at Altitude

VO_{2max} is decreased significantly above an altitude of 1,600 m. For every 1,000 m above that, VO_{2max} drops by approximately 8–11%. At extreme altitudes approaching the summit of Mt. Everest, inspiratory oxygen partial pressure is 43 Torr, an average sea level VO_{2max} of 62 $mLO_2 \cdot kg^{-1} \cdot min^{-1}$ can drop to 15 $mLO_2 \cdot kg^{-1} \cdot min^{-1}$ [50]. For individuals with a sea level VO_{2max} less than 50 $mLO_2 \cdot kg^{-1} \cdot min^{-1}$ would be unable to move as their VO_{2max} would drop to 5 $mLO_2 \cdot kg^{-1} \cdot min^{-1}$ enough only to support resting oxygen requirements. Sustained hyperventilation was crucial to exercise performance during chronic, severe hypoxemia. VO_{2max} was lower after altitude exposure compared with initial sea level values, indicating that exposure had not improved sea-level exercise capacity. VO_{2max} falls progressively with increasing altitude; the diffusion that depends on partial pressure also falls progressively with increasing hypoxia. Therefore, it is suggested that the passive diffusive steps in the lungs and muscles explain most of the decrement in oxygen availability, while changes in the mostly convective processes of ventilation and blood flow contribute little or no impediment to oxygen transport [50]. To estimate the relative role of the different factors limiting VO_{2max}, several resistances to oxygen transport are identified, inversely proportional to: alveolar ventilation, oxygen transport by the circulation, oxygen diffusion from capillary blood to mitochondria, and mitochondrial capacity [51].

Peripheral Versus Central Theories

Long-standing yet unresolved debates center on whether central cardiopulmonary or local skeletal muscle circulatory and metabolic factors limit VO_{2max} [52]. Over the years, two main theories have been proposed to explain the limits of VO_2, for example, *central theory* associated with the systemic and muscle oxygen delivery [53] and the *peripheral theory* in which the working skeletal muscle cells, which account for more than 90% of the energy spent during *severe exercise*, largely determine VO_{2max} [54]. In addition, a *general theory* was also initially advanced postulating that there is no single limiting factor for VO_2.

The classical theory proposes that exercise is limited only after oxygen delivery to the exercising skeletal muscles becomes inadequate, inducing high levels of lactic acid [15, 55]. It holds that exercise is limited when sufficient oxygen cannot be delivered to the skeletal muscle, which is a function of the cardiovascular system [15, 55], and defends that VO_2 is not limited by the utilization capacity. Both cardiopulmonary *oxygen delivery* and *tissue diffusion* limitation are believed to limit VO_{2max} in normal humans during maximal exercise [56]. The studies of Richardson and colleagues [57] demonstrated reduced *cytoplasmic partial pressure* of oxygen at VO_{2peak} during single-legged exercise even when *cardiac output* was submaximal. These results are consistent with a supply limitation to VO_{2max} in trained skeletal muscle, even during *hyperoxia*. Their data also revealed a disproportionate increase in *intracellular oxygen pressure* during hyperoxia, which could mean that the *mitochondrial* limits determining peak muscle VO_2 are approached even at relatively high oxygen pressure in trained skeletal muscle [24]. Thus, a logical starting point in the search for a *central governor* are those studies of cardiopulmonary function during acute *hypoxia* since the possibility that myocardial ischemia will develop is increased during maximal exercise in hypoxia. It is generally accepted that relatively mild hypoxia inhibits mitochondrial oxidative phosphorylation when *mitochondrial* PO_2 falls below a critical level in oxygen-sensing cells, thereby mediating, in part, cell activation [58]. Anaerobic pathways, which produce ATP inefficiently, are then utilized. The main anaerobic metabolites are H^+ and lactic acid ions, which are not easily excreted. They accumulate in the circulation, where they may be quantified in terms of the base deficit and the lactic acid/pyruvate ratio. It has been suggested by Evans et al. that a rise in the cellular AMP/ATP ratio activates three possible AMP-activated protein kinase subunit isoform combinations in pulmonary arterial myocytes, with $\alpha 1\beta 2\gamma 1$ predominant, and thereby, evokes Ca^{2+} signals in oxygen-sensing cells [58].

Numerous studies have shown that VO_{2max} can be modified acutely by altering one or more of the variables considered to limit this measurement. These acute changes occur before structural adaptations, normally requiring several weeks to develop, can occur. Examples of acute modifications in VO_{2max} are increases with acute *red blood cell* transfusion [59]. With *endurance training* over a long (chronic) period, VO_{2max} increases but decreases with *detraining* [60] or with prolonged exposure to high altitude [61]. Structural as well as functional changes in cardiopulmonary and neuromuscular function are more likely to explain these chronic changes.

The *peripheral theory* maintains that VO_2 is limited by lack of sufficient *oxidative enzymes* within the cell's *mitochondria* [20], being the body's ability to utilize the available oxygen that determines VO_2. This theory is supported by numerous studies showing that oxidative enzymes and the number and size of mitochondria increase with *training* paralleling increases in VO_2 [62]. Additionally, these is coupled with increased $(a\text{-}v)O_2$ accounting for improved oxygen utilization and hence training-improved VO_2.

According to this theory, the maximal $(a\text{-}v)O_2$ is determined by the tissues to use oxygen. However, it is important to highlight that even if that would be true, the *central factors* such as *pulmonary capacity* and *cardiac output* should not be neglected. Moreover, based on the VO_2 plateau at peak exercise, speaks in favor of a *central limitation* to VO_2 because although the increasing amount of muscle fibers recruited and the amount of mitochondria able to use oxygen, the VO_2 does not increase [63].

The *central theory* defends that VO_2 is not limited by the utilization capacity, but by the ability of the *cardiopulmonary system* to deliver and release oxygen to active tissues. Supporters [64] of this theory maintain that an increase in blood volume, *maximal cardiac output* due to increased *stroke volume*, and better perfusion of blood into the muscles account for the changes in VO_2 with training. González-Alonso [14] and Calbet [65] reviewed the literature and concluded that *oxygen supply* is the major limiter to maximal oxygen uptake. Studies have shown only a weak relationship between an increase in oxidative enzymes and an increase in VO_2. One of these studies measured the effects of a 6-month swim training program on aerobic function. While oxidative enzymes continued to increase until the end, there was no change in oxygen uptake in the final 6 months of the program. Consequently, this theory postulates that the maximal *(a-v)O_2* is determined by the *hemoglobin* maximal ability to release oxygen and not directly influenced by tissues capacity to use it [66].

From the evidence presented thus far, it would seem that the limitation to *VO_{2max}* might not be a single factor, but a combination of a number of elements of the cardiopulmonary systems. Evidence supporting this notion is the similar VO_{2max} values for exercise that involves large muscle mass and leg work alone. Additional further support for *central limitation* of VO_{2max} during bicycle exercise with large muscle mass (legs and arms) is the fact that the added muscle mass reduces blood flow to the exercising legs by vasoconstriction. This mechanism supports the cardiac output to maintain blood pressure [23].

To conclude, the majority of data presented in today's debate points to oxygen supply and not oxygen utilization at a peripheral level as the broad process that sets VO_{2max} for an individual, under a given set of conditions. Therefore, it can clearly be stated that the limitation to VO_{2max} and thus aerobic capacity is central.

VO_{2max} in Cardiovascular Disease Patients

Beyond the reduced *maximal cardiac output*, pulmonary disorders, also common in patients with advanced heart failure, may also contribute to the lower VO_{2max} usually seen in these patients. Indeed, evaluating findings detected on pre- and postoperative assessments of heart failure patients, who underwent heart transplantation, suggested that following heart transplantation, pulmonary complications are common [67]. These changes that compromise the percentage of saturated hemoglobin in the arterial blood could also contribute to the lowering of *VO_2* in *cardiac patients*. In addition, in cardiac patients, another mechanism to explain the lower *cardiac output* is the medication with beta-blockers. Hawkins et al. [68] suggested that beta-blockers can decrease maximal *heart rate* significantly, being the maximal *cardiac output* decreased by 15–20%, while *stroke volume* increases slightly. Although the decreased cardiac output is partially VO_2 compensated by an increase in (a-v)O_2, the VO_2 declines by 5–15%. Thus, it can be concluded that the decline in VO_2 seen in patients under cardio-selective beta-blocker is caused by diminished blood flow and oxygen delivery [53]. Surprisingly, the exercise intolerance in patients with chronic heart failure shows a weak correlation with the degree of left ventricular dysfunction [11]. This unexpected finding has directed the attention to peripheral changes in chronic heart failure patients. During the last years, several different peripheral factors as determinants of exercise intolerance have been defined, that is, abnormalities in ventilation, reduced endothelium-dependent vasodilatation of peripheral conduit and resistance vessels, and altered skeletal muscle metabolism [69].

Skeletal muscle alterations are characterized by a reduced *oxidative capacity*, a catabolic state with reduced local IGF-I expression and muscle atrophy, chronic inflammation with local expression of the inducible isoform of nitric oxide synthase, and an accelerated rate of programmed cell death (apoptosis) [69]. In opposition to the widely accepted theory of the *central limitation* for *VO_2* in healthy subjects, it is not yet resolved to what extent the *peripheral factors* contributes to the exercise intolerance and lower VO_2 described in these *cardiac patients*.

VO_{2max} Following Training

The extent by which VO_{2max} can change with training also depends on the starting point. Considerable training is required to reach the upper limit for VO_{2max}. However, much less is required to maintain it. In previously sedentary people, training at 60–75% of oxygen uptake, for 30 min, three times a week over 6 months, increases VO_{2max} an average of 15–20% [70]. However, this is an average, and there are large individual variations with increases as wide ranging as 4–93% reported [70]. When volume of exercise is controlled, higher intensities of exercise are more effective for improving VO_{2max} than lower intensities of exercise in healthy, young adults [71]. There are three primary ways to improve maximal oxygen uptake: (a) Since VO_{2max} is based on weight, the individual could just simply lose weight. Then, the individual's VO_{2max} will instantly go up. However, this is not advised as a method of improving maximal oxygen uptake for most runners since losing weight compromise health. (b) The individual can improve VO_{2max} through running more kilometers per week. Going from being sedentary to running 40 km/week can improve VO_{2max} by up to 16%. Moving from 40 to the 80 km/week range can improve it up to another 16%. And moving from 80 to 110 km/week improves it up to 3% more. Beyond 110 km/week, there is minimal to no effect at all on VO_{2max}. One has to keep in mind that with each increase in kilometer, there is a enormous increase in injuries' incidence. There also seems to be a genetic upper limit beyond which further increases in either intensity or volume have no effect on VO_2 [70]. The fitter an individual is to begin with, the less potential there is for an increase and most elite athletes hit this peak early in their career, and (c) the individual can use the anaerobic threshold, speed work, to improve not only VO_{2max} but also its anaerobic threshold. From the standpoint of athletic performance, sometimes running faster is a better mode of exercise to improve VO_{2max}. However, if training is to improve health without participating in competition, it is preferably to increase volume of exercise above the anaerobic threshold than increasing speed. Once a plateau in VO_{2max} has been reached, further improvements in performance are still seen with training. Two major reasons for this are improvements in anaerobic threshold and running economy.

Intense resistive training and anaerobic training have small effect on VO_{2max} [72]. Resistance training alone does not increase VO_{2max} [71] even when short rest intervals are used between sets and exercises [73]. However, others found significant increase though small in VO_{2max}. Study undertaken to determine if heavy resistance training results in an increase in VO_{2max} found a significant 4% increase in VO_{2max} during bicycle exercise following resistive training, but no significant differences were observed when expressed in ($mLO_2 \cdot kg^{-1} \cdot min^{-1}$). Strength training had no effect on VO_{2max} when measured during treadmill exercise. The data suggest that the small increase in leg cycle VO_{2max} may be due to adaptations in oxidative capacity and increased mass of the strength-trained muscles [74]. In a recent study, significant improvements in aerobic capacity and treadmill time to exhaustion can be obtained in older adults as a consequence of either high- or low-intensity resistance exercise. These findings suggest that increased strength, as a consequence of resistance exercise training, may allow older adults to reach and/or improve their aerobic capacity [75].The discrepancy in the results following resistive training may be due to different cohorts and protocols used during the different studies.

Oxygen-Carrying and Release Capacity of the Blood

Most oxygen is carried in the blood as oxyhemoglobin. The small contribution that dissolved oxygen makes to transport is usually negligible. It can be calculated using Henry's law – for each mmHg of oxygen partial pressure (PO_2), there is 0.003 mLO_2 dissolved per 100 mL of blood, absolutely very small. Each gram of pure hemoglobin can carry 1.34 mL of oxygen when it is fully saturated. Therefore, every liter of blood with a hemoglobin concentration of 15 g/100 mL of blood can carry about 200 mLO_2 when fully saturated. Usually, it happens when alveoli's oxygen partial pressure is >100 mmHg. At this oxygen partial pressure, only 3 mLO_2 will dissolve in every liter of plasma. When considering the adequacy of oxygen delivery to the tissues, three factors need to be taken into account: hemoglobin concentration, cardiac output, and oxygenation. Figure 2.12 illustrates that under normal conditions in healthy

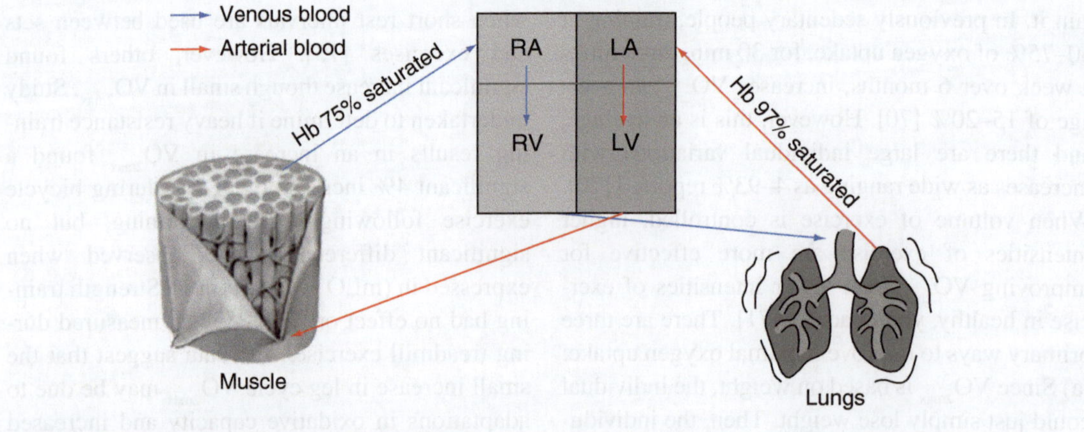

Fig. 2.12 Levels of hemoglobin (*Hb*) saturation (%) in blood leaving the lungs (*red arrows*) and blood arriving to the lungs (*blue arrows*). Deoxygenated blood (*blue arrow*) enters the *right side* of the heart via the vena cava and is ejected through to the lungs where oxygen is replenished and carbon dioxide diffuses out to the lungs. Oxygenated blood (*red arrow*) enters the *left side* of the heart and is subsequently delivered to the body

humans at rest, hemoglobin in blood leaving the lungs is about 97% saturated with oxygen, while deoxygenated blood returning to the lungs is still approximately 75% saturated.

Hemoglobin has an oxygen binding capacity of between 1.36 and 1.37 $mLO_2 \cdot g^{-1}$ [76]. Increased VO_2 by recruited muscles during strenuous exercise reduces the oxygen saturation of venous blood, which already referred might reach less than 10% in a trained athlete [77].

During exercise, the effectiveness of *hemoglobin-oxygen* binding can be affected by body core temperature, *2,3-diphosphoglycerate* (*2,3-DPG*), *partial pressure of* CO_2 (*PCO_2*), or pH (Fig. 2.13). These factors can be viewed as having the effect of shifting or reshaping the oxyhemoglobin curve of a typical healthy person. The standard curve is shifted to the right by an increase in temperature, 2,3-DPG, PCO_2, or a decrease in pH.

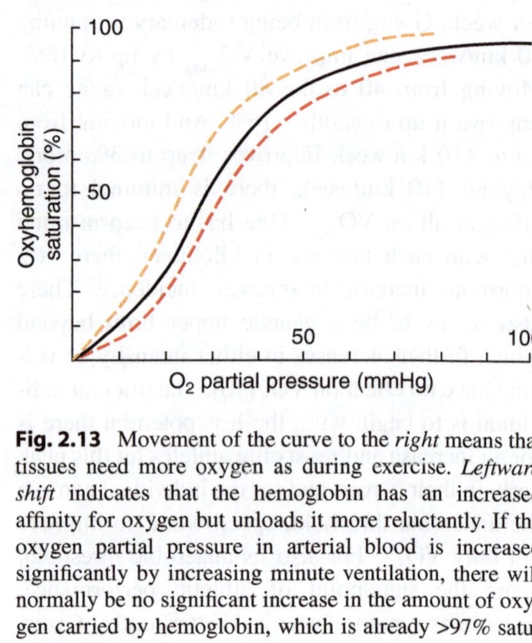

Fig. 2.13 Movement of the curve to the *right* means that tissues need more oxygen as during exercise. *Leftward shift* indicates that the hemoglobin has an increased affinity for oxygen but unloads it more reluctantly. If the oxygen partial pressure in arterial blood is increased significantly by increasing minute ventilation, there will normally be no significant increase in the amount of oxygen carried by hemoglobin, which is already >97% saturated with oxygen

The dissociation curve shifts to the right when CO_2 or H^+ ion concentration is increased. This facilitates increased oxygen release to the tissue. This mechanism allows for the body to adapt the problem of supplying more oxygen to tissues that need it the most. When muscles are undergoing strenuous activity, they generate CO_2 and lactic acid as products of cellular respiration and lactic acid fermentation. In fact, muscles generate lactic acid so quickly that pH of the blood passing through the muscles will drop to around 7.2. As lactic acid releases its protons, pH decreases, which causes hemoglobin to release ~10% more oxygen, that is, the Bohr effect [78]. Conversely, a *leftward shift* increases the affinity, making the oxygen easier for the hemoglobin to pick up [26].

The *Bohr effect* influence of pH/CO_2 on hemoglobin-oxygen affinity and the reciprocal *Haldane effect* which influence of hemoglobin-oxygen saturation on H^+/CO_2 binding originate in the hemoglobin oxy/deoxy conformational change and allosteric interactions between oxygen and H^+/CO_2 binding sites [26]. CO_2 affects the curve in two ways: First, it influences intracellular erythrocyte pH, the Bohr effect; and second, CO_2 accumulation causes carbamino compounds to be generated through chemical interactions. Low levels of *carbamino* compounds have the effect of shifting the curve to the left, while higher levels cause a rightward shift.

Bohr effect states that an increasing concentration of protons and/or CO_2 will reduce the oxygen affinity of hemoglobin [78]. Increasing blood CO_2 levels can lead to a decrease in pH because of the chemical equilibrium between protons and CO_2. This effect facilitates oxygen transport as hemoglobin binds to oxygen in the lungs, but then releases it in the tissues, particularly those tissues in most need of oxygen. When a tissue's metabolic rate increases, its CO_2 production increases, and bicarbonate is formed (see above Eq. 2.7). Although the reaction usually precedes very slowly, the enzyme family, carbonic anhydrase in red blood cells accelerates the formation of bicarbonate and protons. This causes the pH of tissues to decrease, and so, promotes the dissociation of oxygen from hemoglobin to the tissue, allowing the tissue to obtain enough oxygen to meet its demands. Conversely, in the lungs, where oxygen concentration is high, binding of oxygen causes hemoglobin to release protons, which combine with bicarbonate to drive off CO_2 in exhalation. Since these two reactions are closely matched, there is little change in blood pH.

The 2,3-DPG is an organophosphate, created in erythrocytes during glycolysis. It controls the movement of oxygen from red blood cells to body tissues. The production of 2,3-DPG is likely an important adaptive mechanism, because the production increases for several conditions in the presence of diminished peripheral tissue oxygen availability, such as *hypoxemia*, chronic lung disease, anemia, and congestive heart failure, among others [79]. High levels of 2,3-DPG shift the curve to the right, while low levels of 2,3-DPG cause a leftward shift, seen in states such as septic shock, temperature, and hypophosphatemia. Temperature does not have so dramatic effect as the previous factors, but hyperthermia causes a rightward shift, while hypothermia causes a leftward shift.

The increase of the blood hemoglobin content is a common strategy to improve the oxygen transport to working muscles. Blood doping is the practice of artificially increasing a person's volume of total red blood cells through removal, storage, and subsequent infusion. Reinfusion of 900–1,350 mL blood elevates the oxygen-carrying capacity of the blood. This procedure has been shown to increase aerobic power by 4–9% in well designed, double-blind studies [64]. Once again, these studies provide evidence of a cause-and-effect link between *oxygen delivery* and VO_2 during *aerobic exercise*. *During exercise* in normal males, females, and *coronary artery disease patients*, increases in $(a\text{-}v)O_2$ are produced by flow redistribution from metabolically less active tissue to the exercising muscle, *hemoconcentration* from fluid loss into the exercising muscle interstitial space, and increased *oxygen extraction* over the active muscle bed [80].

In *coronary artery disease patients* with low cardiac output, exercise tolerance is reduced despite modulated regional blood distribution and oxygen extraction. Thus, the increase in VO_{2peak} during exercise is more reduced than in normal subjects [81]. However, low cardiac output does not necessarily lead to reduced exercise tolerance. The presence of a unique mechanism regulating $(a\text{-}v)O_2$ in severe cardiovascular disease patients contributes to efficient oxygen delivery to the peripheral tissues thus compensating for the reduced exercise tolerance in those patients. It has been previously reported that the $(a\text{-}v)O_2$ increases proportionally to the VO_{2max} percentage, and this relationship is unaltered regardless of the underlying heart disease and the severity of heart failure [69], for example, at VO_{2max}, $(a\text{-}v)O_2$ should be the maximal, and at 50% of VO_{2max}, $(a\text{-}v)O_2$ should be half the value of maximal $(a-v)O_2$. Decreased oxygen supply due to reduced *cardiac output* is not fully compensated by the increased *oxygen extraction* [82].

Anemia

Anemia comes in various forms, with some types posing greater health problems than others. One of the primary symptoms of anemia is fatigue. Anemia is a condition in which the production and amount of the healthy red blood cells is below normal and is a frequent complication of many diseases, but the mechanisms that link reduced blood oxygen content to the long-term consequences of anemia are incompletely understood. Red blood cells which carry oxygen from the lungs to muscle tissues and organs are synthesized in the bone marrow. Each cell lives for about 120 days in the circulation.

Exercise may easily bring upon the subject *fatigue* and short of breath. Thus, a drop in athletic performance or a general feeling of fatigue may indicate the existence of anemia. Because the blood is iron deficient and carries less oxygen to working muscles, when exercising moderately, the individual may be relatively exercising significantly more strenuous. The maintenance of oxygen supply to the tissues during anemia involves complex cardiovascular adaptations, including an increase in cardiac output, reduced peripheral resistance, and increased oxygen extraction from hemoglobin [83]. Reduced arterial oxygen content by the lower hemoglobin concentration would result in a higher blood flow, as observed with a low arterial partial pressure, and maintenance of oxygen delivery. A low arterial oxygen partial pressure induces an elevation in submaximal muscle blood flow [84]. In addition, hypoxia-inducible factors are associated with the transcriptional activation of genes involved in adaptive mechanisms that increase oxygen delivery and provide alternative metabolic pathways. The normal hemodynamic responses to chronic *anemia* include increased cardiac output, decreased systemic vascular resistance, widened arteriovenous oxygen gradient, and increased plasma volume [85].

Role of the Pulmonary System in VO_2

Pulmonary capacity to *saturate* blood *hemoglobin* content in conditions of high blood flow depends on the lung ability to increase pulmonary surface area and hence diffusing capacity for oxygen in response to an increase in oxygen demand. This has been determined in humans who are native to the Andes who have relatively large lungs [86]. These observations demonstrate a consistent response of an increase in diffusing capacity for oxygen to a chronic reduction in oxygen supply. Data suggest that pulmonary gas exchange may contribute to the limitation of VO_{2max} in highly trained athletes who exhibit exercise-induced reductions in arterial oxygen saturation at sea level [87]. In normal individuals exercising at sea level, the pulmonary system saturates the arterial blood 97% which is to its maximal ability.

During exercise, augmentation in *alveolar ventilation* (V_A) is very important for the diffusion of oxygen from the lung to the blood capillaries while at the same time, blood flow to the capillaries is enlarged. Thus, the ratio of alveolar ventilation over *cardiac output* (Q) or *ventilation/perfusion ratio* (V_A/Q) is increased. At rest, the *dead space/tidal volume ratio* (V_D/V_T) is normally about one-third of the tidal volume. During exercise, in normal subjects, it declines to about one-fifth, the major decrement occurring at the lowest work rates. The V_D/V_T ratio is higher when alveolar ventilation relative to perfusion is nonuniform. When V_D/V_T ratio is increased, minute ventilation is typically inordinately high for the work rate performed. A high V_E at a given exercise CO_2 (high V_E/VCO_2) is indicative of either high V_D/V_T *ratio* or acute or chronic *hyperventilation* [88].

Although there is some support in the literature for pulmonary diffusion capacity being the principal limitation to VO_{2max}, the prevailing opinion is that VO_{2max} is primarily limited by cardiac function. Evidence in support of this comes from experimental manipulation of hemoglobin concentration, cardiac output, and partial pressure of oxygen in arterial blood [89]. From the evidence presented thus far, it would seem that the limitation to VO_{2max} might not be a single factor, but a combination of a number of elements of the cardiopulmonary systems.

Gender Effect on Pulmonary Function

Women exhibit several anatomic and physiologic characteristics that distinguish their responses to exercise from those of men. These factors have been shown to influence the training response and contribute to lower maximal aerobic power in women. Sedentary women may experience greater pulmonary gas exchange impairment during exercise than men; however, data indicate that active women do not experience greater exercise-induced abnormalities in gas exchange than men matched for age, height, aerobic capacity, and lung size. Possibly, fitness level and lung size are more important in determining whether or not pulmonary gas exchange impairment occurs during exercise than sex per se [90].

The basis for *gender* differences in *pulmonary function* and exercise tolerance is primarily from two sources: namely hormones, especially progesterone and estrogen, and in structural/morphological differences [91]. The reproductive hormones, estrogen and progesterone, can influence ventilation, substrate metabolism, thermoregulation, and pulmonary function during exercise. Increased estrogen levels tend to increase fluid retention and therefore increase blood volume [92], which could potentially affect gas exchange in the lung. Pulmonary structural and morphologic differences between genders suggest that women may be an exception as height-matched men have larger diameter airways and larger lung volumes and diffusion surfaces, smaller vital capacity, and maximal expiratory flow rates [93] compared with postpubertal women [94]. The effect that these differences have on gas exchange during exercise is incompletely understood. Women may have a larger alveolar-arterial pressure difference that may be compensated for, in part, by increased V_A.

Under normal conditions, in young healthy fit adult male, functional capacity of the pulmonary system, including the lung and chest wall and the supporting neural control system, exceeds the demands placed on them for flow rate, volume, and oxygen and CO_2 exchange [95]. These factors have been shown to influence the training response and contribute to lower maximal aerobic power in women. It has been suggested that gender differences in *lung diffusing capacity* can be explained by fewer total number of alveoli ends up in a smaller surface area and smaller airway diameter relative to lung size in women results in lower maximum flow rates [93]. These differences probably become significant relatively late in the growth period of the lung [96]. These differences may have an effect on the integrated ventilatory response, respiratory muscle work, and in pulmonary gas exchange during exercise. Specifically, evidence suggests that during heavy exercise, women demonstrate greater expiratory flow limitation, an increased work of breathing, and perhaps greater exercise-induced arterial hypoxemia compared to men. The consequence of these pulmonary effects has the potential to adversely affect aerobic capacity and exercise tolerance in women [91].

It seems that smaller lung volumes and maximal flow rates for women in general, and especially highly fit women, causes increased prevalence of expiratory flow limitation during heavy exercise, a relative hyperinflation, an increased reliance on breathing frequency, and a greater encroachment on the ventilatory preserved [97]. Consequently, tidal volume and V_E are mechanically constrained during maximal exercise in many fit women because the demand for high expiratory flow rates encroaches on the airways' maximum flow-volume envelope [88]. However, it appears that there is no a gender difference in the elastic properties of the lungs [98].

Pulmonary Function at Altitude

At *altitude*, V_E is limited. At 5,200 m, V_E is 120 L · mim^{-1} that ties 2 LO_2 · min^{-1}. This *hypoxic situation* reduces the muscle ability to be *oxygenated* due to the reduced *diffusion capacity* between the oxygen-rich arterial blood and the muscle; thus, hyperventilation ensues. Unfortunately, *hyperventilation* eliminates CO_2 in large quantities, and as a consequence, acid–base imbalance is reached. In addition, hyperventilation can bring to a relatively body's dehydration by losing water through ventilation [99].

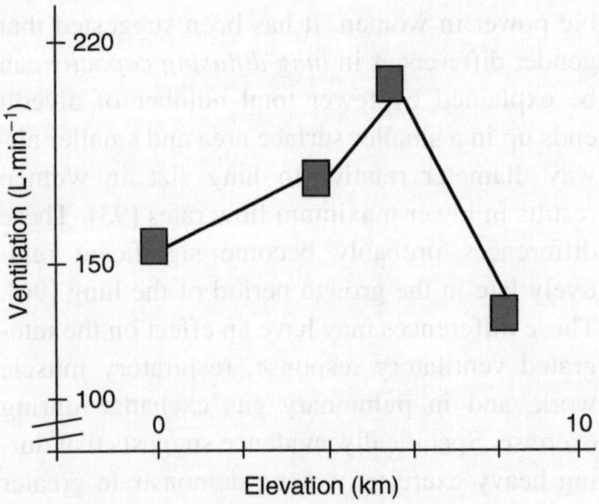

Fig. 2.14 Minute ventilation at different altitudes. At elevation of 6,000 m, maximal minute ventilation is 210 L · min^{-1} while at height of 8,000 m, it drops to 125 L · min^{-1}

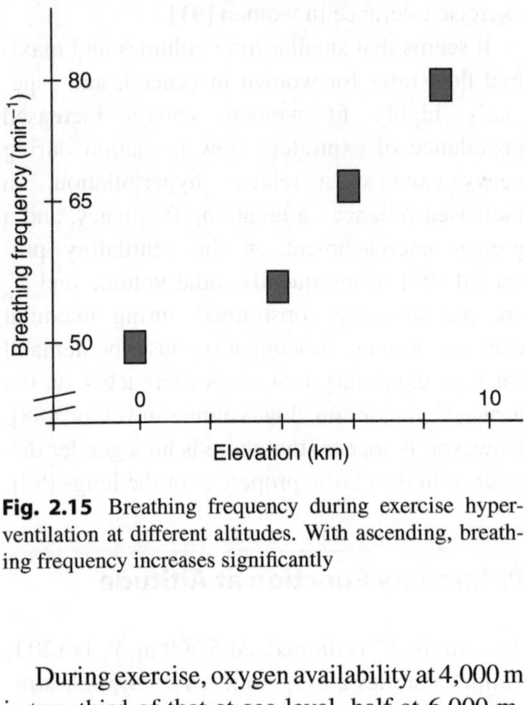

Fig. 2.15 Breathing frequency during exercise hyperventilation at different altitudes. With ascending, breathing frequency increases significantly

During exercise, oxygen availability at 4,000 m is two-third of that at sea level, half at 6,000 m, meaning that at 6,000 m one has to double its V_E and triple it at 8,000 m (Fig. 2.14) compared to the V_E needed at sea level (Avogadro's law). High values for *hyperventilation* are achieved mainly by significantly increase in *breathing frequency* (Fig. 2.15).

Under normal conditions at sea level, diffusion capacity from the alveolar to the blood is not limited. However, at 3,000 m, oxygen partial pressure is 110 mmHg, and therefore, the saturation percentage is 88 in the arterial blood. Though, this is not the reason for the decrease in VO_2 during exercise. It turned out that the reason is the reduced diffusion capacity between the blood and the muscle's cells.

At rest, at sea level, there is a sufficient pressure differences of oxygen partial pressure between arterial blood (100 mmHg) and tissue cells (40 mmHg). This difference of 60 mmHg is enough to maintain an appropriate diffusion from the blood to the muscle [20]. However at an altitude of 2,439 m, arterial oxygen pressure decreases to 60 mmHg, so the pressure gradient drops to about 20 mmHg. In effect, less oxygen diffuses from the oxygen-rich arterial blood to the tissues [100]. In addition, in sedentary individuals, decreased mitochondrial density and volume will reduce VO_2 since the relationships between oxygen uptake and mitochondrial number and size are linear. As mentioned earlier, the oxygen unloading from oxygen-rich arterial blood to the muscle depends also on the velocity of blood flow and on the oxygen disassociation curve direction. In order to overcome the diffusion interference, number of capillaries, mitochondrial size, mitochondrial volume, and myoglobin are increased following training and acclimatization.

Under these conditions, hypoxia will directly affect the vascular tone of the pulmonary resistance vessels and increase ventilation and sympathetic activity via stimulation of the peripheral chemoreceptors [101]. The major effects of acute hypoxia on the lung are shown in Fig. 2.16.

The muscular chemoreceptors send an impulse to the sympathetic nervous system on the hypoxic situation in the muscle. Then, the sympathetic nervous system increases V_E to deliver more oxygen. It is important to realize that the pulmonary system will response to hypoxic situation via the sympathetic nervous system since the lungs cannot be acclimatized to hypoxia in addition to the fact that diffusion capacity is determined genetically. V_E is increased by increasing both tidal volume and breathing frequency as a quick response to hypoxia. *Breathing rate increases at rest and*

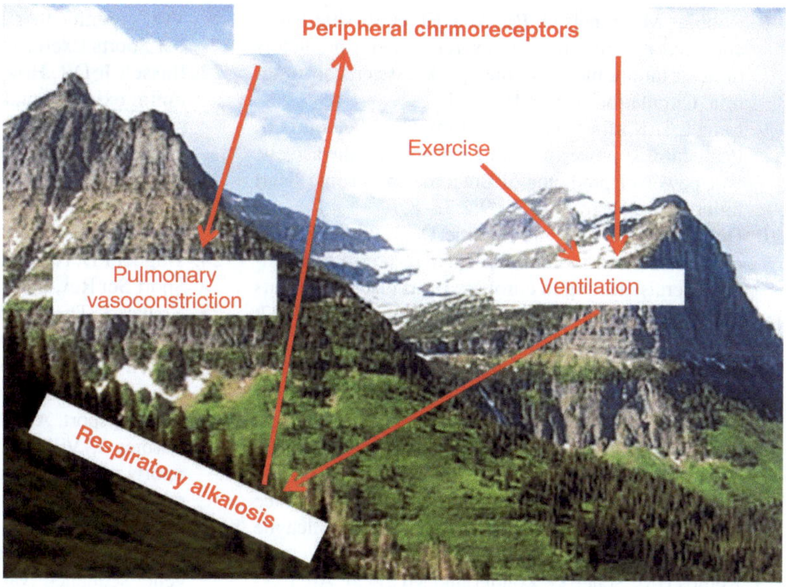

Fig. 2.16 Effect of hypoxia on the pulmonary circulation response at high altitude. Peripheral chemoreceptors are a key factor in the regulation of minute ventilation

during exercise. A smaller number of oxygen molecules per given amount of air means that increased ventilation is required to consume the same amount of oxygen as at sea level [20]. Interactions occur between the direct effects of hypoxia on blood vessels and the chemoreceptor-mediated responses in the systemic and pulmonary circulation. Peripheral chemoreceptor afferent activity rises hyperbolically as hypoxia increases [102]. With exposure over days to weeks, the sensitivity of the peripheral chemoreceptors to hypoxia increases, leading to further enhancement of ventilation.

The Training Effect on the Pulmonary System

The training effect on the pulmonary system is not as found in skeletal muscles and the cardiovascular system. In the lungs at rest, following *training*, no significant changes are observed with regard to maximal voluntary volume (MVV), vital capacity (VC), and forced expiratory volume (FEV). In addition, following exercise training, there is no *training effect* on the *diffusion* of gases. However, functional changes during exercise were noted. Comparing pre- and post-training, at the same absolute workload, V_E was lower due to the increased VO_{2max} and enhanced *cardiac function*, and thus, the demand for V_E is reduced. In addition, f is decreased while V_T is greater than before. By that, the same V_E is achieved with lower breathing energy cost.

References

1. Guyton AC, Hall JE. Textbook of medical physiology. 9th ed. Philadelphia: Saunders; 1996.
2. Vogiatzis I, Zakynthinos S, Boushel R, et al. The contribution of intrapulmonary shunts to the alveolar-to-arterial oxygen difference during exercise is very small. J Physiol. 2008;586:2381–91.
3. Zuurbier M, Hoek G, Oldenwening M, Lenters V, Meliefste K, van den Hazel P, Brunekreef B. Commuters' exposure to particulate matter air pollution is affected by mode of transport, fuel type, and route. Environ Health Perspect. 2010;118:783–9.
4. Johnson BD, Saupe KW, Dempsey JA. Mechanical constraints on exercise hyperpnea in endurance athletes. J Appl Physiol. 1992;73:874–86.
5. Baker SE, Wheatley CM, Cassuto NA, Foxx-Lupo WT, Sprissler R, Snyder EM. Genetic variation of αENaC influences lung diffusion during exercise in humans. Respir Physiol Neurobiol. 2011;179:212–8.
6. O'Neill JO, Young JB, Pothier CE, Lauer MS. Peak oxygen consumption as a predictor of death in patients with heart failure receiving beta-blockers. Circulation. 2005;111:2313–8.
7. Woods PR, Bailey KR, Wood CM, Johnson BD. Submaximal exercise gas exchange is an important prognostic tool to predict adverse outcomes in heart failure. Eur J Heart Fail. 2011;13:303–10.

8. Robbins M, Francis G, Pashkow FJ, et al. Ventilatory and heart rate responses to exercise: better predictors of heart failure mortality than peak oxygen consumption. Circulation. 1999;100:2411–7.
9. Lang CC, Karlin P, Haythe J, Lim TK, Mancini DM. Peak cardiac power output, measured noninvasively, is a powerful predictor of outcome in chronic heart failure. Circ Heart Fail. 2009;2:33–8.
10. Dufour Doiron M, Prud'homme D, Boulay P. Time-of-day variation in cardiovascular response to maximal exercise testing in coronary heart disease patients taking a beta-blocker. Appl Physiol Nutr Metab. 2007; 32:664–9.
11. Sagiv M, Amir O, Goldhammer E, Ben-Sira D, Amir R. Left ventricular contractility in response to upright isometric exercise in heart transplant recipients and healthy men. J Cardiopulm Rehabil Prev. 2008;28: 17–23.
12. Gabbett TJ, Johns J, Riemann M. Performance changes following training in junior rugby league players. J Strength Cond Res. 2008;22:910–7.
13. Kemps HM, Schep G, Zonderland ML, et al. Are oxygen uptake kinetics in chronic heart failure limited by oxygen delivery or oxygen utilization? Int J Cardiol. 2010;142:138–44.
14. González-Alonso J, Calbet JA. Reductions in systemic and skeletal muscle blood flow and oxygen delivery limit maximal aerobic capacity in humans. Circulation. 2003;107:824–30.
15. Bassett DR Jr, Howley ET. Limiting factors for maximum oxygen uptake and determinants of endurance performance. Med Sci Sports Exerc. 2000;32:70–84, Tolle J, Waxman A, Systrom D. Impaired systemic oxygen extraction at maximum exercise in pulmonary hypertension. Med Sci Sports Exec. 2008;40:3–8.
16. Sheel AW, MacNutt MJ, Querido JS. The pulmonary system during exercise in hypoxia and the cold. Exp Physiol. 2010;95:422–30.
17. Van de Veirea NR, Van Laethemb C, Philippéc J, De Winterd O, De Backere G, Vanderheyden M, De Suttere J. V_E/VCO_2 slope and oxygen uptake efficiency slope in patients with coronary artery disease and intermediate peakVO_2. Eur J Cardiovasc Prev Rehabil. 2006;13:916–23.
18. Casaburi R, Patessio A, Ioli F, Zanaboni S, Donner CF, Wasserman K. Reductions in exercise lactic acidosis and ventilation as a result of exercise training in patients with obstructive lung disease. Am Rev Respir Dis. 1991;143:9–18.
19. Koga S, Poole DC, Shiojiri T, Kondo N, Fukuba Y, Miura A, Barstow TJ. Comparison of oxygen uptake kinetics during knee extension and cycle exercise. Am J Physiol Regul Integr Comp Physiol. 2005;288: R212–20.
20. Wilmore JH, Costill DL. Physiology of sport and exercise: rate of reaction. 3rd ed. Champaign: Human Kinetics; 2005.
21. Billat V, Beillot J, Jan J, Rochcongar P, Carre F. Gender effect on the relationship of time limit at 100% VO_{2max} with other bioenergetic characteristics. Med Sci Sports Exerc. 1996;28:1049–55.
22. Bassett Jr DR, Howley ET. Limiting factors for maximum oxygen uptake and determinants of endurance performance. Med Sci Sports Exerc. 2000; 32:70–84.
23. Bassett Jr DR, Howley ET. Maximal oxygen uptake: "classical" versus "contemporary" viewpoints. Med Sci Sports Exerc. 1997;29:591–603.
24. Wagner PD. New ideas on limitations to VO_{2max}. Exerc Sport Sci Rev. 2000;28:10–4.
25. Noakes T. The lore of running. 4th ed. Oxford: Oxford University Press; 2003.
26. Jensen FB. Red blood cell pH, the Bohr effect, and other oxygenation-linked phenomena in blood O_2 and CO_2 transport. Acta Physiol Scand. 2004;182: 215–27.
27. Barbier J, Ville N, Kervio G, Walther G, Carre F. Sports-specific features of athlete's heart and their relation to echocardiographic parameters. Herz. 2006;31:531–43.
28. Argyropoulos G, Stütz AM, Ilnytska O, et al. KIF5B gene sequence variation and response of cardiac stroke volume to regular exercise. Physiol Genomics. 2009;36:79–88.
29. Bouchard C, Dionne FT, Simoneau JA, Boulay MR. Genetics of aerobic and anaerobic performances. Exerc Sport Sci Rev. 1992;20:27–58.
30. Shadel GS, Clayton DA. Mitochondrial DNA maintenance in vertebrates. Ann Rev Biochem. 1997; 66:409–35.
31. Hagberg JM, Moore GE, Ferrell RE. Specific genetic markers of endurance performance and VO_{2max}. Exerc Sport Sci Rev. 2001;29:15–9.
32. Bouchard C, Rankinen T, Chagnon YC, et al. Genomic scan for maximal oxygen uptake and its response to training in the HERITAGE Family Study. J Appl Physiol. 2000;88:551–9.
33. Amir O, Amir R, Yamin C, et al. The ACE deletion allele is associated with Israeli elite endurance athletes. Exp Physiol. 2007;92:881–5.
34. Scott CB. Re-interpreting anaerobic metabolism: an argument for the application of both anaerobic glycolysis and excess post-exercise oxygen consumption (EPOC) as independent sources of energy expenditure. Eur J Appl Physiol Occup Physiol. 1998;77: 200–5.
35. Jones A, Woods DR. Skeletal muscle RAS and exercise performance. Int J Biochem Cell Biol. 2003;35: 855–66.
36. Danser AH, Schalekamp MADH, Bax WA, et al. Angiotensin-converting enzyme in the human heart. Effect of the deletion/insertion polymorphism. Circulation. 1995;92:1387–8.
37. Rankinen T, Perusse L, Gagnon J, et al. Angiotensin-converting enzyme ID polymorphism and fitness phenotype in the HERITAGE Family Study. J Appl Physiol. 2000;88:1029–35.
38. Gordon S, Davis BS, Carlson CJ, et al. Ang II is required for optimal overload-induced skeletal muscle

hypertrophy. Am J Physiol Endocrinol Metab. 2001; 280:E150–9.

39. Cassis L, Helton M, English V, et al. Angiotensin II regulates oxygen consumption. Am J Physiol Regul Integr Comp Physiol. 2002;282:R445–53.
40. Endo MY, Kobayakawa M, Kinugasa R, et al. Thigh muscle activation distribution and pulmonary VO_2 kinetics during moderate, heavy, and very heavy intensity cycling exercise in humans. Am J Physiol Regul Integr Comp Physiol. 2007;293:R812–20.
41. Ben-Sira D, Sagiv M. The effect of gender on left ventricular systolic function at Peak Wingate Anaerobic Test. Eur J Appl Physiol. 1977;75:549–53.
42. Astrand P-O, Rodahl K, Dahl HA, Stromme SB. Textbook of work physiology: physiological bases of exercise. 4th ed. Champaign: Human Kinetics; 2003.
43. Pardaens K, Van Cleemput J, Vanhaecke J, Fagard RH. Peak oxygen uptake better predicts outcome than submaximal respiratory data in heart transplant candidates. Circulation. 2000;101:1152–7.
44. Lindqvist P, Mörner S, Henein MY. Cardiac mechanisms underlying normal exercise tolerance: gender impact. Eur J Appl Physiol. 2012;112(2):451–9. Epub 2011 May 17.
45. Batterham A, George K, Mullineaux D. Allometric scaling of left ventricular mass by body dimensions in males and females. Med Sci Sports Exerc. 1997;29:181–6.
46. Nybo L, Jensen T, Nielsen B, et al. Effects of marked hyperthermia with and without dehydration on VO_2 kinetics during intense exercise. J Appl Physiol. 2001;90:1057–64.
47. Febbraio MA, Snow RJ, Stathis CG, Hargreaves M, Carey MF. Effect of heat stress on muscle energy metabolism during exercise. J Appl Physiol. 1994;77: 2827–31.
48. Drinkwater E. Effects of peripheral cooling on characteristics of local muscle. Med Sport Sci. 2008; 53:74–88.
49. Comeau MJ, Potteiger JA, Brown LE. Effects of environmental cooling on force production in the quadriceps and hamstrings. J Strength Cond Res. 2003; 17:279–84.
50. West JB. American medical research expedition to Everest. High Alt Med Biol. 2010;11:103–10.
51. di Prampero PE. Factors limiting maximal performance in humans. Eur J Appl Physiol. 2003;90:420–9.
52. Wagner PD. Muscle O_2 transport and O_2 dependent control of metabolism. Med Sci Sports Exerc. 1995; 27:47–53.
53. Noakes TD, Peltonen JE, Rusko HK. Evidence that a central governor regulates exercise performance during acute hypoxia and hyperoxia. J Exp Biol. 2001; 204:3225–34.
54. Whipp BJ, Higgenbotham MB, Cobb FC. Estimating exercise stroke volume from asymptotic oxygen pulse in humans. J Appl Physiol. 1996;81:2674–9.
55. Tolle J, Waxman A, Systrom D. Impaired systemic oxygen extraction at maximum exercise in pulmonary hypertension. Med Sci Sports Exec. 2008;40:3–8.
56. Vella CA, Robergs RA. A review of the stroke volume response to upright exercise in healthy subjects. Br J Sports Med. 2005;39:190–5.
57. Richardson RS, Leigh JS, Wagner PD, Noyszewski EA. Cellular PO_2 as a determinant of maximal mitochondrial O_2 consumption in trained human skeletal muscle. J Appl Physiol. 1999;87:325–31.
58. Evans AM, Mustard KJW, Wyatt CN, et al. Does AMP-activated protein kinase couple inhibition of mitochondrial oxidative phosphorylation by hypoxia to calcium signaling in O_2-sensing cells? J Biol Chem. 2005;280:41504–11.
59. Gledhill N. The influence of altered blood volume and oxygen transport capacity on aerobic performance. Exerc Sport Sci Rev. 1985;13:75–93.
60. Duncker DJ, Bache RJ. Regulation of coronary blood flow during exercise. Physiol Rev. 2008;88:1009–86.
61. Green HJ, Roy B, Grant S, et al. Increases in submaximal cycling efficiency mediated by altitude acclimatization. J Appl Physiol. 2001;89:1189–97.
62. Brink-Elfegoun T, Holmberg HC, Ekblom MN, Ekblom B. Neuromuscular and circulatory adaptation during combined arm and leg exercise with different maximal workloads. Eur J Appl Physiol. 2007; 101:603–11.
63. Barker AR, Williams CA, Jones AM, Armstrong N. Establishing maximal oxygen uptake in young people during a ramp cycle test to exhaustion. Br J Sports Med. 2011;45:498–503.
64. Mortensen SP, Damsgaard R, Dawson EA, Secher NH, González-Alonso J. Restrictions in systemic and locomotor skeletal muscle perfusion, oxygen supply and VO_2 during high-intensity whole-body exercise in humans. J Physiol. 2008;586:2621–35.
65. Calbet JA, Rådegran G, Boushel R, Saltin B. On the mechanisms that limit oxygen uptake during exercise in acute and chronic hypoxia: role of muscle mass. J Physiol. 2009;587:477–90.
66. Nielsen HB. Arterial desaturation during exercise in man: implication for O_2 uptake and work capacity. Scand J Med Sci Sports. 2003;13:339–58.
67. Nanas SN, Terrovitis JV, Charitos C, et al. Ventilatory response to exercise and kinetics of oxygen recovery are similar in cardiac transplant recipients and patients with mild chronic heart failure. J Heart Lung Transplant. 2004;23:1154–9.
68. Hawkins MN, Barnes Q, Purkayastha S, Eubank W, Ogoh S, Raven PB. The effects of aerobic fitness and beta1-adrenergic receptor blockade on cardiac work during dynamic exercise. J Appl Physiol. 2009;106: 486–93.
69. Sillanpää E, Häkkinen A, Nyman K, et al. Body composition and fitness during strength and/or endurance training in older men. Med Sci Sports Exerc. 2008;40: 950–8.
70. Costill DL. Inside running: basics of sports physiology. Indianapolis: Benchmark Press; 1986.
71. Gormley SE, Swain DP, High R, Spina RJ, Dowling EA, Kotipalli US, Gandrakota R. Effect of intensity of

aerobic training on VO_{2max}. Med Sci Sports Exerc. 2008;40:1336–43.
72. Gergley JC. Comparison of two lower-body modes of endurance training on lower-body strength development while concurrently training. J Strength Cond Res. 2009;23:979–87.
73. Kraemer WJ, Patton JF, Gordon SE, et al. Compatibility of high-intensity strength and endurance training on hormonal and skeletal muscle adaptations. J Appl Physiol. 1995;78:976–89.
74. Van Zant RS, Bouillon LE. Strength cycle training: effects on muscular strength and aerobic conditioning. J Strength Cond Res. 2007;21:178–82.
75. Vincent KR, Braith RW, Feldman RA, Kallas HE, Lowenthal DT. Improved cardiorespiratory endurance following 6 months of resistance exercise in elderly men and women. Arch Intern Med. 2002;162:673–8.
76. Costanzo LS. Physiology. Hagerstwon: Lippincott Williams & Wilkins; 2007.
77. Mortensen SP, Dawson EA, Yoshiga CC, Dalsgaard MK, Damsgaard R, Secher NH, González-Alonso J. Limitations to systemic and locomotor limb muscle oxygen delivery and uptake during maximal exercise in humans. J Physiol. 2005;566:273–85.
78. Murray, RK, Granner DK, Mayes PA, Rodwell VW. (2003). Harper's Illustrated Biochemistry (LANGE Basic Science) (26th ed). McGraw-Hill Medical. pp. 44–45.
79. Grippi MA. Pulmonary pathophysiology. Philadelphia: JB Lippincott Company; 1995.
80. Tanaka H, Seals DR. Endurance exercise performance in Masters athletes: age-associated changes and underlying physiological mechanisms. J Physiol. 2008; 586:55–63.
81. Lang CC, Agostoni P, Mancini DM. Prognostic significance and measurement of exercise-derived hemodynamic variables in patients with heart failure. J Card Fail. 2007;13:672–9.
82. Sun XG, Hansen JE, Garatachea N, Storer TW, Wasserman K. Ventilatory efficiency during exercise in healthy subjects. Am J Respir Crit Care Med. 2002;166:1443–8.
83. Eckardt KU. Anaemia in end-stage renal disease: pathophysiological considerations. Nephrol Dial Transplant. 2001;16 Suppl 7:2–8.
84. Koskolou MD, Roach RC, Calbet JA, Rådegran G, Saltin B. Cardiovascular responses to dynamic exercise with acute anemia in humans. Am J Physiol. 1997;273:H1787–93.
85. Mancini DM, Kunavarapu C. Effect of erythropoietin on exercise capacity in anemic patients with advanced heart failure. Kidney Int. 2003;64:S48–52.
86. Huang YC, O'Brien SR, MacIntyre NR. Intrabreath diffusing capacity of the lung in healthy individuals at rest and during exercise. Chest. 2002;122:177–85.
87. Keslacy S, Matecki S, Carra J, Borrani F, Candau R, Prefaut C, Ramonatxo M. Effect of inspiratory threshold loading on ventilatory kinetics during constant-load exercise. Am J Physiol Regul Integr Comp Physiol. 2005;289:R1618–24.
88. Wasserman K, Hansen JE, Sue DY, Stringer WW, Whipp BJ. Principles of exercise testing and interpretation. 4th ed. Philadelphia: Lippincott, Williams and Wilkins Publications; 2005.
89. Hoppeler H, Weibel ER. Structural and functional limits for oxygen supply to muscle. Acta Physiol Scand. 2000;168:445–56.
90. Olfert IM, Balouch J, Kleinsasser A, Knapp A, Wagner H, Wagner PD, Hopkins SR. Does gender affect human pulmonary gas exchange during exercise? J Physiol. 2004;557:529–41.
91. Harms CA. Does gender affect pulmonary function and exercise capacity? Respir Physiol Neurobiol. 2006;151:124–31.
92. Stager JM, Tanner DA. Swimming: 2nd edition; An International Olympic Committee Publication. Oxford: Blackwell Science Ltd.; 2005.
93. Guenette JA, Witt JD, McKenzie DC, Road JD, Sheel AW. Respiratory mechanics during exercise in endurance-trained men and women. J Physiol. 2007;581: 1309–22.
94. Harms CA, Rosenkranz S. Sex differences in pulmonary function during exercise. Med Sci Sports Exerc. 2008;40:664–8. Harms CA, Rosenkranz S. Sex differences in pulmonary function during exercise. Med Sci Sports Exerc. 2008;40:664–8.
95. Umar S, van der Laarse A. Nitric oxide and nitric oxide synthase isoforms in the normal, hypertrophic, and failing heart. Mol Cell Biochem. 2010;333:191–201.
96. Zavorsky GS, Walley KR, Russell JA. Red cell pulmonary transit times through the healthy human lung. Exp Physiol. 2003;88:191–200.
97. McClaran SR, Harms CA, Pegelow DF, Dempsey JA. Smaller lungs in women affect exercise hyperpnea. J Appl Physiol. 1998;84:1872–81.
98. Rohrbach MC, Perret C, Kayser B, Boutellier U, Spengler CM. Task failure from inspiratory resistive loaded breathing: a role for inspiratory muscle fatigue? Eur J Appl Physiol. 2003;90:405–10.
99. Ng LJ, Sih BL, Stuhmiller JH. An integrated exercise response and muscle fatigue model for performance decrement estimates of workloads in oxygen-limiting environments. Eur J Appl Physiol. 2011 Jul 19. [Epub ahead of print].
100. Grocott MP, Martin DS, Levett DZ, McMorrow R, Windsor J, Montgomery HE, Caudwell Xtreme Everest Research Group. Arterial blood gases and oxygen content in climbers on Mount Everest. N Engl J Med. 2009;360:140–9.
101. Bartsch P, Gibbs R. Effect of altitude on the heart and the lungs. Circulation. 2007;116: 2191–202.
102. Marshall JM. Peripheral chemoreceptors and cardiovascular regulation. Physiol Rev. 1994;74:543–94.

3 Cardiac Output

Cardiac Output in Normal Subjects

The total amount of blood flow circulating through the heart, lungs, and all the tissues of the body represents the *cardiac output*. Cardiac output responses to exercise at sea level depend mainly on the type of *exercise* performed, *metabolic demand*, and *fitness level*. Modes of exercise include *dynamic aerobic*, *dynamic anaerobic*, and *isometric* or resistive bout. Cardiac output is affected by the phase of respiration with intrathoracic pressure changes influencing diastolic heart filling and therefore cardiac output. Breathing in reduces intrathoracic pressure, filling the heart and increasing cardiac output, while breathing out increases intrathoracic pressure and reduces heart filling and cardiac output. This respiratory response is called stroke volume variation and can be used as an indicator of cardiovascular health and disease. These respiratory changes are important, particularly during mechanical ventilation, and cardiac output should therefore be measured at a defined phase of the respiratory cycle, usually end-expiration [1]. Most individual tissues determine their own flow in proportion to their metabolic rate. The skin is a notable exception where the priority is thermal rather than metabolic. Brain, heart, skeletal muscle, and the splanchnic area all vary their blood flows according to local tissue metabolic rate. Summation of peripheral blood flows constitutes venous return and hence cardiac output [2]. The significant increase in VO_2 during *dynamic aerobic exercise* forces the heart to increase *cardiac output* (*Q*) and to dilate the arterioles (autoregulation). During *dynamic aerobic exercise* such as walking, running, swimming and cycling, oxygen demand by the working muscles increases proportionally to intensity (Fig. 3.1) and by diverting blood from the liver, kidneys, and digestive tract. *During submaximal dynamic aerobic* exercise at the same absolute load, *cardiac output* will be similar in trained and untrained subjects. However, the way to achieve that cardiac output differs significantly between these two subjects. In *untrained subjects*, the increase in cardiac output is achieved mainly by a significant increase in *heart rate* and a moderate increase in *stroke volume* (SV), while in *trained subject*, the increase is due to a significant increase in stroke volume and *heart rate* (HR).

This is not the case with *isometric* and *anaerobic exercises* where the increase in VO_2 is not

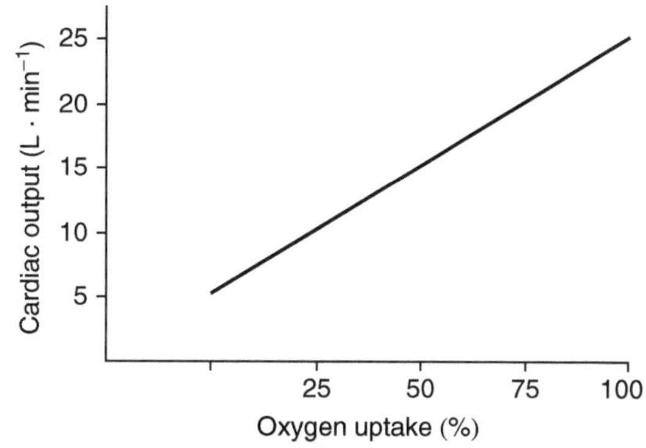

Fig. 3.1 With increase in metabolic demand, cardiac output increases linearly with oxygen uptake

M.S. Sagiv, *Exercise Cardiopulmonary Function in Cardiac Patients*,
DOI 10.1007/978-1-4471-2888-5_3, © Springer-Verlag London 2012

significant. Therefore, compared to aerobic exercise, *cardiac output* will be significantly lower, during isometric exercise and anaerobic exercise with the lowest values during isometric exercise.

Note that during isometric bouts, there is no *autoregulation* mechanism, due to compression of vessels undergoing muscle contraction. The same is true during *anaerobic exercise* regarding the autoregulation mechanism, because anaerobic effort is characterized by exposing the subjects to a very high degree of sudden strenuous all-out exercise [3]. Therefore, there is a need to consider such effects in individuals with impaired cardiovascular function [4]. The total volume of blood in the circulatory system of an average person is about 5 L (5,000 mL). Since *at rest cardiac output* equals also 5 L · min^{-1}, it means that the entire volume of blood within the circulatory system is pumped by the heart each minute. During *vigorous aerobic exercise*, *cardiac output* can increase up to eightfold or 25–40 L · min^{-1} [5].

The *maximal heart rate* of sedentary persons is approximately 220 beats · min^{-1} at maximal work; in trained, it is slightly lower, 215–220 beats · min^{-1}. This gives during aerobic exercise a *cardiac output* of about 25 L · min^{-1} for the sedentary individual, 30–35 L · min^{-1} for the well-trained, and 35–40 L · min^{-1} for world-class athletes (Fig. 3.2).

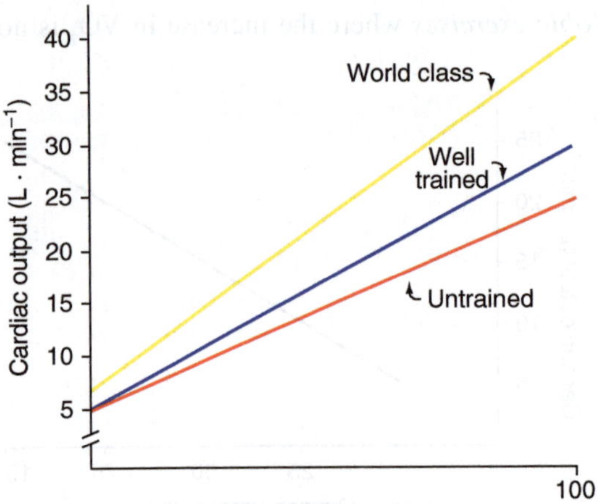

Fig. 3.2 Cardiac output values for different fitness levels: untrained, well-trained, and world-class athlete

When exercising *aerobically* at any given intensity, more oxygen must be delivered to the working muscle. Measuring the responses of an individual running at a 12 km · h^{-1} pace before and after 3 months of regular exercise, it will reveal that the metabolic cost of effort at the same intensity will be unchanged with the assumption that no improvement in movement efficiency happened.

Therefore, *cardiac output* will be also the same. However, just as during rest, the heart will deliver more blood with each beat, that is, the same cardiac output will be achieved with lower *heart rate* and larger *stroke volume* [6].

Previous investigations have indicated that *cardiac output* values for *adolescents* at VO_{2peak} are low compared to young adults during *maximal aerobic exercise* [7]. The explanation for the *lower cardiac output* in both males and females adolescent groups at VO_{2peak} might be related to the *smaller ventricular cavities*, increased *afterload* and lower VO_{2max} [8]. The changes in *left ventricular volumes* during exercise may be due to reduced *contractility*, diastolic and systolic left ventricular functions, and loading conditions [8]. The extent that enhanced ventricular function contributes to superior aerobic fitness of trained athletes compared to sedentary adolescents is unclear. Recent study [7] revealed no differences between young trained adolescents and nonathlete adolescents in cardiac output responses to progressive exercise, implying that greater aerobic fitness in these athletes reflected volume expansion of the cardiovascular system without contribution of enhanced systolic or diastolic ventricular function. Such findings should be considered limited to the context of young trained adolescents with limited duration of athletic training. No significant differences are obtain for *stroke volume*, *cardiac output*, and left ventricular dimensions when they are scaled to body surface area at rest and whatever the exercise intensity. The patterns of stroke volume, as well as its underlying mechanisms, are not age-related during an upright maximal exercise test [9].

The Interplay Between Heart Rate and Stroke Volume

The contribution of stroke volume and heart rate to *cardiac output* varies at *three different stages* of aerobic exercise intensities: (a) from rest to 40% of VO_{2max}, (b) between 40% and 90% of VO_{2max}, and (c) from 90% to VO_{2max} (Fig. 3.3).

During the *first intensity* from rest to 40% of VO_{2max}, *cardiac output* is increased mainly by *augmented stroke volume* (Fig. 3.4) along with a *moderate* increase in *heart rate*, in *untrained individuals*. When 40% of VO_{2max} is reached in sedentary subjects, *stroke volume* attains its maximal value. During the *second load*, between 40% and 90% of VO_{2max}, any further increase in *cardiac output* is met only by increased *heart rate* (Fig. 3.5), based on that the PWC170 test was suggested. The primary purpose of the PWC170 test is to predict the power output or VO_2 at a projected heart rate of 170 beats · min^{-1}. However, in well-trained individuals and *world-class athletes*, stroke volume increases with the increment of workload up to VO_{2max} [10]. Highly trained endurance athletes are able to make progressively increasing usage of the Frank-Starling effect throughout incremental exercise.

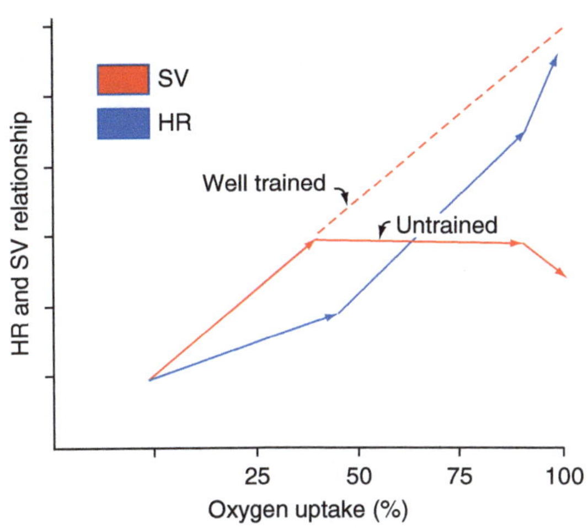

Fig. 3.3 The inverse relationships between hearts rate (HR, *blue line*) and stroke volume (SV *red line*) in three different workloads: 0–40%, 40–85%, and 85–100% of maximal work capacity. If stroke volume increases markedly, heart rate will increase moderately and vice versa

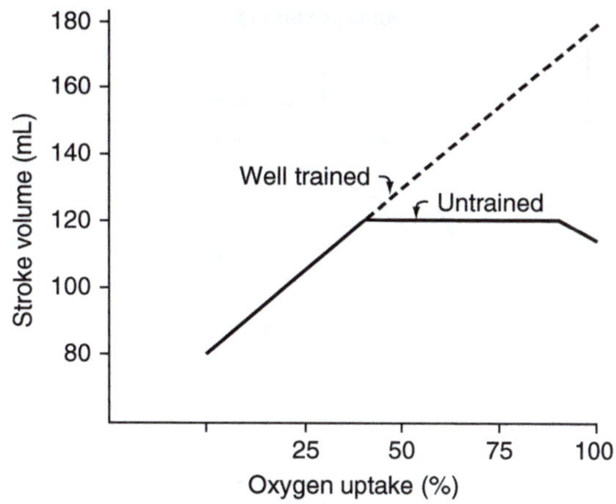

Fig. 3.4 Stroke volume values in trained and untrained individuals during submaximal and at peak dynamic aerobic exercise. In untrained individual, stroke volume increases up to 40% of maximal oxygen uptake, while in well-trained and top athletes, it increases up to maximal oxygen uptake

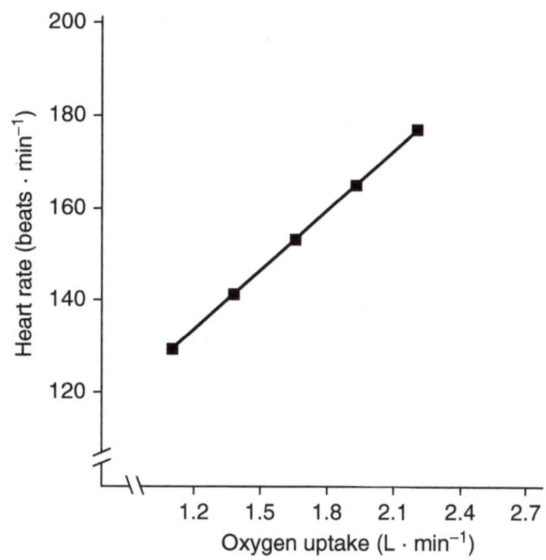

Fig. 3.5 Linear changes in heart rate with increasing workload between 120 and 180 beats · min^{-1}. Based on these relationships, the PWC170 test is utilizes to estimate maximal oxygen uptake

The Frank-Starling mechanism describes the ability of the heart to change its force of contraction and hence stroke volume in response to changes in venous return. In other words, if the end-diastolic volume increases, there is a

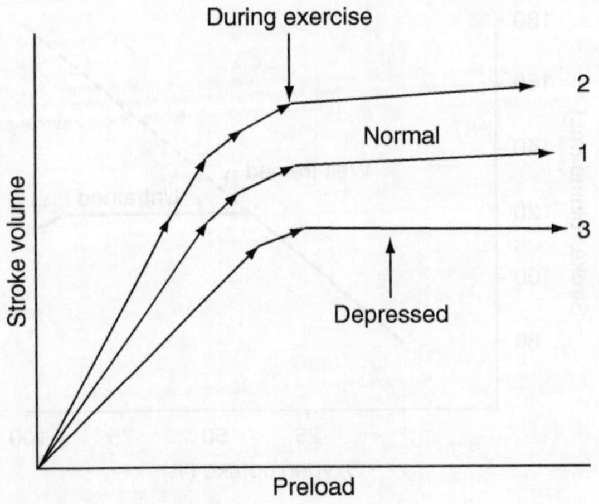

Fig. 3.6 In the figure on *top*, three different *curves* illustrating the *Frank–Starling law of the heart*, the *y*-axis often describes the stroke volume, stroke work, or cardiac output. The *x*-axis often describes end-diastolic volume, right atrial pressure, or pulmonary capillary wedge pressure. The normal *curve* (*line 1*) representing 10 mmHg filling pressure in the left ventricular and normal stroke volume, the depressed curve (*line 3*) representing higher filling pressure in the left ventricular to achieve equal amounts of stroke volume, which can be observed in cases of diastolic heart failure, and exercise positive inotropic *curve* (*line 2*) showing that more stroke volume can be ejected with similar filling pressures

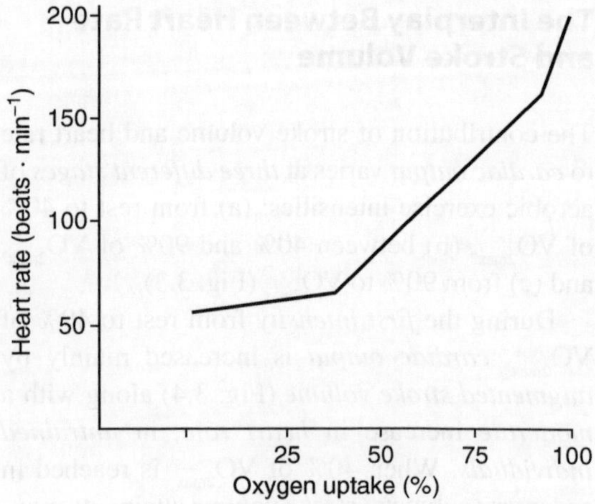

Fig. 3.7 Heart rate-workload relationship for three different workloads: 0–40%, 40–85%, and 85–100% of maximal oxygen uptake, with varying degrees of cardiac function during a progressive exercise test

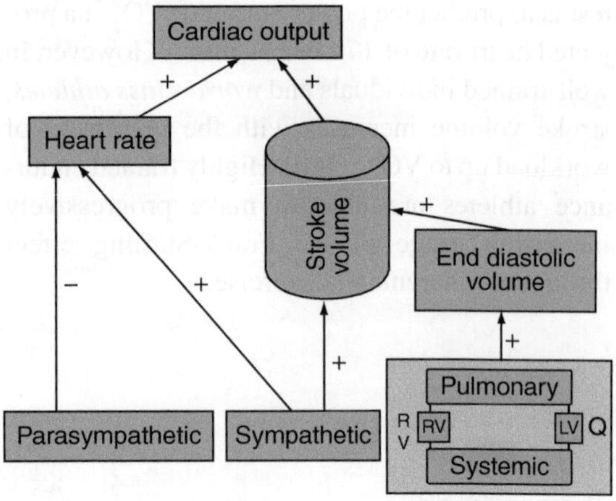

Fig. 3.8 Factors such as parasympathetic with negative effect (–), sympathetic, venous return (*VR*), end-diastolic volume, heart rate, and stroke volume all with positive effects (+) controlling cardiac output (*Q*) at rest and during exercise. *RV* right ventricular, *LV* left ventricular

corresponding increase in stroke volume (Fig. 3.6). The Frank-Starling mechanism can be explained on the basis of preload. As the heart fills with more blood than usual, there is an increase in the load experienced by each muscle fiber. This stretches the muscle fibers, increasing the affinity of troponin C to Ca^{2+} ions causing a greater number of cross-bridges to interact with actin and thus increase contractility.

Evidence indicates that endurance-trained athletes are able to increase their stroke volume throughout incremental upright exercise, probably due to a progressively greater effect of the Frank-Starling mechanism. This is contrary to the widely held belief that stroke volume reaches a plateau at a submaximal heart rate irrespective of fitness level, owing to a limitation in the time for diastolic filling [11].

During the *third load*, between 90% and VO_{2max}, in sedentary subjects, cardiac output increases as a result of a sharp increase in heart rate due to slight decreased stroke volume, owing to the shorter left ventricular filling time, and thus smaller left ventricular end-diastolic volume (Fig. 3.7).

Therefore, in *untrained individuals*, during dynamic exercise at the third load, working muscles will rely more and more on the anaerobic pathway to produce ATP, with elevated levels of *lactic acid*. This in turn will increase fatigue. Figure 3.8 summarizes the factors controlling

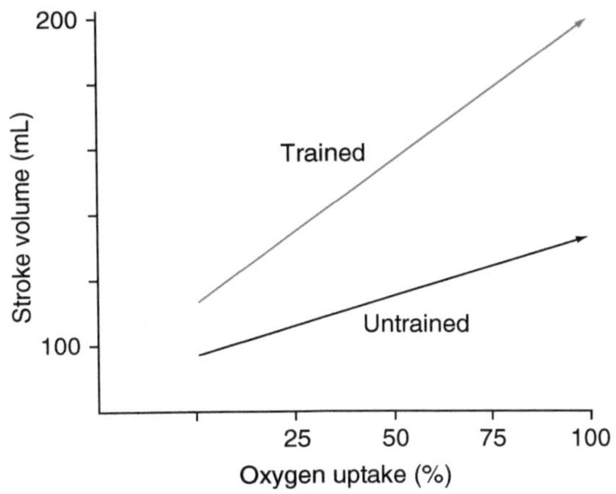

Fig. 3.9 Values for stroke volume at rest and peak aerobic exercise in well-trained and untrained healthy subjects. Untrained individual attains values around 140 mL for each stroke volume while well-trained and top athletes can obtain 200 mL

cardiac output at rest and during exercise during *aerobic exercise*.

Figure 3.9 reveals that in *untrained* individuals, stroke volume at rest averages 80 mL · beat^{-1} and it increases up to 130 mL · beat^{-1} during intense physical activity. In *elite athletes* resting, stroke volume averages 110 mL · beat^{-1} and in Olympic cross-country skiers, stroke volume can increase at peak exercise up to 200 mL · beat^{-1} [12].

During aerobic exercise at a given *cardiac output*, the *interplay* between *heart rate* and *stroke volume* is inversely related (Fig. 3.3). If stroke volume increases markedly, heart rate will increase moderately. Under the same given cardiac output, *stroke volume* will increase only slightly if *heart rate* increase significantly.

The relationship between heart rate and stroke volume is best defined at the end of the filling stage, which is expressed as left ventricular *end-diastolic volume*. Ventricular volume depends on filling time, which is dependent of beats · min^{-1}. Increased heart rate reduces diastolic period, and thus filling time as in untrained individuals. Therefore, for *cardiac output* to increase during vigorous exercise, it is reasonable to argue that there is a progressive utilization of myocardial contractility, tachycardia, and the Frank-Starling mechanism. Very little information exists regarding the cardiovascular responses to changes in postural position during incremental to maximal exercise in endurance-trained athletes. Previously, it has been suggested that when comparing erect vs. supine exercises, *peak diastolic filling rate*, end-diastolic volume, and *stroke volume* are consistently lower throughout incremental exercise in the upright position, reflecting differences in the effective filling volume of the myocardium. Investigators have shown that there are minor changes in stroke volume during incremental exercise in the supine position in healthy individuals [13], indicating that the myocardium may approach its limits for ventricular filling during supine exercise.

At rest, stroke volume and resting *heart rate* of the average person are approximately 70 mL · beat^{-1} and 70 beats · min^{-1}, respectively. This gives us about 5 L · min^{-1} resting cardiac output, determined by oxygen demand at rest which is approximately 250 mLO_2 · min^{-1} and also by the need for high blood flow to the kidneys for filtration purposes. It does not change appreciably with *endurance training*. However, the manner in which the heart delivers this resting demand does change following aerobic training.

Supine Exercise

Postural position has a significant effect on the relative contribution of heart rate, myocardial contractility, and the Frank-Starling mechanism to the increase in cardiac output during exercise conditions [11]. During supine bicycle exercise in sedentary individuals, *cardiac output* increases linearly with the increase in VO_2. During the supine position increased, end-diastolic volume, stroke volume, and peak diastolic filling rate are increased reflecting an increase in *preload*. Thus with increase in exercise workload, stroke volume has a small contribution, and therefore, it relies mainly on the increase of *heart rate* [14]. It is believed that the supine position prevents blood from pooling in the lower extremities enhancing venous return. Linear regression analysis suggested by Warburton et al. revealed that in top athletes, stroke volume increases in a linear

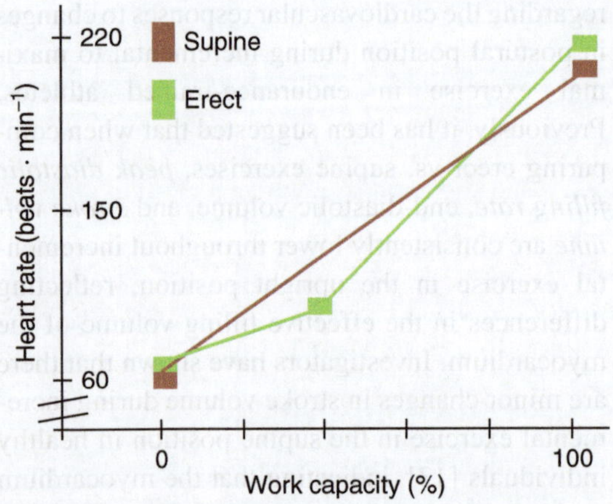

Fig. 3.10 Heart rate response at maximal effort: a comparison between erect exercise (*green*) and supine exercise (*brown*)

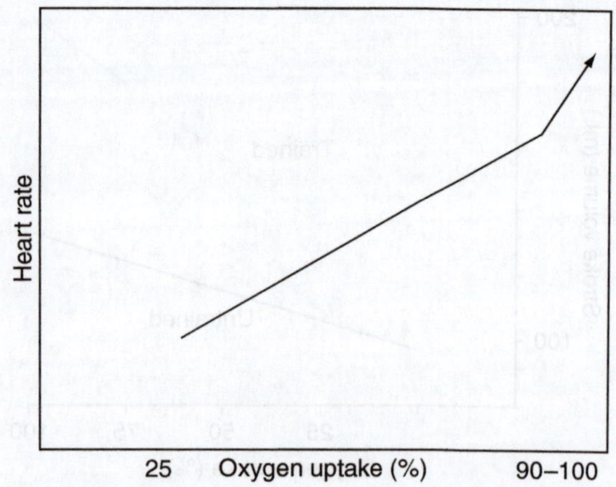

Fig. 3.11 Oxygen uptake and heart rate relationship during supine exercise. Note that up to 90% heart rate is linear to oxygen uptake. From 90% and up, there is a sharp increase in heart rate

fashion throughout incremental exercise in both the supine and upright positions. The highest level for *stroke volume* was reached during *maximal exercise* in both the supine and upright positions. In absolute terms, stroke volume was significantly larger in the supine than the upright position [11].

Maximal heart rate is higher in the erect position due to the smaller stroke volume compared to the lower maximal heart rate in the erect condition (Fig. 3.10).

Supine exercise results in a significantly larger cardiac output than *upright exercise* at rest and throughout incremental exercise. Cardiac output increased throughout incremental exercise in both exercise positions.

The contribution of *stroke volume* and *heart rate* to cardiac output during *supine dynamic exercise* varies during two different stages of exercise intensities: (a) from rest to 90% of VO_2 and (b) from 90% to VO_{2max}. During the *first load*, from rest to 90% VO_{2max}, *cardiac output* is increased mainly by increased *heart rate* along with a small increase in stroke volume. During supine exercise, such as swimming, stroke volume also increases, but usually by only about 20–40%, not nearly as much as in an upright position such as in cross-country skiing. Such a difference depends on body position; when the body is in the supine position, blood does not pool in the lower extremities. Because of this, blood returns more easily to the heart, which means that resting stroke volume values are much higher in the supine position than in the upright position and, hence lower heart rate. Thus, the increase in stroke volume with maximal exercise is not as great in the supine position as in the upright position of cross-country skiing. Interestingly, the highest stroke volume attainable in supine exercise is only slightly greater than the resting value. The majority of the stroke volume increase during low to moderate levels of work appears to be compensating for the force of gravity.

During the *second load*, between 90% to VO_{2max}, *cardiac output* increases as a result of a sharp increase in heart rate due to slightly decrease in stroke volume, owing to smaller left ventricular end-diastolic volume (Fig. 3.11), as an outcome of short ventricular filling time [14]. Therefore, during supine dynamic exercise at loads above 90% maximal oxygen uptake, working muscles will rely more and more on the anaerobic pathway to produce ATP, with elevated levels of lactic acid. This in turn will increase fatigue.

During *sitting dynamic exercise*, such as bicycle, *cardiac output* values are 8–9% less than those attained during standing exercise on a treadmill. These differences in cardiac output are attributed to the smaller muscle mass involved during sitting exercise and consequently to the lower VO_2.

Control of Heart Rate

There are two different factors involved in heart rate management: intrinsic and extrinsic controls. Intrinsic regulation of heart rate is the result of the unique nature of cardiac tissue – it is self-regulating and maintains its own rhythm without direction. Extrinsic controls are those that come from both hormonal responses as well as the commands from the nervous system: the central nervous system and the autonomic nervous system. Extrinsic regulation can cause the heart rate to change rapidly because of chemicals that circular in the blood or by direct action of nerves that go to the heart. The cardiovascular control center is located in the ventrolateral medulla. In that center, heart rate is reduced if activated by the cardio inhibitory center in the medulla or increases if activated by the cardio accelerator. The heart rate is primarily a function of the balance between sympathetic and parasympathetic input to the heart. Other important factor is exercise: with increased skeletal muscle, metabolism increases the total oxygen demands, leading to increased heart rate. Two other minor factors also influence heart rate: (a) chemical reactions proceed faster at elevated temperatures. Fever may cause an increase heart rate solely from the effect of temperature, and (b) increased changes in extracellular ionic environment (hyperkalemia, hypokalemia, acidosis) may also alter heart rate.

At rest in humans, the parasympathetic influence dominates and the resting heart rate is slower than in a totally denervated heart. At rest and *during exercise*, *heart rate* is controlled by the autonomic nervous system. Heart rate is the result of physical and emotional influences mediated through the autonomic nervous system. At rest, sympathetic and parasympathetic nervous stimulations are in balance. During exercise, parasympathetic stimulation decreases and sympathetic stimulation increases. Several factors can alter sympathetic nervous system input. These influences include excitement, fear, anticipation, temperature alterations, respiratory maneuvers, and exercise.

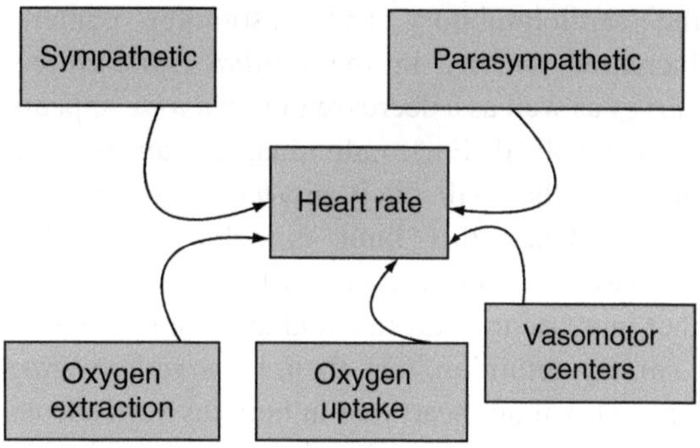

Fig. 3.12 Summary of the variables affecting heart rate at rest and during exercise. While the sympathetic nervous system increases heart rate, the parasympathetic system attenuates it

Both the vagal and the sympathetic nerves are constantly stimulating the SA node. Sympathetic stimulation has a positive chronotropic effect so that if it is increased, the result will be an increase in heart rate, while an increase in vagal tone has a negative *chronotropic* effect on *heart rate* (Fig. 3.12). Studies have shown that *exercise training*, in general, *reduces sympathetic* activity and/or increases *parasympathetic* tonus either in human or laboratory animals. In healthy middle-aged and older men, all sedentary, strenuous, and prolonged *endurance training* elicited reductions in heart rate at rest, due to increase cardiac *vagal tone* [4].

Alterations in *autonomic nervous system* have been correlated with reduction in *heart rate* and blood pressure, either in normal subjects or hypertensive subjects. However, the underlying mechanisms by which physical exercise produces *bradycardia* and reduces blood pressure have not been fully understood. It seems that the role of receptor and *transduction signaling pathways* on the heart and blood vessels influences the heart's response to *exercise training* [15].

Heart rate increases at the start and sometimes in anticipation for exercise. The rapid onset of *tachycardia* is probably due to impulses from the cerebral cortex relayed via the hypothalamus to the cardioinhibitory and vasomotor centers. Increased activity in the *cardiac sympathetic nerves* as well as a decrease in *vagal tone* appears to be involved. Each individual has an exercise intensity that will elicit his *maximum cardiac output*. Once this limit is achieved, further increases in work intensity will result in no further increase in heart rate and anaerobic metabolism. By definition, this, then, is *maximum heart rate*. Maximum heart rate in humans varies from individual to individual and decreases with age. Therefore, the only way to know precisely what a specific person's maximal heart rate is to conduct a *maximal exercise stress test*. Without such precise knowledge, professionals often use the *Karvonen formula* (220 minus ages), to approximate maximum heart rate [16]. This formula will generally give results within plus or minus 10 beats · min^{-1} of reality.

True maximum heart rate may not be achieved in some forms of exercise that do not employ a large muscle mass, or if the person is unfamiliar with the mode of exercise employed. For example, one person may have a true maximum heart rate of 195 beats · min^{-1} in uphill running, but only 191 beats · min^{-1} in a *cycling test*, and 187 beats · min^{-1} while *swimming*. These latter *heart rates* are termed *peak heart rates* and should be used as a basis for determining training intensity for a specific exercise mode. The important thing to remember is that *maximal heart rate* does not increase after aerobic training. It stays the same or might even decrease just slightly. However, maximal *stroke volume* increases therefore *maximal cardiac output* increases in response to aerobic exercise. This is the primary reason for the increase in VO_{2max} Baroreceptors are groups of neurons located in the carotid arteries, the arch of aorta, and the right atrium. At rest and during exercise, these neurons sense changes in oxygen concentration. When oxygen concentration in the blood is decreased, parasympathetic activity decreases and sympathetic activity increases. In addition, these neurons sense changes in pressure in the vascular system. An increase in blood pressure during exercise results in a decrease in parasympathetic activity, when the sympathetic activity overrides the parasympathetic activity. *Baroreceptors* and *chemoreceptor* supply information to the cardiovascular control areas in the brain. Numerous animal and human experiments have provided supportive evidence of arterial baroreflex resetting *during exercise*. Also, it has been demonstrated that both the feed-forward mechanism of central command that plays an essential role in shaping and refining the brain's representation of sensory stimulus attributes [17] and the feedback mechanism associated with skeletal muscle afferents (the exercise *pressor response*) play both independent and interactive roles in the resetting of the arterial baroreflex with exercise. Others suggested that central command and the cardiopulmonary baroreceptors may play a role in this movement of the operating point on the *baroreflex heart rate* [18].

The *autonomic nervous system* responds to pressure sensors in the cardiovascular system via the baroreceptors [19], which technically are *mechanoreceptors*. These major stretch receptors are located in the proximal aorta and in the area of the carotid sinus. Additional stretch receptors are found in the great veins, atria, and pulmonary artery and in other areas of the cardiovascular system.

At *rest* and during *exercise*, the autonomic nervous system also responds to levels of CO_2 sensors through *chemoreceptors*. Portion of the changes related to the heart performance during exercise are similar to those that result from stimulation of the sympathetic nervous pathways to the heart. Thus, it can be that an increase in sympathetic nervous activity occurs during exercise and is an important factor in *heart rate* response [19]. There is considerable evidence that parameters thought to reflect the complex interaction between the autonomic nervous system and the cardiovascular system during exercise can provide significant prognostic information. Specific variables of great importance include heart rate response to exercise (reserve), heart rate recovery after exercise, and multiple components of heart rate variability both at rest and with exercise. Poor *heart rate* response to exercise has been strongly associated with *sudden cardiac death*, and heart rate recovery from a standard exercise test has been shown to be predictive of mortality. In addition, there are limited studies evaluating the components of heart rate variability at rest and during exercise and their prognostic significance. Research continues seeking to refine these exercise measurements and further define their prognostic value. Future findings should augment the power of the exercise test in risk-stratifying cardiovascular patients [20].

Parasympathetic may influence the high frequency-peak shift during strenuous exercise. *Heart rate* variability and the usual indices of sympathetic activity do not accurately reflect changes in autonomic modulation during exhaustive exercise [21]. From the control center located in the ventrolateral medulla, the two channels of the autonomic nervous system originate the sympathetic and parasympathetic components. The sympathetic components increase heart rate by releasing the neural hormone catecholamines – epinephrine and norepinephrine. These hormones are cardioaccelerators. The parasympathetic nervous system located in the brain stem and upper or sacral portion of the spinal cord slows heart rate. The parasympathetic releases the neurohormone acetylcholine, which inhibits heart rate. During *aerobic exercise*, *norepinephrine* levels increase threefold. It seemed that exercise induces a significant response of the sympathetic nervous system [22]. The cardiac muscle cells of the ventricular myocardium are richly enervated by sympathetic nerve fibers. Release of norepinephrine by these fibers during *exercise* causes an increase in the *strength* of *myocardial contraction*, thus increasing *stroke volume*. *Norepinephrine* is thought to increase the intracellular concentration of calcium in myocardial cells, thus facilitating faster *actin/myosin cross bridging* interaction. Also, a general sympathetic response by the body will induce the release of epinephrine from the adrenal medulla. Epinephrine, like norepinephrine, will stimulate an increase in the strength of *myocardial contraction* and thus increase again *stroke volume* [23].

Factors Affecting Stroke Volume

In general, *stroke volume* is controlled by end-diastolic volume, average aortic blood pressure, and the strength of left ventricular contraction. At rest and during exercise, *stroke volume* size depends mainly on venous return, which affects the force of ventricular contraction. As a result, stroke volume increases as suggested by the *Frank-Starling law*: "Energy of contraction is proportional to the initial length of cardiac muscle fiber," that is, the force of cardiac contraction increases in proportion to the degree of diastolic stretch of its muscle fibers (*end-diastolic volume*). In healthy subjects, end-diastolic volume often referred to as the preload. If the end-diastolic volume increases, the stroke volume increases. With an increased end-diastolic volume, a slight stretching of the cardiac muscle fibers occurs, which increases the force of contraction. Thus, any increase in contractility will augment stroke volume and ejection fraction. The sliding filament hypothesis has been used to explain the fundamental property of the cardiac muscle. It has been found that maximal generated contraction force is manifested when the sarcomere is stretched at the end of diastole between 2 and 2.2 nm.

Sympathetic stimulation constricts the veins that drain skeletal muscle. This causes greater blood to flow to the arterials. The muscle pump is the rhythmic contraction and relaxation of skeletal muscle that compresses the veins and thus drains the skeletal muscle. This causes greater blood flow back to the heart, that is, *venous return*. The muscle pump is very important during both resting and *aerobic exercise* conditions. During exercise, the *respiratory pump* also increases venous return. The pressure within the chest decreases and abdominal pressure increases with inhalation, thus facilitating blood flow back to the heart. Because of the increased respiratory rate and depth of breathing during exercise, this is an effective way to increase venous return. This increase in *venous return* in turn increases *left ventricular end-diastolic volume* and hence augments *stroke volume*, as in the *Frank-Starling law*. At the same time, the increase in sympathetic discharge increases inotropic stimulation to the heart which increases ventricular contractility (Fig. 3.13). Strength of ventricular contractility is increased by the secretion of epinephrine and

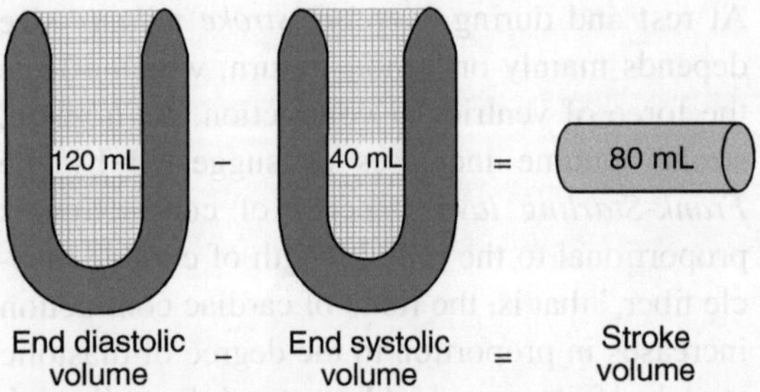

Fig. 3.13 Describes left ventricular volumes affecting stroke volume. Stroke volume is the difference between left ventricular end-diastolic volume and left ventricular end-systolic volume

norepinephrine which increases calcium concentration within the cardiac muscle fiber. Epinephrine and norepinephrine allow for greater calcium entry through the calcium channels in cardiac muscle fiber membranes. This allows for greater myosin and actin interaction and an increase in force production. Inotropy is the term applied to changes in heart muscle performance independent of alterations in preload and afterload. Inotropy varies with a variety of factors, including increases associated with increased frequency of contraction and the effect of post-extrasystolic potentiation, as well as catecholamine, glucagon, and inotropic drugs, and decreases with *myocardial ischemia*, *heart failure*, and depressant agents including almost all anesthetics.

Blood ejected to the aorta is the result of differences in pressure developed in the left ventricle and that existing in the aorta often referred as *afterload*. The blood pressure in the aorta represents a barrier to the blood being ejected from the left ventricle. The *stroke volume* is inversely proportional to the aortic blood pressure. During aerobic exercise, the afterload is reduced, which allows for an increase in stroke volume. Following the ejection of *stroke volume*, about 30–50 mL of blood is left in each ventricle at the end of systole (*end-systolic volume*), which is dependent of the afterload and *state of left ventricular contractility*. Increase in *afterload* will reduce *stroke volume* unless there is sufficient augmentation in left ventricular contractility to match the increase in afterload.

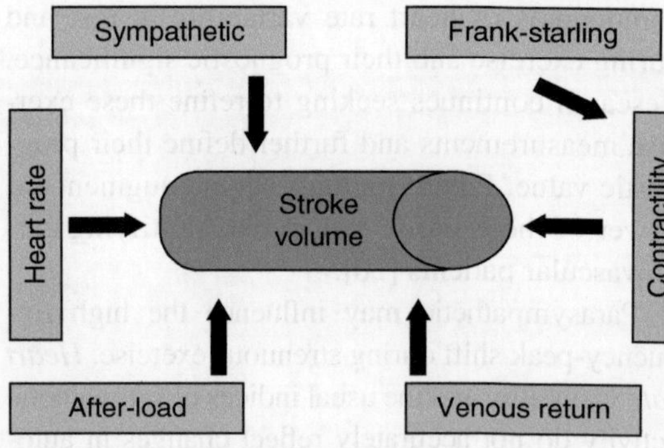

Fig. 3.14 Factors controlling stroke volume at rest and during exercise factors such as Frank-Starling law, venous return, heart rate, contractility, and afterload

Stroke volume in sedentary individuals during dynamic aerobic exercise in the supine position is almost 160 compared to 130 mL during erect dynamic aerobic exercise. The *differences* in stroke volume during dynamic exercise between *erect and supine* can be attributed to the decreased resting stroke volume normally found in the erect position [11]. This *orthostatic effect* is compensated for by increase in the muscle pump and heart rate.

In response to endurance exercise, the heart adapts by increasing *stroke volume* at rest, during *submaximal exercise* and during *maximal exercise*. There is some debate as to whether stroke volume increases because *heart rate* decreases (*increasing diastolic filling time*) or because of an increase in left ventricular volume due to *eccentric hypertrophy* of the heart muscle. Based on available data, both factors probably contribute. Both changes also rapidly revert toward normal with the cessation of training (Fig. 3.14). One other important change that takes place is increased *blood volume*, which helps to take advantage of the increased *filling capacity* of the heart and facilitates *stroke volume* increase. This adaptation occurs fairly rapidly with training, but is also the first adaptation lost if stop training for a week or two.

Understanding the Fick equation is of principal importance for appreciating the utility of the stroke volume prediction. Since $(a\text{-}v)O_2$ do not change dramatically during steady state exercise, the final equation for the estimation of stroke volume was suggested by Whipp et al. [24] as follows (Eq. 3.1):

$$\text{SVexe}(\%) = 5\left(\Delta\text{VO}_2 / \Delta\text{HR}\right)100 \quad (3.1)$$

Whereas SVexe = stroke volume during exercise, VO_2 = oxygen uptake, HR = heart rate, Δ = delta, 5 = a constant number.

Thus, during exercise, *stroke volume* is significantly related to oxygen pulse ($p<.05$) but not to $(a\text{-}v)O_2$ [25], However, this relationship is not valid, in patients with lung disease, anemia, or hyperemia; normal subjects at high altitude or subjects who desaturate during exercise, such as some highly trained athletes [24].

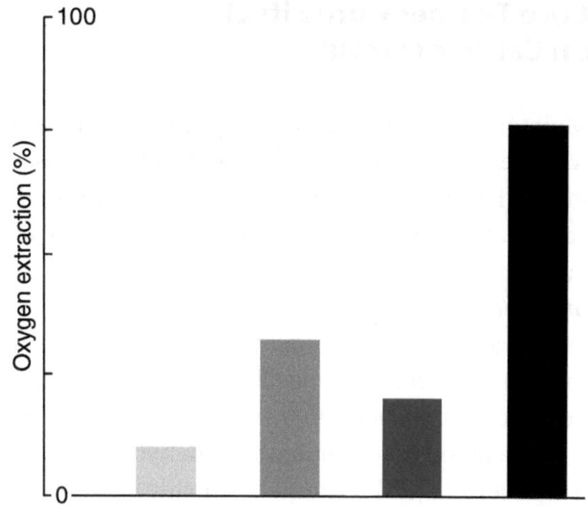

Fig. 3.15 Describes the percentage of oxygen extracted at rest for (from *left to right*) the skin, skeletal muscles, kidney, and myocardium

Oxygen Extraction and Cardiac Output

In healthy subjects, *during maximal aerobic exercise*, a large amount of the available *oxygen is extracted* from blood perfusing the working muscles. At rest, for a subject with approximately $15\ g \cdot dL^{-1}$ of 98% saturated hemoglobin, the oxygen content of arterial blood is approximately $200\ mLO_2 \cdot L^{-1}$. In the exercising legs, blood flow and oxygen delivery leveled off at 73–88% of VO_{2peak} accompanying a rise in *systemic oxygen extraction* to 84 ± 2%, particularly in well-trained athletes. This brings about a fall in oxygen content to about 20–30 $mLO_2 \cdot L^{-1}$ in the venous blood [26]. However, these high percentages of oxygen extraction are not applied to sedentary individuals, whose maximal percentage of oxygen extraction rounds 70–75% of blood oxygen content [27]. Consequently, particularly in athletes, there is little oxygen left to be extracted out of the blood during *heavy exercise*. Hence, the dominant mechanism for the *increase in* VO_2 with training must be an increase in *cardiac output* and oxygen delivery.

Anaerobic metabolism becomes increasingly important during periods of ischemia resulting from an inadequate blood flow that fails to meet the energy demands of tissues. If tissues are subject to ischemia, they try to compensate by extracting more oxygen from the blood. Tissue groups such as muscle typically use at rest only a third of the oxygen available to them (Fig. 3.15), and therefore are able to increase oxygen extraction up to maximal exercise. Conversely, the myocardium extracts most of the available oxygen from the blood even during periods when the body is at rest. The heart, then, has very little physiological reserve to respond to episodes of high energy demand. Rather, the myocardium depends almost entirely on increased coronary blood flow to satisfy high energy demand. Low *cardiac output* can cause cardiac ischemia – perhaps more so for the myocardium than other organs because of the heart's already high rate of oxygen extraction. A vicious cycle ensues. Cardiac ischemia forces a shift toward anaerobic metabolism from the much more efficient aerobic metabolism. With less energy available and increased intercellular acidity, the left ventricular contractility weakens, causing a further reduction in *stroke volume* and *cardiac output*.

Under physiological conditions, VO_2 is independent of oxygen delivery. In order to maintain a constant VO_2, the body can respond by increasing $(a\text{-}v)O_2$ corresponding to a reduction of venous oxygen content and/or by increasing cardiac output.

Core Temperature Effect on Cardiac Output

Maintaining homeostasis is of prime importance when exercising in both hot and cold environments. Failing to do so will result in a decrease in cardiac performance and an increase in the risk of developing potentially fatal situations. *Exercise in the heat* can cause a severe challenge to human cardiovascular control, and thus the provision of oxygen to exercising muscles and vital organs, because of enhanced *thermoregulatory* demand for skin blood flow coupled with dehydration and hyperthermia [28]. External (climatic) and internal (metabolic) heat sources influence body temperature. Ambient temperature, humidity, air movement, and radiant heat from the sun, as well as warm and cold surfaces, contribute to climatic heat stress. *Intense exercise* may increase the metabolic energy expenditure 20–25 times over resting levels. *Metabolic heat* is produced by exercise; however, only 25% of the energy produced is converted into mechanical power; the remainder 75% is heat, which the body must dissipate [29]. In fact, the body is able to respond to a heat load through a variety of physiologic mechanisms mainly through sweat rate, cardiac, and skin blood flow shifts. Cardiovascular strain is characterized by reductions in *cardiac output*, skin and working muscle blood flow, and muscle oxygen delivery accompanies marked dehydration and hyperthermia during prolonged and intense exercise [28].

Exercise in the *warm ambient* places substantial demand on the cardiovascular system, due to the transport of heat generated by muscle contraction to the external environment. To achieve this during exercise in the heat, a large portion of *cardiac output* is taken up by the skin and the exercising muscles. As the volume of blood in circulation is limited, exercise poses a complex problem: An increase in *blood flow* to one of these areas automatically decreases blood flow to the others. This can lead to potentially problematic situations.

The effect of exercise on the cardiovascular induced from hypohydration during heat stress revealed that cardiac output is reduced at severe hypohydration levels and with increased exercise intensity. Thus, cardiovascular strain from high skin blood flow requirements combined with blood volume reductions induced by hypohydration is an important contributor to impaired performance [30]. Under these conditions, in order to have action potential, mineral concentration should be within the physiological range. Any abnormal changes in calcium, potassium, and sodium concentrations will shorten the refractory period which in turn will increase *heart rate*. Such changes can occur with the loss of a significant amount of water in *hot environment* following *prolonged exercise*. People who become hyperthermic during exercise display large increases in heart rate and reductions in stroke volume. During prolonged exercise, cardiovascular drift is characterized by a progressive decline in *stroke volume*. It seems that during prolonged exercise in a neutral environment, the decline in stroke volume under normothermic and mildly hyperthermic conditions is related to the increase in *heart rate* rather than a progressive increase in cutaneous blood flow as body temperature rises [31, 32]. In order to maintain adequate *cardiac output* while shunting blood to the skin, the cardiovascular system has to make some significant adjustments. The subsequent redistribution of blood reduces the overall volume of *venous returns* to the heart, which reduces the *end-diastolic volume*, which in turn, reduces stroke volume. The reduction in *stroke volume* and thus cardiac output beyond the regulatory adjustments to increases in blood oxygen content will result in a fall in systemic oxygen delivery. The lower stroke volume could therefore be a critical factor in the development of fatigue with dehydration and concomitant hyperthermia during exercise in the heat [33]. Therefore, increased body *core temperature* at rest and during *submaximal exercise* will elevate *heart rate* in order to decrease body core temperature by increasing *skin blood flow*. Figure 3.16 compares heart rate response in two different ambient temperatures. During events performed at intensities eliciting VO_{2max}, the superimposition of heat stress causes an earlier decline in exercising muscle blood flow, presumably due to lower cardiac output and

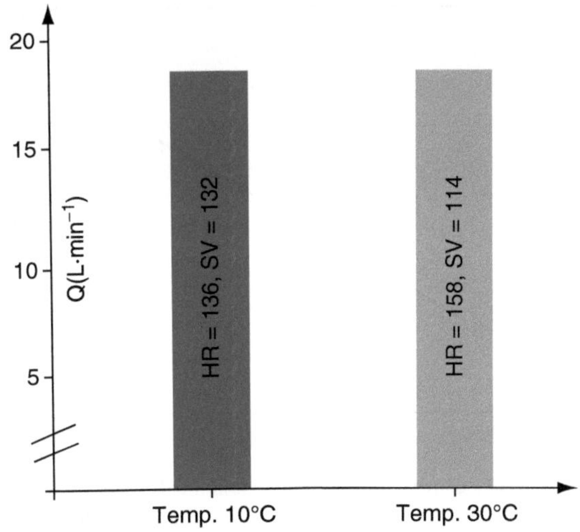

Fig. 3.16 Cardiac output is the same (18 L · min^{-1}) in two different ambient temperatures (Temp): 30°C and 10°C. At an ambient of 30°C, cardiac output is achieved mainly by significant increase in heart rate (*HR*) and moderate stroke volume (*SV*), while at an ambient of 10°C, stroke volume is larger with moderate increase in heart rate

perfusion pressures, leading to a more rapid suppression in systemic and working muscles oxygen delivery and VO_2 compared to non-heat stressed conditions [34].

Following heat acclimatization, adaptations to the heat stress occur by enabling the many adjustments made in both sweating and blood flow. The rate of sweating during activity will occur earlier and will increase, resulting in a lower skin temperature. Because heat loss is facilitated by blood, less blood needs to flow to the skin for body heat transfer; therefore, smaller *cardiac output* will be needed to continue muscular function. In addition, the sweat produced is more diluted following training in the heat in an acclimatized individual, which will conserve the body's mineral stores.

Thus far, the physiological mechanisms for heat dissipation and bodily reactions to heated environment were discussed; however, it is obvious that the external environment is not always warmer than internal temperatures. Heavy exercise and cold and windy environments alter body temperature outside the normal range. In these instances, whole new adaptations and reactions take place to maintain normal body temperature and optimal *cardiac output* function. At rest, after 1 h of cold exposure, to low ambient temperatures (4.5–6.5°C) minimally clad subjects showed increases of V_E, VO_2, and *cardiac output.* During exercise in the cold ambient, VO_2 and cardiac output are greater than during the same workload at normal temperature. Cardiovascular responses to cold temperatures are characterized by peripheral vasoconstriction except for the head and increase of flux in deep veins. The increased *cardiac output* during cold exposure is achieved by an increase of stroke volume rather than heart rate. Hypothermia causes *bradycardia,* in contrast to changes in *heart rate* during aerobic and isometric exercises at normal ambient temperatures. Reduced sympathetic nerve activity in the cold has effects on arteriolar resistance, resulting in increased central blood volume. These changes result in an increase in *stroke volume* and cardiac output [35]. The difference between *heart rate* and stroke volume at increased levels of cardiac output during exercise at normal temperatures and during rest and exercise in cold conditions may be explained by changes of arterial baroreceptor input and of blood catecholamine levels

Cardiac Output During Isometric Exercise

It is well accepted that *resistive* training program results in an increase in muscular *strength* [36]. *Isometric exercise* is an activity in which muscle undergo no change in length with contraction. As a result, no physical work is done despite an increase in the metabolic rate. Isometric exercise is a long-lasting muscle contraction in which intramuscular pressure is increased, thereby resulting in compression of the blood vessels and mechanical occlusion of blood flow. It has been observed that contractions at 20–30% of maximal voluntary contraction can be maintained for 3–5 min. It has been assumed that in normal subjects, *resistive training* could be very demanding due to the dramatic increase in systolic, diastolic, and mean arterial blood pressures, that is, *pressor response* which is mediated by a slight increase in *cardiac output*, but not to the level observed during dynamic aerobic exercise and, no change from rest in total peripheral resistance and sometimes it is increased [37], this might have a significant effect on *cardiac output* especially on *stroke volume* [37]. When large muscle mass was utilized in static contraction, blood pressure and heart rate increased proportionately.

Cardiovascular response during isometric exercise in young, *elderly*, *adolescents*, and *coronary artery disease patients*, males and females, are in general similar [38–40]. In normal subjects, *isometric* exercise causes a small increase in cardiac output resulting almost entirely from an increase in *heart rate*, which increase to approximately 140 beats · min^{-1}. Two mechanisms could be responsible for the role that muscle mass and degree of tension play in the reflex increase in heart rate, the central command, and the exercise pressor reflex. The central command theory involves activation of higher brain centers on the volition and initiation of muscular contraction. The exercise pressor reflex theory suggests that there is a reflex stimulus originating in nerve endings in the contracting muscle, activated either by chemical substances presumably released during the contraction or by physical deformation. Thus during sustained isometric contractions, the greater the number of motor units activated, the greater the activation of afferent nerve fibers. This suggests that the increase in heart rate is related to the muscle mass and the percentage of maximal force developed. The increase in cardiac output, however, is modest 12 L · min^{-1} (Fig. 3.17), compared to 25 L · min^{-1} during aerobic exercise [40].

Additional mechanism suggested for the increase in *heart rate* during isometric exercise is the suppression of the *baroreflex* during *static contractions*, and thus allowing the maintenance of relatively high heart rate [41]. However, others [42] have suggested that the heart rate response can be attributed to changes in *vagal* tone and not to the *baroreflex sensitivity* during isometric exercise.

The normal response of *stroke volume* during *isometric exercise* with large muscle mass such as *dead-lift* maneuver show no change from resting values or even decrease slightly [39]. In order to maintain appropriate stroke volume, the left ventricular end-systolic dimension may significantly decrease and fractional shortening increase during large muscle mass compared to small muscle mass such as handgrip exercise [39].

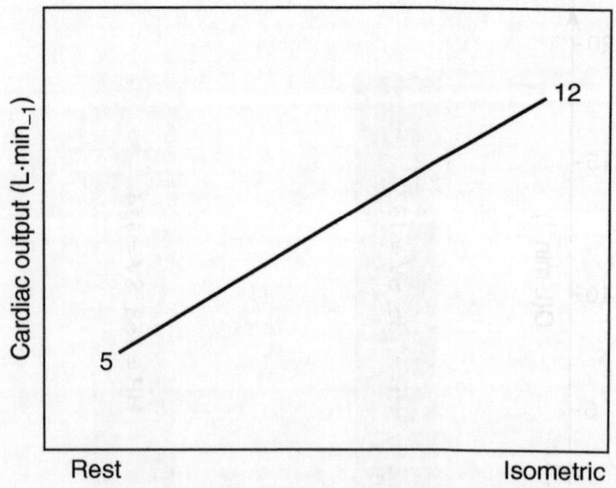

Fig. 3.17 Cardiac output response in healthy individuals to isometric bout utilizing large muscle mass such as the dead-lift maneuver. Cardiac output values are significantly lower during isometric bout compared to values at maximal aerobic exercise

These responses are due to the nature of the dead-lift maneuver in which postural muscle tension while standing may gradually increase intrathoracic and abdominal pressure. This is not the case during *isometric handgrip* utilizing small muscle mass, in which the normal response is an increase in left ventricular dimensions and no change in ejection fraction phase indices, in both trained and untrained normal subjects [39]. The relatively unchanged or decreased stroke volume (Fig. 3.18) that has been reported during resistance exercise is due to a combination of decreased preload, increased afterload, and enhanced contractility. *Preload* may be lower than baseline because of decreased *venous return*. Venous return is likely decreased due to *mechanical occlusion* of the muscle during contraction and the performance of the *Valsalva maneuver* [43]. In summary, during isometric bout, *heart rate* increases at the start largely due to decreased cardiac vagal tone and some contribution by increased cardiac sympathetic stimulation. Total peripheral resistance increased partly due to contracted muscles.

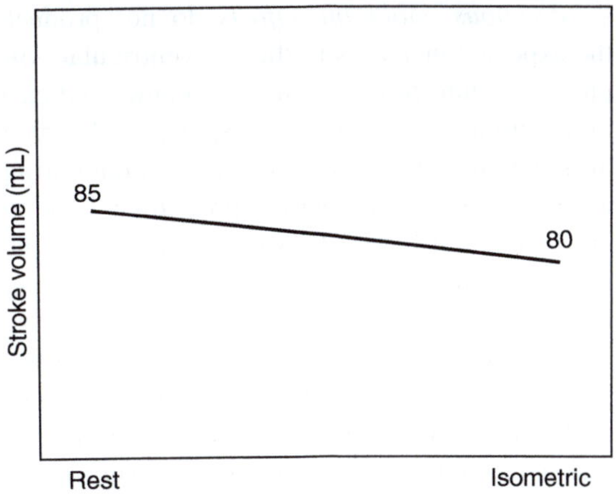

Fig. 3.18 Stroke volume response in healthy subjects from rest to isometric dead-lift maneuver utilizing large muscle mass

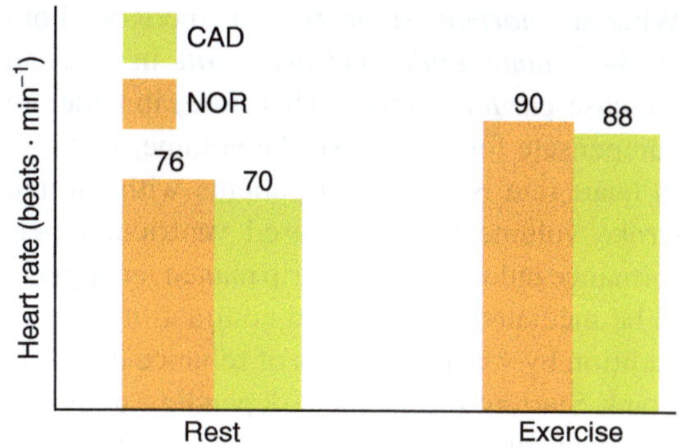

Fig. 3.19 Heart rate responses at rest and during dead-lift isometric exercise in coronary artery disease patients (*CAD*) and normal subjects (*NOR*). Coronary artery disease patients increased their heart rate from rest to exercise by 14 beats · min^{-1} while normal increased it by 18 beats · min^{-1}

Both systolic blood pressure and diastolic blood pressure increase sharply; however, stroke volume remains relatively unchanged.

At a *voluntary contractions* equal or greater than 20–30% of maximal voluntary contraction, the intramuscular pressure exceeds the intravascular pressure in the contracting muscle and significantly reduces localized blood flow, causing muscle ischemia and hypoxia [44]. Therefore, *isometric exercise* is usually discouraged in *coronary artery disease* patients as of the potential adverse effects of increased *afterload* and associated *ischemia* on left ventricular function [45]. During *resistive exercise, coronary artery disease patients* show the same *pressor response* as *normal subjects*.

Figure 3.19 reveals that coronary artery disease patients increase *heart rate* from resting values by 14 beats · min^{-1} at peak dead-lift isometric exercise lower but not significant than that seen in normal subjects which increased their heart rate from rest by 18 beats · min^{-1} [39]. This increase in heart rate is dominant mechanism for the slight increased cardiac output [39]. Despite the increased cardiac output, blood flow to the noncontracting muscles does not significantly increase, probably because of reflex vasoconstriction. The *isometric* exercise slight increase in cardiac output (Fig. 3.20) results almost entirely from an increase in heart rate, which increase to approximately 140 beats · min^{-1}. The increase in cardiac output, however, is modest 9–10 L · min^{-1} [39], compared to 20 L · min^{-1} during aerobic exercise [46].

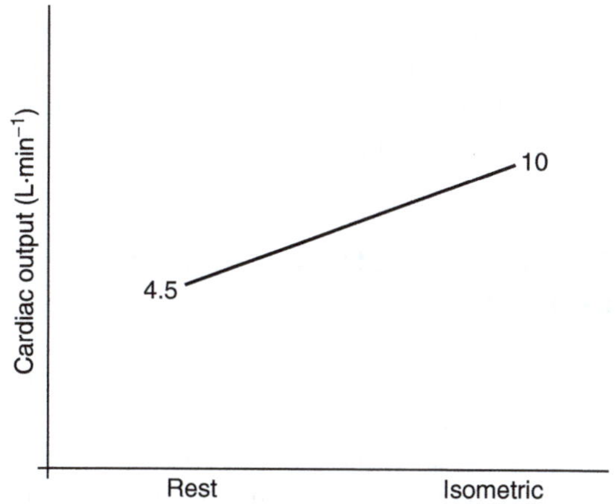

Fig. 3.20 Cardiac output response to isometric bout utilizing large muscle mass such as the dead-lift maneuver in coronary artery disease patients. Cardiac output values are significantly lower in coronary artery disease patients during isometric bout compared to values attained by normal individuals (see Fig. 3.17)

The increase in *heart rate* in the *coronary artery disease patients* is probably explained by the limited ability of the patient to increase *stroke volume*. It remains largely unchanged except at high levels of tension (>50% maximal voluntary contraction), wherein it may decrease.

Whereas *normal subjects* can increase both *stroke volume mildly* and *heart rate* in order to increase *cardiac output*. Therefore, in order to compensate for the low stroke volume, increase in heart rate is greater in patients with limited stroke volume [47]. Increased ventricular performance induced by handgrip maneuver appears to be mediated by increased contractility, but in addition by varying degrees of reliance upon the Frank-Starling mechanism, depending upon the adequacy of inotropic to increase contractility reserve to meet the stress imposed by isometric exercise.

Following mild to moderate-intensity *isometric exercise*, in *coronary artery disease patients*, results in a lower *rate-pressure product* (heart rate times systolic blood pressure), which is an indirect index of myocardial oxygen demand compared to maximum treadmill aerobic exercise. However, while gaining strength, no alterations in heart rate, stroke volume, and thus in cardiac output are noted [44].

Cardiac Output During Anaerobic Exercise

Anaerobic exercise is characterized by exposing the subject to a very high degree of sudden *strenuous all-out exercise*. It places special demands on the cardiovascular system and skeletal muscles. In order to improve the athlete's physical performance, the athlete devotes a large portion of the training program to speed and strenuous exercise [48]. This kind of effort brings about *oxygen debt*, which increases blood lactate concentration in direct associated with increase in maximum performance [49]. It has been assumed that this type of activity is potential dangerous for *elderly* and *cardiac patients*, due to hypoxia and seemingly inappropriate blood pressure response. This has the effect of placing a large load on the left ventricular which have a significant effect on *left ventricular systolic function*, and hence on *cardiac output* [50]. During anaerobic exercise, *stroke volume* in young subject remains unchanged compared to the resting values while it decreases in elderly [46].

Strenuous anaerobic efforts do not produce the expected increases in the left ventricular volumes, *ejection fraction*, stroke volume, and cardiac output compared to responses observed during aerobic-type effort. Cardiac output during anaerobic exercise increases approximately up to 16–17 L · min^{-1} [51]. This may suggest that the increase in left ventricular *inotropic state* during the strenuous bouts is not adequate to increase left ventricular volumes, and hence ejection fraction and *stroke volume* [52]. In addition, it is suggested that during all-out exercise, total peripheral resistance and *afterload* values are lower than at rest; however, these variables were not reduced to the level observed at peak aerobic exercise (Fig. 3.21). Such inadequate reduction in *total peripheral resistance* and *afterload* could be responsible for the relatively small augmentation in left ventricular function found during the *strenuous anaerobic exercise* [51].

The end result is a lower *cardiac output* than that expected at VO_{2max}. An additional explanation for the relatively lower cardiac output during *anaerobic exercise* may be related to the short duration of the exercise bout. Thus, insufficient time do not allow an appropriate adjustment of the *circulatory system* such as impeded venous return. This, coupled with lower values of *heart rate*, compared to the maximal heart rates that

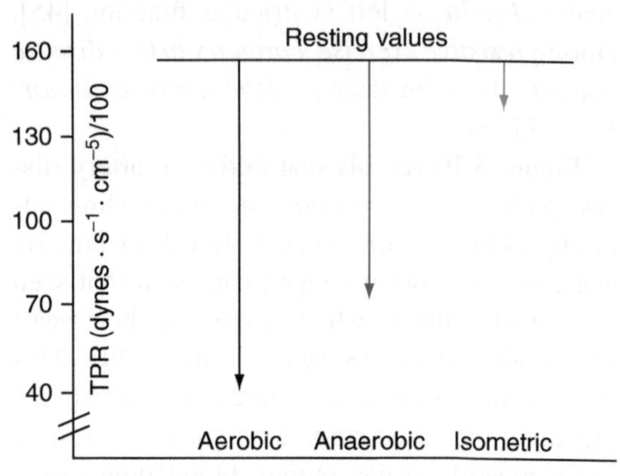

Fig. 3.21 Different values for total peripheral resistance (*TPR*) during different modes of exercise: aerobic, anaerobic, and isometric. The maximal reduction in total peripheral resistance is obtained during aerobic exercise, while the lowest reduction is obtained during isometric exercise

healthy subjects can reach during *dynamic exercise* when achieving VO_{2max} result in a lower *cardiac output*.

Because *anaerobic exercise* increases the *adrenergic state*, one would expect the *acceleration time* and *peak velocity of aortic flow* to increase [43]. However, during anaerobic exercise, a significant decrease in both acceleration time and peak aortic velocity is noted may be, due to the inverse relationship between left ventricular afterload and performance [53]. Therefore, at maximal exercise, when the ability of ventricular ejection would be expected to be completely utilized, an increase in *afterload* might be a potential factor that opposes systolic emptying. The decreased *aortic Doppler indices* during the anaerobic exercise may be due to the elevated systolic and diastolic blood pressures, and thus *mean arterial blood pressure* [54], demonstrating that during *sudden strenuous exercise* in healthy subjects, left ventricular end-systolic and diastolic *radionuclide counts* were increased. Thus, *ejection fraction* was reduced.

The assumed lack of the *autoregulation mechanism* during *anaerobic exercise* may explain the reduced *stroke volume*. Therefore, the ventricle has to eject against a relatively high pressure opposing left ventricular ejection. This coupled with lower values of *heart rate* compared to the maximal heart rates; these subjects can reach during dynamic exercise when achieving VO_{2max} ends up with a low *cardiac output*.

Stroke volume and *Doppler-derived indices* values during *anaerobic exercise* are similar to those seen during *isometric exercise* [37]. This may be due to the high exercise intensity likely associated with greater magnitude of α- and β-adrenergic stimulation than that in low-intensity exercise [55]. Thus, while increasing contractility, it causes a *vasoconstriction*, which in turn may influence the *end-systolic pressure-volume relationship*.

In summary, *cardiac output* increases during *isometric*, *anaerobic*, and *aerobic* exercises with the lower values during *isometric exercise* and the highest at VO_{2max} during aerobic exercise. Figure 3.22 emphasizes the differences in *cardiac output* during the different mode of exercises.

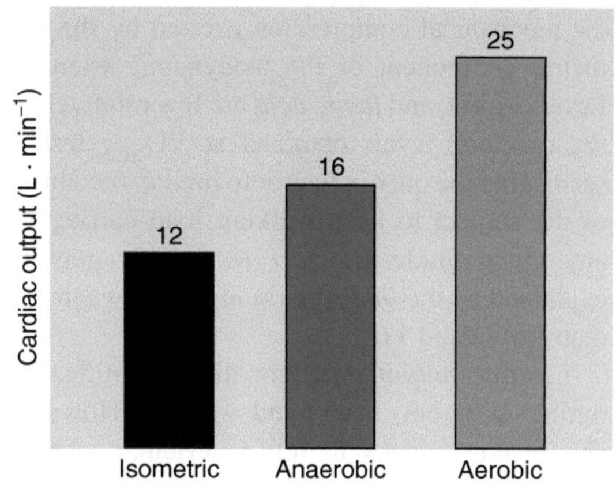

Fig. 3.22 Cardiac output values during different mode of exercises: isometric, anaerobic, and aerobic. The highest values are seen during aerobic exercise while, the lowest is obtained during isometric exercise

Cardiac Output During Isodynamic Exercise

Isodynamic exercise such as backpack carriage or load carriage is a form of exercise which *combines dynamic* and *isometric* components or combined volume and pressure load. The effect of the isometric stress on the dynamic exercise of a graded exercise test in normal subjects was examined in previous studies, revealing that at the same absolute VO_2, the *isometric component* augmented significantly *afterload* and *heart rate*, more than those found during dynamic exercise alone [56].

Previously, it has been shown that *prolonged isodynamic exercise* at constant speed and grade with different backpack carriage loads did not change the steady state of left ventricular systolic function and hemodynamic throughout 240 min of efforts [3].

During *isodynamic exercise*, changes in *grade* of walking are the most important factor determining *cardiac output* response, that is, with increase in grade, VO_2 is elevated, without any relationship to speed or load [56]. Blood flow to the working muscles during *isodynamic* exercise is sufficient to avoid heavy reliance on anaerobic pathway as a source of energy. This is mediated mainly by the *autoregulation mechanism* despite the mechanical compression exerted by the isometric component of the isodynamic exercise. Levels of *VO_2* and *lactic acid* are low relatively to the maximal levels obtained at VO_{2peak} test; it seems that the only indicator to predict the ability of the subject to keep walking load carriage at any given grade is *heart rate*. This may be explained by the *linear relationship* between cardiac output and *VO_2*.

Cardiac output does not differ significantly during different loads and speeds. However, significant changes in left ventricular systolic function are observed with the change in grade. It seems that with changes in grade, there is a large reduction in central blood volume following large increase in intrathoracic and abdominal pressures along with higher increment in mean arterial blood pressure, due to the change in body position, that is, bending forward in order to keep balance, with the elevation of the grade. The reduced central blood volume and higher *afterload* in turn alter *venous return* by disturbing the pressure flow relationship of the venous system, and by increasing systemic venous resistance. Thus, *stroke volume* decreases; however, *cardiac output is* increased with increase in grade due to augmentation in *heart rate*. This suggest that *total peripheral resistance* reduction with continuing isodynamic exercise may have some importance in augmenting *cardiac output* in the face of reduced *left ventricular systolic function* and increased *mean arterial blood pressure* during steady state exercise.

Ischemic responses indicated by 0.1 mV ST depression were absent in patients with coronary artery disease during *isodynamic* exercises. This is in contrast to performing dynamic exercise alone at similar rate-pressure product [57]. Attenuation of ST depression during isodynamic exercise may be attributed to a combination of increased diastolic perfusion pressure, decreased heart rate, and possibly to reductions in venous return and ventricular diastolic wall tension due to increased intrathoracic and abdominal pressure. In addition, exercise-induced myocardial ischemia is markedly attenuated on the more gradually increasing workload of the individualized ramp ergocycle (isodynamic) compared with the dynamic treadmill protocol. This effect is unexplained by energy expenditure (VO_2) or myocardial rate-pressure product [47].

During *isodynamic* and *dynamic* exercises at the same relatively workloads, there are no significant differences between the two modes of exercise in ejection fraction, heart rate left ventricular end-diastolic and -systolic volumes and stroke volume, and thus *cardiac output* [56]. The similar *cardiac output* responses during isodynamic and dynamic exercises are different from what one would expect to find with an increased adrenergic state during isodynamic exercise due to the isometric component. It appears that the autoregulation mechanism on one hand kept mean arterial blood pressure during isodynamic exercise at a relatively low level compared to isometric maneuver [39].

Cardiac Output in Coronary Artery Disease Patients

Compared to healthy subjects, values for *cardiac output* during aerobic exercise at *VO_{2peak}* are low in *coronary artery disease patients*. In *coronary artery disease patients* while determining their *VO_2* and hemodynamic values at rest and during maximal treadmill exercise, *maximal cardiac output* is reduced significantly approximately by 5–6 L · min^{-1} compared to matched healthy sedentary subjects (Fig. 3.23). The lower cardiac output in coronary artery disease patients at *peak aerobic exercise* is related to the medications, limited *maximal heart rate*, *stroke volume*, *left ventricular contractility*, and to the inappropriate adjustment of the circulation [37, 51].

The determinants of *cardiac output* during aerobic exercise in patients with *coronary artery disease* are multifactorial and incompletely understood in patients with symptomatic left ventricular dysfunction, with much less information regarding asymptomatic left ventricular dysfunction [58]. Exercise performance and its hemodynamic differ in patients with symptomatic and asymptomatic *left ventricular dysfunction*. *Asymptomatic* coronary artery disease *patients*

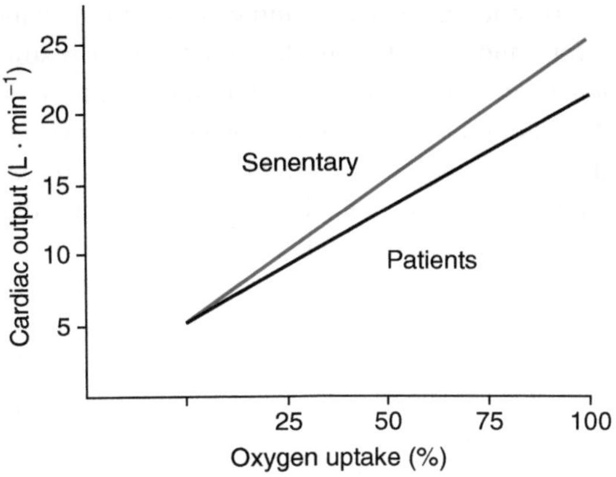

Fig. 3.23 Differences in cardiac output between coronary artery disease patients and sedentary healthy subjects at peak aerobic exercise

have greater increases in *heart rate*, systolic blood pressure, left ventricular *ejection fraction*, and *cardiac output* than *symptomatic* coronary artery disease *patients*.

The reduction in *maximal heart rate* is a greater factor in the reduction of cardiac output than *stroke volume*. As compared with healthy controls, *cardiac output* is more frequently preserved in young than older coronary artery disease patients with short disease duration, although the left ventricular response to exercise is already reduced [59].

During *endurance dynamic* exercise, the normal response is an increase in stroke volume and heart rate and hence *cardiac output*. Patients with ischemic myocardial disease respond to the stress of endurance exercise by *cardiac dilatation* to maintain increase in *stroke volume* at increased heart rates. Following 6 months of *aerobic training* in 42 patients with anterior myocardial infarction, relationships between heart rate variability and different prognostic markers such as *stroke volume* and *functional capacity*, as well as the comparison of their time courses, are not fully elucidated. It has been suggested that the percent increase in *heart rate* variability between the first week of training and 6 months was greater among those cardiac patients with the lowest basal *ejection fraction* and *stroke volume* [60].

Isometric Exercise in Coronary Artery Disease Patients

At a *voluntary contraction* equal to or greater than 20–30% of maximal voluntary contraction, the intramuscular pressure exceeds the intravascular pressure in the contracting muscle and significantly reduces localized blood flow, causing muscle ischemia and hypoxia [44]. Therefore, *isometric exercise* is usually discouraged in *coronary artery disease* patients as of the potential adverse effects of increased *afterload* and associated *ischemia* on left ventricular function [45]. During *resistive exercise*, *coronary artery disease patients* show the same *pressor response* as *normal subjects*.

Increase in heart rate is dominant mechanism for the slight increased cardiac output [39]. Despite the increased cardiac output, blood flow to the noncontracting muscles does not significantly increase, probably because of reflex vasoconstriction. The *isometric* exercise slight increase in cardiac output results almost entirely from an increase in heart rate, which increase to approximately 140 beats · min^{-1}. The increase in cardiac output, however, is modest 9–10 L · min^{-1} [39], compared to 20 L · min^{-1} during aerobic exercise [46].

The increase in *heart rate* in the *coronary artery disease patients* is probably explained by the limited ability of the patient to increase *stroke volume*. It remains largely unchanged except at high levels of tension (>50% maximal voluntary contraction), wherein it may decrease. Whereas *normal subjects* can increase both *stroke volume mildly* and *heart rate* in order to increase *cardiac output*. Therefore, in order to compensate for the low stroke volume, increase in heart rate is greater in patients with limited stroke volume [47]. Increased ventricular performance induced by handgrip maneuver appears to be mediated by increased contractility, but in addition by varying degrees of reliance upon the Frank-Starling mechanism, depending upon the adequacy of inotropic to increase contractility reserve to meet the stress imposed by isometric exercise.

Following mild to moderate-intensity *isometric exercise*, in *coronary artery disease patients*, results in a lower *rate-pressure product* (heart rate times systolic blood pressure), which is an indirect index of myocardial oxygen demand compared to maximum treadmill aerobic exercise. However, while gaining strength, no alterations in heart rate, stroke volume, and thus in cardiac output are noted [44].

Aerobic Training Effect on Cardiac Output

In response to *maximal exercise aerobic training*, the augmentation in VO_{2max} in trained elderly and young adults is mainly due to the adaptive increases in *cardiac output* and to the lesser extent to the $(a\text{-}v)O_2$ [61, 62]. The increase in *maximal cardiac output* during maximal aerobic exercise in trained elderly and young adults is the result of a large increase in stroke volume increased due to a significant increase in *left ventricular end-diastolic volume*, while *left ventricular end-systolic volume* decreased [52]. These significant changes in *left ventricular volumes* at VO_{2max} exercise seen result from an integrated mechanism that involves changes in *contractility* and *afterload*.

Longitudinal studies have shown that the training-induced increase in oxygen uptake results primarily from an increase in *maximal cardiac output* rather than a widening of the systemic $(a\text{-}v)O_2$. Indeed, it is estimated that 70–85% of the training-induced increase in VO_2 is explained by the increase of maximal *cardiac output* [63]. Capelli et al. [63] examined VO_2 in sedentary individuals after 20 days of bed rest and 50 days of training. The *difference* in VO_2 between the deconditioned and trained states resulted mostly from a significant differences in *cardiac output*.

Earlier, in a similar study, Ekblom et al. [64] found that 16 weeks of physical training increased VO_2 from 3.15 to 3.68 $L \cdot min^{-1}$. This improvement in VO_2 resulted from an 8.0% increase in cardiac output (from 22.4 to 24.2 $L \cdot min^{-1}$) and a 3.6% increase in $(a\text{-}v)O_2$ (from 138 to 143 $mL \cdot L^{-1}$).

In sedentary individuals, after 6 months of *endurance training*, resting *heart rate* may decrease to 55 beats $\cdot$ min^{-1}. At the same time, resting *stroke volume* increases to about 90 mL (heart rate X stroke volume stays the ~same before and after training). So a *reduced* resting *heart rate* is a hallmark of endurance training. In elite endurance *athletes*, resting heart rate is often in the 30s and low 40s. Since *resting oxygen demand* still has not changed, this means that these athletes have high resting *stroke volume*. Thus, the resting heart of the athlete is more efficient. It performs the same work with fewer heart beats and less myocardial energy demand.

Following *dynamic aerobic exercise*, heart rate is decreased at rest and during submaximal exercise, and thus, the heart of well-trained individual is at least 25% more efficient. At peak exercise, maximal heart rate does not increase after training. It stays the same or might even decrease slightly. In untrained individuals, maximal heart rate is achieved at peak exercise. It might seem that *untrained individuals* have an advantage overtrained individuals in their ability to attain higher maximal heart rate than trained individual. However, the opposite is true, the trained individuals and world-class athletes have significant advantage over the untrained individuals, since the reduction in *maximal heart rate* in the *trained individuals* and world-class athletes is slightly while the decrease in resting heart rate is significant. Therefore, the trained individual and world-class athletes are able to increase from rest to peak exercise their heart beats much more than that of the untrained individuals (Fig. 3.24).

The reduced heart rate in the trained subjects increases relatively to the untrained individuals' *left ventricular filling time* during submaximal and maximal exercise. Consequently, at peak exercise, the slightly reduced heart rate attenuates the reduction of *stroke volume*. Thus, the greater increase in the number of heart beats from rest to peak exercise coupled with the increase in filling time, that is, stroke volume, will increase maximal cardiac output which is the primary reason for the increase in VO_{2max}. *Following training*, during submaximal dynamic aerobic exercise at the same absolute load, *cardiac output* will be similar in *trained* and *untrained subjects*. However, the way to achieve that cardiac output differs significantly between these two subjects.

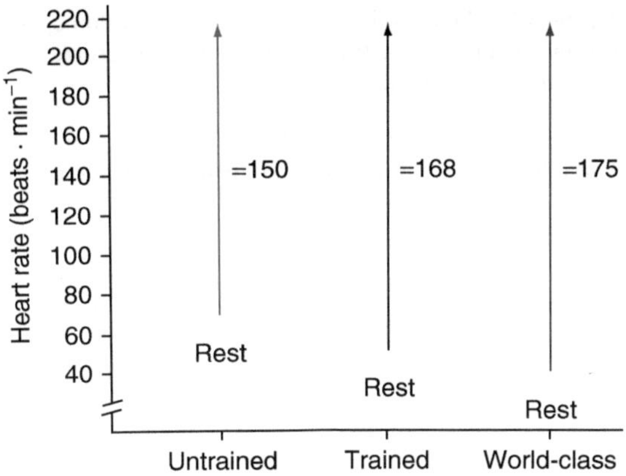

Fig. 3.24 Maximal heart rate values following aerobic exercise training in untrained, trained, and world-class individuals. Although maximal heart rate is slightly lowered in world-class, still, trained individual and world-class athletes are able to increase from rest to peak exercise their heart beats much more than that of the untrained individuals

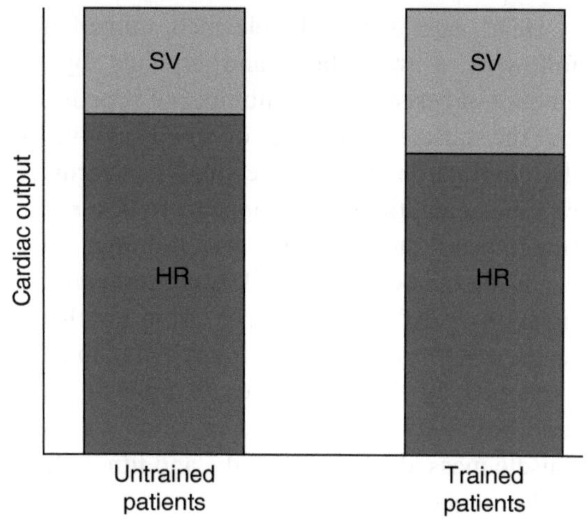

Fig. 3.26 At the same cardiac output, untrained coronary artery disease patients rely more on heart rate and less on the limited stroke volume. With training, heart rate is lower and stroke volume increases (mild)

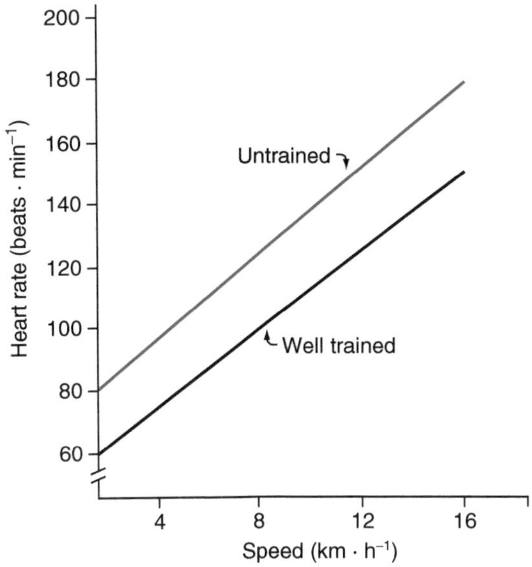

Fig. 3.25 Heart rate response following prolonged dynamic aerobic exercise training program, with training heart rate in the trained individual compared to untrained individual, is lower at the same absolute workload

In *untrained subjects*, the increase in cardiac output is achieved mainly by a significant increase in *heart rate* (Fig. 3.25) and a moderate increase in *stroke volume*, while in *trained subject*, the increase in cardiac output is due to an increase in *stroke volume* and *heart rate* (Fig. 3.26).

Isometric Training and Cardiac Output Adaptations

In general, there is no dramatic change in *cardiac output*, *heart rate*, and *stroke volume* following *isometric exercise training*. However, it may change left ventricular physiologically and morphologically. Training with repetitive static exercise derives little benefit from an increase in oxygen transport capacity, so that VO_{2max} is increased only minimally or not at all. Some of these adaptations can occur in *cardiac* or *hypertensive patients* with no concomitant cardiovascular complications. In both healthy individuals and those with *cardiovascular disease*, the manner in which resistance training is performed may dictate the extent to which these adjustments take place. Specifically, training that involves frequent repetitions of moderate weight and hence contains dynamic components seems to produce the most beneficial results [65].

Heart rate decreases for maximal work and recovery from short-term weight training.

Heart rate is acutely elevated immediately following a work bout and affected by the amount of resistance, the number of repetitions, and the muscle mass large or small involved in the contraction [65]. Interestingly, in terms of chronic adaptations, there appears to be a reduction in heart rate from resistance training, which is considered beneficial [66]. Long-term adaptations observed in the research, from no change up to a 11% decrease in *heart rate*, may be explained by the differences in intensity, volume, rest between sets, use of small vs. large muscle mass, duration of study, and fitness level of the subjects.

Summary of the changes in *cardiac output* at rest, during submaximal and maximal efforts following aerobic, anaerobic, and isometric training, is presented in Tables 3.1, 3.2, and 3.3.

Table 3.1 reveals that *at rest* following aerobic training, heart rate decreases, stroke volume increases while VO_2 and cardiac output remain unchanged. Subsequent to *anaerobic training*, heart rate decreases, while VO_2, stroke volume, and cardiac output remain unchanged. *Isometric training* causes no change in oxygen uptake, heart rate, stroke volume, and cardiac output.

Table 3.2 shows that during *submaximal aerobic exercise* following aerobic training, heart rate decreases, stroke volume increases while VO_2 and cardiac output remains unchanged. Subsequent to resistive training, there is no change in VO_2, heart rate, stroke volume, and cardiac output.

Table 3.3 suggests that during *maximal aerobic effort*, aerobic training brings about increase in VO_2 and decrease in maximal *heart rate*, and thus increases left ventricular filling time. As an effect of training, stroke volume increases significantly. This *stroke volume* increase can be achieved by increasing left ventricular dimensions, filling time, or by improving left ventricular contractility, and as a consequence, *cardiac output* is increased. The increased contractile state is a result of decreased left ventricular end-systolic volume and increased left ventricular ejection fraction.

Subsequent to *anaerobic training*, during anaerobic bouts heart rate, stroke volume and cardiac output remain unchanged. Following isometric training during *maximal exercise*, isometric bout heart rate remains unchanged while stroke volume and cardiac output may decrease or unchanged.

Table 3.1 Changes in heart rate, stroke volume, and cardiac output at rest following aerobic, anaerobic, and isometric exercise programs

	Mode of exercise		
Variable	Anaerobic	Isometric	Aerobic
Heart rate	↓	→	↓
Stroke volume	→	→	↑
Cardiac output	→	→	→
Oxygen uptake	→	→	→

Table 3.2 Changes in heart rate, stroke volume, and cardiac output during submaximal efforts following aerobic and isometric exercise programs

	Mode of exercise	
Variable	Isometric	Aerobic
Heart rate	→	↓
Stroke volume	→	↑
Cardiac output	→	→
Oxygen uptake	→	→

Table 3.3 Changes in cardiovascular at peak efforts following dynamic aerobic, anaerobic, and isometric exercise programs

	Mode of exercise		
Variables	Anaerobic	Isometric	Aerobic
Heart rate	↓	→	↓
Stroke volume	→	→ ↓	↑
Cardiac output	→	→ ↓	↑
Oxygen uptake	→	→	→

Aerobic Exercise Training in Coronary Artery Disease

Following intense endurance exercise training, an increase in left ventricular *stroke volume* and in *stroke work* during exercise in patients with coronary artery disease is noted. Stroke volume during upright exercise that required 35–65% of VO_{2max} was 18% higher after training. As a result, left ventricular stroke work (mean blood pressure · stroke volume) also increases by 18%. This is due to cardiac rather than peripheral adaptations. The increase in VO_{2max} in the trained group paralleled an increase in *maximal cardiac output*. The augmentation in VO_{2max} in trained coronary artery disease patients is mainly due to the adaptive increases in *cardiac output* and to the lesser extent to the $(a\text{-}v)O_2$ [61]. The increase in *maximal cardiac output* during maximal aerobic exercise in trained elderly as well as in young adult patients is the result of a large increase in *left ventricular end-diastolic volume*, while *left ventricular end-systolic volume* decreased slightly consequently, *stroke volume* is increased [67]. These significant changes in *left ventricular volumes* at VO_{2max} exercise seen result from an integrated mechanism that involves changes in *contractility* and *afterload* [67]. Following *aerobic training*, at the same percentage of VO_{2max}, mean blood pressure is the same before and after training; as a result, left ventricular *stroke work* increased suggesting that in patients with coronary artery disease, prolonged, intense training induces a moderate increase in *cardiac output* [67]. Consequently, VO_{2max} is reduced more than the reduction seen in *cardiac output* due to lower *peripheral extraction* in the coronary patients.

Heart rate decreases at rest and during exercise due to the improvement in *venous return* and *stroke volume*. However, the sum of heart rate and stroke volume stays the same before and after training, since resting and exercise oxygen demand still has not changed. Thus, the resting heart of the trained patient is more efficient. It performs the same work with fewer beats and less myocardial energy demand (Fig. 3.25).

Table 3.4 Changes in heart rate, stroke volume, and cardiac output at rest following aerobic and isometric exercise programs in coronary artery disease patients

	Mode of exercise	
Variable	Aerobic	Isometric
Heart rate	→	→
Stroke volume	↑	↓
Cardiac output	→	↓
Oxygen uptake	→	→

Table 3.5 Changes in heart rate, stroke volume and cardiac output during submaximal efforts following aerobic and isometric exercise programs in coronary artery disease patients.

	Mode of exercise	
Variable	Isometric	Aerobic
Heart rate	↑	→
Stroke volume	↓	→
Cardiac output	↑	→
Oxygen uptake	→	→

In summary of the changes in coronary artery disease, patients for cardiac output at rest, during submaximal and maximal efforts following aerobic and isometric training, are presented in Tables 3.4, 3.5, and 3.6. Table 3.4 reveals that *at rest* following *aerobic training*, *coronary artery disease patients* may decrease heart rate and may increase stroke volume while cardiac output and VO_2 remain unchanged. In coronary artery disease patients, no *anaerobic training* is recommended, and therefore, no data is available on the effects of anaerobic training on cardiac output in coronary artery disease patients. *Isometric training* causes no change in VO_2 and *heart rate* while *stroke volume* and *cardiac output* decrease slightly in coronary artery disease patients.

Table 3.6 Changes in cardiovascular at peak efforts following dynamic aerobic and isometric exercise programs in coronary artery disease patients

	Mode of exercise	
Variable	Isometric	Aerobic
Heart rate	→	→
Stroke volume	↓	→
Cardiac output	↑	→↓
Oxygen uptake	→	→↓

Table 3.5 shows that during *submaximal exercise* following *aerobic training* heart rate decreases, VO_2 and stroke volume are increased while cardiac output remains unchanged. Subsequent to isometric training, there is no change in VO_2, heart rate, stroke volume, and cardiac output.

Table 3.6 suggests that during *maximal aerobic effort*, aerobic training brings about a decrease in heart rate and increase in VO_2, stroke volume, and cardiac output. Following isometric training during *maximal exercise*, isometric bout heart rate remains unchanged while stroke volume and cardiac output may decrease or unchanged.

References

1. Guyton AC, John E. Textbook of medical physiology. 11th ed. Philadelphia: Elsevier Inc; 2006.
2. Wolff CB. Normal cardiac output, oxygen delivery and oxygen extraction. Adv Exp Med Biol. 2007;599: 169–82.
3. Sagiv M, Ben-Sira D, Sagiv A, Werber G, Rotstein A. Left ventricular responses during prolonged treadmill walking with heavy load carriage. Med Sci Sports Exerc. 1994;26:285–8.
4. Wilson LB, Andrew D, Craig AD. Activation of spinobulbar lamina I neurons by static muscle contraction. J Neurophysiol. 2002;87:1641–5.
5. Wilmore JH, Costill DL. Physiology of sport and exercise. 3rd ed. Champaign: Human Kinetics; 2005.
6. O'Leary DS. Heart rate control during exercise by baroreceptors and skeletal muscle afferents. Med Sci Sports Exerc. 1996;28:210–7.
7. Rowland TW, Garrard M, Marwood S, Guerra ME, Roche D, Unnithan VB. Myocardial performance during progressive exercise in athletic adolescent males. Med Sci Sports Exerc. 2009;41:1721–8.
8. Obert P, Mandigouts S, Nottin S, Vinet A, N'Guyen LD, Lecoq AM. Cardiovascular responses to endurance training in children: effect of gender. Eur J Clin Invest. 2003;33:199–208.
9. Nottin S, Vinet A, Stecken F, Nguyen LD, Ounissi F, Lecoq AM, Obert P. Central and peripheral cardiovascular adaptations during a maximal cycle exercise in boys and men. Med Sci Sports Exerc. 2002;34: 456–63.
10. Zhou B, Conlee RK, Jensen R, Fellingham GW, George JD, Fisher AG. Stroke volume does not plateau during graded exercise in elite male distance runners. Med Sci Sports Exerc. 2001;33:1849–54.
11. Warburton DE, Haykowsky MJ, Quinney HA, Blackmore D, Teo KK, Humen DP. Myocardial response to incremental exercise in endurance-trained athletes: influence of heart rate, contractility and the Frank-Starling effect. Exp Physiol. 2002;87:613–22.
12. Warburton DE, Gledhill N. Counterpoint: stroke volume does not decline during exercise at maximal effort in healthy individuals. J Physiol Appl. 2008;104:274–6.
13. Kanstrup IL, Marving J, Gagsboll N, Lonborg-Jensen H, Hoilund-Carlsen PF. Left ventricle haemodynamics and vaso-active hormones during graded supine exercise in healthy male subjects. Eur J Appl Physiol. 1995;72:86–94.
14. Sampath S, Derbyshire JA, Ledesma-Carbayo MJ, McVeigh ER. Imaging left ventricular tissue mechanics and hemodynamics during supine bicycle exercise using a combined tagging and phase-contrast MRI pulse sequence. Magn Reson Med. 2011;65:51–9.
15. Sandercock GR, Hardy-Shepherd D, Nunan D, Brodie D. The relationships between self-assessed habitual physical activity and non-invasive measures of cardiac autonomic modulation in young healthy volunteers. J Sports Sci. 2008;26:1171–7.
16. Camarda SR, Tebexreni AS, Páfaro CN, Sasai FB, Tambeiro VL, Juliano Y, Barros Neto TL. Comparison of maximal heart rate using the prediction equations proposed by Karvonen and Tanaka. Arq Bras Cardiol. 2008;91:311–4.
17. O'Connell MN, Falchier A, McGinnis T, Schroeder CE, Lakatos P. Dual mechanism of neuronal ensemble inhibition in primary auditory cortex. Neuron. 2011;69:805–17.
18. Portier H, Louisy F, Laude D, Berthelot M, Guezennec CY. Intense endurance training on heart rate and blood pressure variability in runners. Med Sci Sports Exerc. 2001;33:1120–5.
19. Raven PB, Fadel PJ, Ogoh S. Arterial baroreflex resetting during exercise: a current perspective. Exp Physiol. 2006;91:37–49.
20. Freeman JV, Dewey FE, Hadley DM, Myers J, Froelicher VF. Autonomic nervous system interaction with the cardiovascular system during exercise. Prog Cardiovasc Dis. 2006;48:342–62.

21. Pichon AP, de Bisschop C, Roulaud M, Denjean A, Papelier Y. Spectral analysis of heart rate variability during exercise in trained subjects. Med Sci Sports Exerc. 2004;36:1702–8.
22. Zuckerman-Levin N, Zinder O, Greenberg A, Levin M, Jacob G, Hochberg Z. Physiological and catecholamine response to sympathetic stimulation in turner syndrome. Clin Endocrinol (Oxf). 2006;64: 410–5.
23. Zanesco A, Antunes E. Effects of exercise training on the cardiovascular system: pharmacological approaches. Pharmacol Ther. 2007;114:307–17.
24. Whipp BJ, Higgenbotham MB, Cobb FC. Estimating exercise stroke volume from asymptotic oxygen pulse in humans. J Appl Physiol. 1996;81:2674–9.
25. Bhambhani Y, Norris S, Bell G. Prediction of stroke volume from oxygen pulse measurements in untrained and trained men. Can J Appl Physiol. 1994;19: 49–59.
26. Mortensen SP, Dawson EA, Yoshiga CC, Dalsgaard MK, Damsgaard R, Secher NH, González-Alonso J. Limitations to systemic and locomotor limb muscle oxygen delivery and uptake during maximal exercise in humans. J Physiol. 2005;566:273–85.
27. Ogawa T, Spina RJ, Martin 3rd WH, Kohrt WM, Schechtman KB, Holloszy JO, Ehsani AA. Effects of aging, sex, and physical training on cardiovascular responses to exercise. Circulation. 1992;86:494–503.
28. González-Alonso J, Crandall CG, Johnson JM. Cardiovascular challenge of exercising in the heat. J Physiol. 2008;586:45–53.
29. Brukner P, Khan K. Clinical sports medicine. 2nd ed. Sydney: McGraw-Hill; 2002.
30. Montain SJ, Sawka MN, Latzka WA, Valeri CR. Thermal and cardiovascular strain from hypohydration: influence of exercise intensity. Int J Sports Med. 1998;19:87–91.
31. Coyle EF, González-Alonso J. Cardiovascular drift during prolonged exercise: new perspectives. Exerc Sport Sci Rev. 2001;29:88–92.
32. Trinity JD, Pahnke MD, Lee JF, Coyle EF. Interaction of hyperthermia and heart rate on stroke volume during prolonged exercise. J Appl Physiol. 2010;109: 745–51.
33. González-Alonso J, Mora-Rodríguez R, Coyle EF. Stroke volume during exercise: interaction of environment and hydration. Am J Physiol Heart Circ Physiol. 2000;278:H321–30.
34. González-Alonso J, Dalsgaard MK, Osada T, Volianitis S, Dawson EA, Yoshiga CC, Secher NH. Brain and central haemodynamics and oxygenation during maximal exercise in humans. J Physiol. 2004;557:331–42.
35. Pendergast DR, Lundgren CE. The underwater environment: cardiopulmonary, thermal, and energetic demands. J Appl Physiol. 2009;106:276–83.
36. McArdle WD, Katch FI, Katch VL. Essentials of exercise physiology. 2nd ed. Philadelphia: Lippincott Williams & Wilkins; 2000.
37. Sagiv M, Sagiv M, Ben-Sira D. Weight lifting training and left ventricular function in adolescent subjects. J Sports Med Phys Fitness. 2007;47:329–34.
38. Rowland T, Heffernan K, Jae SY, Echols G, Krull G, Fernhall B. Cardiovascular responses to static exercise in boys: insights from tissue Doppler imaging. Eur J Appl Physiol. 2006;97:637–42.
39. Sagiv M, Hanson P, Besozzi M, Nagle F. Left ventricular responses to upright isometric handgrip and dead-lift in men with coronary artery disease. Am J Cardiol. 1985;55:1298–302.
40. Sagiv M, Metrany R, Fisher N, Fishman ZE, Kellerman JJ. Comparison of hemodynamic and left ventricular responses to increased after-load in healthy males and females. Int J Sports Med. 1991;12:41–5.
41. Dipla K, Zafeiridis A, Koidou I, Geladas N, Vrabas IS. Altered hemodynamic regulation and reflex control during exercise and recovery in obese boys. Am J Physiol Heart Circ Physiol. 2010;299:H2090–6.
42. Takahashi M, Matsukawa K, Nakamoto T, Tsuchimochi H, Sakaguchi A, Kawaguchi K, Onari K. Control of heart rate variability by cardiac parasympathetic nerve activity during voluntary static exercise in humans with tetraplegia. J Appl Physiol. 2007;103:1669–77.
43. Bryg RJ, Lewen NK, Williams GA, Labovitz AJ. Effects of isometric handgrip exercise on Doppler-derived parameters of aortic flow in normal subjects. Am J Cardiol. 1989;63:1410–2.
44. Williams MA, Haskell WL, Ades PA, et al. Resistance exercise in individuals with and without cardiovascular disease: 2007 update. A scientific statement from the American Heart Association Council on Clinical Cardiology and Council on nutrition, physical activity, and metabolism. Circulation. 2007;116:572–84.
45. Pollock ML, Franklin BA, Balady GJ, et al. Resistance exercise in individuals with and without cardiovascular disease. Benefits, rationale, safety, and prescription an advisory from the Committee on Exercise, Rehabilitation, and Prevention, Council on Clinical Cardiology, American Heart Association. Circulation. 2000;101:828–33.
46. Sagiv M, Sagiv M, Meckel Y, Ben-Sira D, Amir R. Effects of different sprint cycling bouts on left ventricular function in top cyclists. J Sports Med Phys Fitness. 2008;48:360–5.
47. Noel M, Jobin J, Marcoux A, Poirier P, Dagenais G, Bogaty P. Comparison of myocardial ischemia on the ergocycle versus the treadmill in patients with coronary heart disease. Am J Cardiol. 2010;105:633–9.
48. Friedmann B, Frese F, Menold E, Bärtsch P. Effects of acute moderate hypoxia on anaerobic capacity in endurance-trained runners. Eur J Appl Physiol. 2007;101:67–73.
49. James DV, Sandals LE, Draper SB, Wood DM. Relationship between maximal oxygen uptake and oxygen uptake attained during treadmill middle-distance running. J Sports Sci. 2007;25:851–8.
50. Sagiv M, Ben-Sira D, Sagiv M, Goldhammer E. Left ventricular function at peak all-out anaerobic exercise in older men. Gerontology. 2005;51:122–5.

51. Sagiv M, Ben-Sira D, Goldhammer E, Soudry M. Left ventricular contractility and function at peak aerobic and anaerobic exercises. Med Sci Sports Exerc. 2000;32:1197–201.
52. Goodman JM, Liu PP, Green HJ. Left ventricular adaptations following short-term endurance training. J Appl Physiol. 2005;98:454–60.
53. Dawson EA, Shave R, Whyte G, et al. Preload maintenance and the left ventricular response to prolonged exercise in men. Exp Physiol. 2007;92:383–90.
54. Sagiv M, Ben-Sira D, Goldhammer E. Direct vs. indirect blood pressure measurement at peak anaerobic exercise. Int J Sports Med. 1999;20:275–8.
55. Krzemiński K, Kruk B, Nazar K, Ziemba AW, Cybulski G, Niewiadomski W. Cardiovascular, metabolic and plasma catecholamine responses to passive and active exercises. J Physiol Pharmacol. 2000;51: 267–78.
56. Sagiv M, Ben-Gal S, Ben-Sira D. Effects of gradient and load carried on human haemodynamic responses during treadmill walking. Eur J Appl Physiol. 2000;83:47–50.
57. Noël M, Jobin J, Poirier P, Dagenais GR, Bogaty P. Different thresholds of myocardial ischemia in ramp and standard bruce protocol exercise tests in patients with positive exercise stress tests and angiographically demonstrated coronary arterial narrowing. Am J Cardiol. 2007;99:921–4.
58. Kronenberg MW, Konstam MA, Edens TR, Howe DM, Dolan N, Udelson JE. Factors influencing exercise performance in patients with left ventricular dysfunction. SOLVD Investigators. Studies of Left Ventricular Dysfunction. J Card Fail. 1998;4:159–67.
59. Colao A, Cuocolo A, Marzullo P, et al. Impact of patient's age and disease duration on cardiac performance in acromegaly: a radionuclide angiography study. J Clin Endocrinol Metab. 1999;84: 1518–23.
60. Monmeneu JV, Chorro FJ, Bodí V, et al. Relationships between heart rate variability, functional capacity, and left ventricular function following myocardial infarction: an evaluation after one week and six months. Clin Cardiol. 2001;24:313–20.
61. Motohiro M, Yuasa F, Hattori T, et al. Cardiovascular adaptations to exercise training after uncomplicated acute myocardial infarction. Am J Phys Med Rehabil. 2005;84:684–91.
62. González-Alonso J, Mortensen SP, Jeppesen TD. Haemodynamic responses to exercise, ATP infusion and thigh compression in humans: insight into the role of muscle mechanisms on cardiovascular function. J Physiol. 2008;586:2405–17.
63. Capelli C, Antonutto G, Kenfack MA, et al. Factors determining the time course of $VO_{2(max)}$ decay during bedrest: implications for $VO_{2(max)}$ limitation. Eur J Appl Physiol. 2006;98:152–60.
64. Ekblom B, Astrand PO, Saltin B, Stenberg J, Wallserom B. Effect of training on circulatory response to exercise. J Appl Physiol. 1968;24: 518–28.
65. Longhurst JC, Stebbins CL. The power athlete. Cardiol Clin. 1997;15:413–29.
66. Stone MH, Fleck SJ, Triplett NT, Kraemer WJ. Health- and performance-related potential of resistance training. Sports Med. 1991;11:210–31.
67. Vasiliauskas D, Benetis R, Jasiukeviciene L, Grizas V, Marcinkeviciene J, Navickas R, Leimoniene L. Exercise training after coronary angioplasty improves cardiorespiratory function. Scand Cardiovasc J. 2007; 41:142–8.

Cardiac Output Redistribution 4

The Autoregulation Mechanism

In general, flow through a tissue bed is a direct function of the *pressure difference* across the bed and the resistance of the vascular bed. All other things being equal, the higher the *driving pressure* (arterial pressure), the greater the blood flow. The cardiovascular system is a closed-loop system in which billions of vessels interact with each other, and it enables the control of the systemic arterial pressure and varying organ flow through autoregulatory mechanisms [1]. The *autoregulation mechanism* is characterized by its vasodilatation effect on the small arteries and arterioles, in spite of the domination of the sympathetic nervous system. Autoregulation is a manifestation of local *blood flow regulation*. It is defined as the intrinsic ability of an organ to maintain a constant blood flow despite changes in perfusion pressure (Fig. 4.1). An important feature of resting skeletal muscle is that it appears to be substantially vasoconstricted. This has been attributed to high baseline sympathetic tone. During exercise, *accumulation of local metabolites* appears to mediate increased *blood flow* and thus, oxygen delivery. Such reactive *hyperemia* may be impaired in disease states, for example, in cardiac failure.

Arterioles are the smallest arteries and are the most important in regulating blood flow into the various capillary beds through smooth muscle bands in the arterioles and at the entrance to *capillaries*. The change in blood vessel diameter brought by the autoregulation mechanism is the result of imbalance between muscle oxygen demand–supply. Arteriolar diameter is controlled by contraction or relaxation of *vascular smooth muscle*. The level of tone generated by a vascular smooth muscle cell depends on several factors, including its length and tension, local levels of metabolites and signaling molecules, communications with other cells via gap junctions, and neural inputs. Given that arterioles are the main effectors of blood flow regulation, a crucial aspect of the metabolic response is the need for arterioles to receive information about the metabolic status of the tissue that they supply [2].

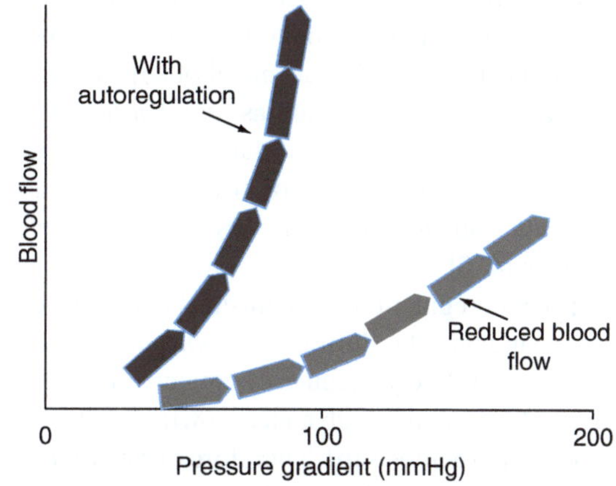

Fig. 4.1 The reduced blood flow curve changes slightly in the face of a large increase in perfusion pressure. The autoregulation (*darker curve*) maintains a constant blood flow despite changes in perfusion pressure

It has been previously suggested that the term autoregulation should also include variation of blood flow in proportion to metabolic rate and the compensatory changes in blood flow which occur

M.S. Sagiv, *Exercise Cardiopulmonary Function in Cardiac Patients*,
DOI 10.1007/978-1-4471-2888-5_4, © Springer-Verlag London 2012

in the face of varying arterial oxygen content [3]. If the pressure perfusing the arteries of almost any organ is varied, flow through the organ changes very little. This is termed autoregulation. Autoregulation only occurs between certain pressure limits: If the pressure drops too low or is too high, autoregulation fails, and organ perfusion is compromised; at low pressures, perfusion drops, and at high pressures, excessive flow occurs. The autoregulatory response occurs in the absence of neural and hormonal influences and therefore is intrinsic to the organ. *Autoregulation* is important in maintaining *coronary* and *arteriole blood flow*, which tends to be kept constant by involving *metabolic controls* that originate from the surrounding tissue linked to tissue metabolism or other *biochemical pathways* such as *metabolites*, *bradykinin*, and mechanisms that originate from inside of the arteriolar smooth muscles such as *myogenic* and *endothelial* factors during *dynamic exercise* [4, 5].

The autoregulation mechanism is not activated in working muscles during *anaerobic* and *isometric exercises*, likely because of greater concentrations of vasoactive substances owing to tissue hypoxia and acidosis [6]. Therefore during *anaerobic exercise*, diastolic blood pressure is elevated and total peripheral resistance is modestly reduced compared with *aerobic*-type effort [7]. For example, during aerobic effort, if from any reason *blood flow* to an organ is reduced, the autoregulation mechanism then acts to restore normal blood flow.

The blood flow to the exercising muscles will be regulated through the arterioles, leading blood in proportion to its needs, and is controlled *intrinsically* by modifying the diameter of local arterioles. This mechanism *during exercise* (Fig. 4.2) keeps on one hand diastolic blood pressure values similar or lower than that at rest, while on the other hand, the elevated systolic blood pressure increases blood flow to the working muscles [8].

Following long-term *exercise training*, *autoregulation* develops over weeks or months, an increase in the size of existing blood vessels and an increase in the number of vessels in a specific area – a process called *angiogenesis*. *Shear stress*-induced intussusceptive angiogenesis gives rise to longitudinal splitting of *blood capillaries*. The cells of the vessel wall can regulate angiogenesis by producing *growth factors*, proteolytic enzymes, extracellular matrix components, cell adhesion molecules, and *vasoactive factors*. This property enables preexisting blood vessels to generate new vessels in the absence of exogenous angiogenic stimuli [9].

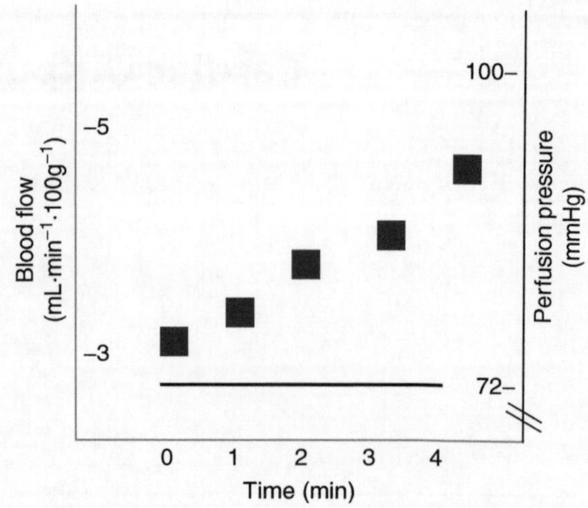

Fig. 4.2 Relationship between blood flow and perfusion pressure. Pressure is somehow kept constant (70–72 mmHg). Following 4 min of exercise, the autoregulation mechanism increases blood flow from 3.3 to 4.7 mL · min^{-1} · 100 g^{-1}

Blood Flow During Exercise

Total blood flow to an organ varies according to metabolic requirements, but is relatively insensitive to arterial pressure. Local control of blood flow ensures matching of perfusion to spatially varying oxygen demand, thereby achieving efficient oxygen delivery [10]. Systemic blood flow affects cardiopulmonary hemodynamic responses. The control of blood flow during exercise is extremely important to ensure that blood and oxygen are transported to the tissues that need them most. Blood flow to tissues is dependent on the relationship between blood pressure and the resistance provided by the blood vessels. *During exercise* in rats, *blood flow* to skeletal muscles varies with level of activity and *fiber type*. The capacity for blood flow is fairly proportional to the differences in oxidative capacity among fiber types [11]. Regular endurance training has been shown to increase mitochondrial *volume densities* in slow twist and fast twist of skeletal muscle fibers [12]. This adaptation is consistent with an increased oxidative capacity following endurance training. In fact, numerous changes within the skeletal muscle's cell act to convert toward a more oxidative profile following endurance training. The *local blood flow* is controlled by chemical factors, metabolites, paracrines, physical factors such as heat or cold, stretch effects on endothelial membrane, active hyperemia, and reactive hyperemia. The paracrine regulation is mainly regulated by nitric oxide, histamine release, and prostacyclin. *Nitric oxide* diffuses to smooth muscle and causes vasodilation by reducing calcium entry into smooth muscle. Muscular autoregulation occurs almost entirely in response to decreased oxygen concentrations. With increased demand for oxygen by the working muscles, it is crucial to increase *blood flow* to the *working muscles* [13]. Therefore, during exercise, vascular *smooth muscle tone* plays a fundamental role in regulating *blood pressure*, *blood flow*, *microcirculation*, and other cardiovascular functions.

The cellular and *molecular mechanisms* by which vascular smooth muscle contractility is regulated are not completely elucidated [14]. Many studies suggest that metabolic, myogenic, and endothelial mechanisms are responsible for this vasodilation. As resistance decreases, blood flow increases despite the presence of reduced perfusion pressure (Fig. 4.3). Blood flow *at rest* is equal to the change in pressure divided by the resistance of the vessels (Eq. 4.1).

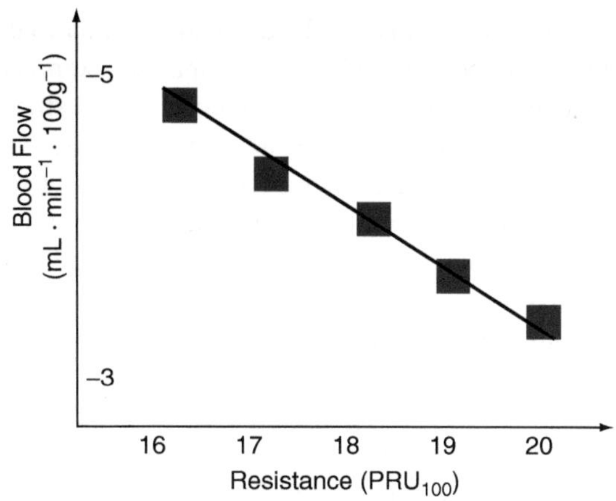

Fig. 4.3 Relationship between resistance and blood flow. When resistance value is high as 20 PRU100, blood flow is 3.3 mL · min^{-1} · dL^{-1}, while when resistance equals to 16 PRU100, blood flow is 4.7 mL · min^{-1} · dL^{-1}

$$BF = P/R, \qquad (4.1)$$

where BF = blood flow, P = pressure, and R = resistance.

Blood flow *during exercise* is regulated by changing blood pressure and altering the peripheral resistance of the vessels, so blood flow to the working muscles increases. *Autoregulatory resistance* is mediated through the *smooth muscles* in the arterioles and precapillary sphincters. The slow, intermittent flow of blood through the capillaries reflects the action of the *precapillary sphincters* in response to *local autoregulatory* controls. Blood flow is also increased during exercise by decreasing the resistance of the vessels in the systemic circulation of active skeletal muscle. Resistance is determined by (Eq. 4.2):

$$\text{Resistance} = (\text{length of tube} \cdot \text{viscocity of blood}) / \text{radius}^4 \qquad (4.2)$$

Changing the radius of the vessels has the most profound effect on blood flow. Doubling the radius of a blood vessel decreases resistance by a factor of 16. Decreasing the radius of a blood vessel by half increases resistance by a factor of 16. The arterioles have the most control over blood flow in the systemic circulation.

Metabolic Theory of Blood Flow Regulation

Methods of blood flow regulation to the exercising muscles are not being understood, but certain factors have been recognized. One school of thought about the autoregulation mechanism is the *metabolic theory*. Traditional explanations for the hyperemia which accompanies exercise have invoked the metabolic theory of vasodilation, whereby contractile activity in the active muscle gives rise to metabolic byproducts [15]. Metabolic controls of autoregulation are most strongly stimulated by a shortage of oxygen at the tissues. Vascular responses to metabolic conditions are clearly necessary for metabolic regulation of blood flow and the development of functional hyperemia. Oxygen is a crucial metabolite, and arterioles in vivo react to oxygen levels, constricting as surrounding oxygen levels are increased [2]. This approach is based on arterial muscle metabolism that creates a local feedback in order to keep levels of oxygen supply as demanded by the muscles. Thus, the resistance to blood flow is regulated by *metabolites* such as *adenosine and potassium* [16]. With increased *oxygen delivery* demand, blood flow to the working muscles is increased, by the *autoregulation mechanism*. This suggested that the sensing of oxygen levels occurs in downstream vessels or in the parenchyma and initiates responses that are conducted to the arteriole. However, it has been shown that arterioles are insensitive to changes in local oxygen level within a normal physiological range. In addition, this mechanism does not exist in the arteries and arterioles leading blood to the internal organs: kidneys, liver, and digestive system [17]. This in turn enables to divert more blood to the exercising muscle. Figure 4.4 reveals that local regulatory mechanisms in arteries, leading blood to the brain, myocardium, skeletal muscles, and skin, act without the influence of extrinsic control mechanisms: sympathetic nerves and circulating hormones.

At the onset of *dynamic endurance exercise*, the demand for oxygen by the working muscles increases; however, the ability to supply that *oxygen* is limited due to the *vasoconstriction* of the arterioles owing to the *sympathetic nervous system* activity. The imbalance created between muscle oxygen demand and supply of the muscle results in anaerobic work of the smooth muscles and skeletal muscles. This in turn will reduce ATP production of the smooth muscles, while the

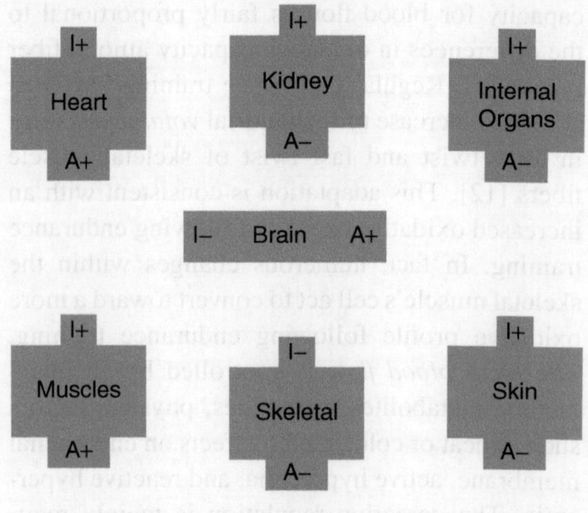

Fig. 4.4 Blood flow regulation mechanisms in the various organs of the body during dynamic aerobic exercise. The positive sign (*I*+) means with the influence of the sympathetic nervous system or, without its influence (*I*–). The positive sign (*A*+) means that the autoregulation mechanism is active, while (*A*–) means that there is no autoregulation effect

amount of AMP will increase. AMP diffuses into the interstitial space, where it can induce arteriolar dilation and reenter the arteriole cell. It is either phosphorylated to AMP by adenosine kinase or deaminated to AMP by adenosine deaminase, or it can enter the capillaries and leave the tissue [18]. AMP is formed by 52 nucleotidase from AMP, which itself is form from ATP and ADP. Adenosine is believed to be the major substance that influences metabolically induced arteriole vasodilatation [18].

At the same time, the increase in CO_2 will change *acid–base* balance, blundering entry and exit of electrolytes from the smooth muscle cells. This will increase the levels of *potassium* in the extracellular fluid. It was hypothesized that the increased levels of adenosine and potassium in the extracellular fluid will cause enlargement of the arteriole, and increase in blood flow and oxygen supply. This mechanism is on the go as long as the muscle's metabolic demand is above what is usual [19]. Oxygen tension, acid–base balance, potassium, osmotic pressure, and ATP-sensitive potassium channels also contribute to the metabolic regulation of flow.

Myogenic Theory of Blood Flow Regulation

Myogenic mechanism increases the stretch of arterial smooth muscle, such as might be seen by increasing arterial pressure, and myogenic mechanism has the effect of causing contraction of the smooth muscle. In other words, when stretched, the smooth muscle contracts, producing an increase in vascular resistance, thereby minimizing an increase in blood flow. *During endurance exercise*, the autoregulation of blood flow, the maintenance of almost steady blood flow in the face of variations in arterial pressure, is characteristic of many tissue types particularly the smooth muscle of blood vessels in small *arteries* and *arterioles*. If the pressure within a vessel is suddenly increased, the vessel responds by contracting smooth muscle of small arteries and arterioles (*myogenic mechanisms*). Myogenic control involves physical forces caused by *blood flow* and *blood pressure* acting on the walls of blood vessels. Flowing blood generates *shear stress* tangential to the endothelial cell surface. The pressure exerted by the blood against the walls of the blood arteries depends mainly on the artery's length, radial thickness, and force exerted (Fig. 4.5). It varies with the strength of the heartbeat, elasticity of arterial walls, blood volume and viscosity, person's health, age, and fitness. Circumferential stretch is caused by the action of blood pressure. In addition, localized response of vascular smooth muscle to passive *stretch-reflex* contraction when stretched to decrease flow and *reflex relaxation* when stretch is reduced to *vasodilate* and increase flow. Arterioles are directly exposed to the effects of the artery metabolites, which diffuse into the interstitial space. The vasodilator metabolites cause smooth muscle cell relaxation and vasodilatation, and thus increased flow.

This maintains a relatively constant flow locally when pressure fluctuates. This in turn diminishes pressure within the small arteries and arterioles and causes relaxation and vasodilation. However, the myogenic mechanism has not been clearly identified in all vascular beds, but it has been noted in the splanchnic and renal circulations, and may be present to a small degree in skeletal muscle [20].

Nitric Oxide and Kinins Influence on Blood Flow

Endothelial cells produce nitric oxide (NO), a rapidly diffusing labile substance which relaxes adjacent vascular smooth muscle. Nitric oxide is released basally and contributes to the regulation of vascular tone by acting as a functional antagonist to sympathetic neural constriction. In addition, *nitric oxide* is spontaneously released in response to deformation of the endothelial cell membrane, indicating that changes in pulsatile flow and wall *shear stress* are likely physiological stimuli [15]. Nitric oxide is released by the arterial endothelium in response to elevation of the pressure gradient along the long axis of the vessel, that is, increased "shear stress." Nitric oxide produces dilation locally in the smooth muscle adjacent to its point of synthesis. This mechanism has been postulated to explain some autoregulation-like changes in blood flow.

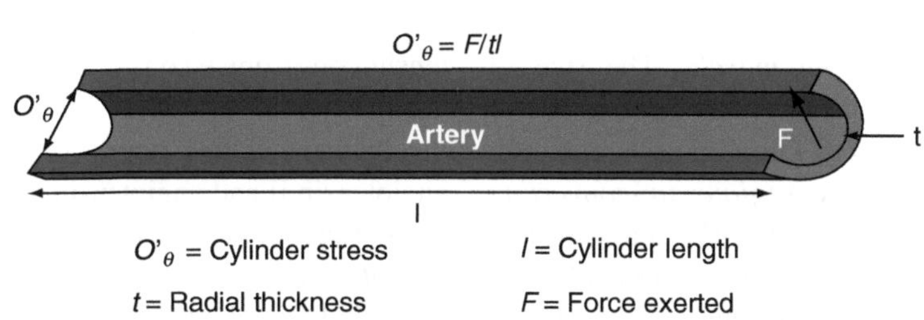

Fig. 4.5 Factors affecting vessel's stress: artery's length, radial thickness, and force exerted. Artery stress (O'_θ) equals to force exerted circumferentially on an area of the cylinder wall (*F*) divided by length (*l*) and radial thickness (*t*)

However, since autoregulation can still occur in a blood vessel from which the endothelium has been removed, it is unlikely that nitric oxide can fully explain the autoregulation phenomenon. The increased exposure to *shear stress* on the vessels throughout the entire body by the systolic blood pressure response during aerobic may upregulate the production of *nitric oxide* synthase and increase the release of *endothelium-derived* nitric oxide [15, 21]. The released nitric oxide induced by the shear stress of increased blood flow opposes adrenergic vasoconstriction, thus limiting the potential reduction in organ perfusion during augmented *sympathoadrenal* drive. In pathological states, endothelial dysfunction may lead to unopposed adrenergic vasoconstriction and subsequent periarteriolar resistive vessel dysfunction [22].

Two other known stimuli for release of nitric oxide are *hypoxia* and flow-mediated dilatation. It is believed that hypoxia initiates *hyperemia*, and flow-mediated dilatation sustains and amplifies it. *Nitric oxide* is believed to be involved through the ability of the *endothelium* to sense changes in perfusion pressure through pressure-sensitive ion channels. The arterial endothelium comprises cells resting on a basement membrane, which have autocrine, paracrine, and endocrine functions [23].

Shear stress applied to the luminal surface of endothelial cells is thought to be transmitted throughout the cell as well as to cell junctions and cellular adhesions. It was suggested previously that *kinins* may play a major role in the *vasodilatation* needed *during exercise*. Kinins are very potent vasodilating peptides which reduce blood pressure by lowering *peripheral vascular resistance*. Plasma and vascular kinins regulate and modulate the control of blood flow by the *endothelium* of vascular *smooth muscle*. The role of kinins in vasomotion is determined by the rate of the peptide production by kininogenases and their degradation by kininases. *Angiotensin-converting enzyme* (*ACE*) splits *bradykinin* into inactive fragments and by that reduces the action of kinins. Therefore, acute increases in plasma kinin levels during exercise indicate that the metabolism of the peptides is fine tuned to the systemic or local metabolic demands [24, 25].

Rennin-Angiotensin System

Clinical and experimental studies have demonstrated a major role of the *rennin-angiotensin system* (*RAS*) in the functional and structural changes of the large arteries. The rennin-angiotensin system is important for regulating *blood pressure* and *extracellular fluid*. The concept of the rennin-angiotensin system has recently evolved from a classical systemic endocrine system to an appreciation of local rennin-angiotensin system functions similar to a local anesthetic drug (procaine) of the amino ester group, including in the vascular wall [26].

Angiotensin-converting enzyme is a key component in the rennin-angiotensin system, generating the *vasoconstrictor angiotensin II* and degrading vasodilator *kinins* [27]. *Angiotensin-converting enzyme* is widely expressed in human tissues, including skeletal muscle, and may play a metabolic role during exercise [28]. Angiotensin II, the predominant biological product of rennin-angiotensin system, has been known for its effects on metabolism and is a recognized growth factor necessary for the hypertrophy of skeletal muscle in response to mechanical load [29]. Most of its known physiological and pathophysiological activities are mediated through the *angiotensin II type 1 receptor* (*AT1R*), which is the dominant receptor in the cardiovascular system [30]. Data suggest that increased angiotensin-converting enzyme activity leads not only to augmented production of angiotensin II, but also to a reduction in *angiotensin peptide* [31, 32], which is known to cause *vasodilating* effects [28]. Thus, it is conceivable that the angiotensin-converting enzyme genotype positively contributes to *endurance performance* by its involvement in fine tuning of the levels of both angiotensin II and angiotensin [31, 32].

A functional polymorphism of the human *angiotensin-converting enzyme gene* has been identified in which the absence (deletion – D allele), rather than the presence (insertion – I

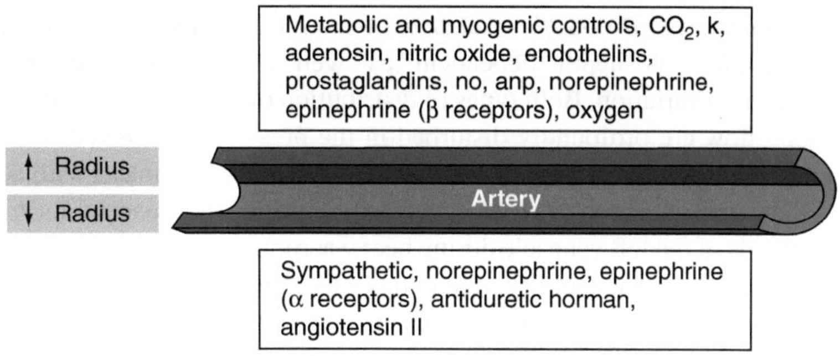

Fig. 4.6 Factors influencing the regulation of blood vessels perfusion. They include metabolic, endothelial, humoral, autoregulatory, myogenic, extravascular compressive, and neural control mechanisms

allele), of a 287-bp Alu repeat element in intron 16 is associated with higher enzyme activity in both serum and tissue [33, 34], resulting in greater production of *angiotensin II* and *aldosterone* and a decreased half-life of *bradykinin* [35].

The most extensively studied polymorphism in the AT1R gene is the A1166C variant [36]. This polymorphism has been linked to enhanced physiological responses of angiotensin II resulting in increased vasoconstrictor activity [37]. Angiotensin II has been shown to regulate VO_2 and affect muscle energy expenditure as well [38]. *Angiotensin-converting enzyme* genotype has been shown to affect exercise and glucose load responses. Figure 4.6 summaries the autoregulation major factors influencing the blood flow by intrinsic and extrinsic factors.

Myocardial Blood Flow

Mechanisms of autoregulation may vary substantially between organs. There is evidence that coronary autoregulation is, for example, quite different from brain autoregulation [39]. Control of coronary blood flow differs depending on the type of vessel being considered – arteries, large arterioles, or smaller arterioles. Coronary capillaries also appear to make a significant contribution to coronary vascular resistance. As if this is not enough, transmural variations occur. Exercise is the most important physiological stimulus for increased myocardial oxygen demand and, thus, blood flow in the coronaries. The requirement of exercising muscle for increased blood flow necessitates an increase in *cardiac output* that results in increases in the three main determinants of myocardial oxygen demand: *heart rate*, *myocardial contractility*, and ventricular work [19]. Coronary blood flow is dependent upon arterial pressure, diastolic time, and small vessel resistance. The system is regulated to achieve a low-flow high oxygen extraction and low myocardial oxygen partial pressure. The myocardium is an aerobic muscle rich in mitochondria and aerobic enzymes. Since the heart is a very aerobic organ, it needs oxygen for the efficient production of ATP and PC from fatty acids and, to a smaller extent, glucose and very little lactic acid. Therefore, the coronary circulation is autoregulated so that the heart receives the right flow of blood and hence sufficient supply of oxygen [19]. Hence, appropriate adjustment of coronary vascular resistance is critical for the cardiac response to exercise. If a sufficient flow of oxygen is met and the resistance in the coronary circulation rises perhaps due to vasoconstriction, then the coronary perfusion pressure increases proportionally, to maintain the same flow. In this way, the same flow through the coronary circulation is maintained over a range of pressures. This part of coronary circulatory regulation occurs over a plateau, reflecting the constant blood flow at varying coronary perfusion pressure and resistance. This setting is sensitive to change in oxygen needs. Regulation of blood flow occurs primarily through local intrinsic regulation, most likely through production of vasodilatation metabolites in response to minimal degrees of ischemia. Local regulation appears to dominate over remote regulation in most circumstances. Blood *flow distribution* to the *myocardium* is depth dependent as well as regional in variation. Both types of distribution of blood flow are profoundly disturbed in the presence of obstructive *coronary atherosclerosis*.

The approximately sixfold increase in oxygen demands of the left ventricle during heavy aerobic exercise is met principally by augmenting ~ fivefold coronary blood flow, as hemoglobin concentration and *oxygen extraction* already 70–80% at rest increase only modestly in most species [19]. The myocardium has a very limited *anaerobic capacity*, and the heart is dependent on a continuous supply of oxygen from the coronary circulation.

At rest, the myocardium extracts ~75% of the oxygen delivered by coronary blood flow compared with 25% extraction in the skeletal muscles. Thus, there is little extraction reserve when myocardial VO_2 is augmented several fold during exercise. Therefore, the relationship between myocardial VO_2, coronary blood flow, and the extraction of oxygen from the blood, $(a\text{-}v)O_2$, is unique.

The human heart weight is on average 300 g in man and 200 g in females [40]. The resting coronary blood flow averages $250\ mL \cdot min^{-1} \cdot 300\ g^{-1}$ ($0.8\ mL \cdot min^{-1} \cdot g^{-1}$ of heart muscle) and has one of the highest energy demands per tissue mass of all human organs [41]. This relationship is an application of the *Fick principle* (Eq. 4.3):

$$MVO_2 = CBF \cdot (a - v)O_2 \qquad (4.3)$$

where MVO_2 = myocardial oxygen uptake, CBF = coronary blood flow, and $(a\text{-}v)O_2$ = arterial-venous oxygen content difference.

Approximately, 80% of the heart's VO_2 is related to its mechanical work, while 20% is used to maintain the basic cellular metabolism. Therefore, myocardial blood flow must be closely matched to myocardial oxygen demand in the normal heart. Because of this, cardiac energy metabolism is extremely sensitive to reductions in perfusion caused by coronary artery disease. Coronary blood flow is tightly coupled to *myocardial* VO_2 to maintain a consistently high level of myocardial oxygen extraction. This requires tight control of coronary blood flow, because an increase in myocardial oxygen demand, as occurs *during exercise*, cannot be obtained by a significant further increase in *oxygen extraction* [42]. Nevertheless, cardiac function is inextricable linked with adequate tissue oxygenation, and because of its high metabolic rate and oxygen extraction, the heart is ultimately dependent on oxygen delivery by a profuse coronary vascular supply. That coronary blood flow is regulated mainly by the *autoregulation mechanism*, and by coronary capillaries also which appear to make a significant contribution to coronary vascular resistance. Control of coronary blood flow differs depending on the type of vessel being considered – arteries, large arterioles, or smaller arterioles. Coronary capillaries also appear to make a significant contribution to coronary vascular resistance. The major factor controlling the resistance of the coronary microcirculation appears to be local production of vasodilatation metabolites [16]. If a sufficient flow of oxygen is met and the resistance in the coronary circulation rises (perhaps due to vasoconstriction), then the coronary perfusion pressure increases proportionally, to maintain the same flow. In this way, the same flow through the coronary circulation is maintained over a range of pressures. This can be seen during isodynamic exercise where blood pressure is increased due to the isometric component and, thus, increase coronary blood flow in coronary artery disease patients manifested by the reduced ECG's ST segment [8].

Energy production in the normally functioning heart is primarily dependent on oxidative phosphorylation, with <5% of ATP production resulting from glycolytic metabolism [43]. As mentioned earlier, the normal oxygen concentration in arterial blood is about $20\ mLO_2 \cdot dL^{-1}$, normal function of the heart requires *at rest* about $6\text{–}8\ mLO_2 \cdot dL^{-1} \cdot min^{-1}$ myocardial tissue, and it increases during exercise by fivefold in the transition from rest to exercise [44]. This high level of oxygen extraction is facilitated by a high capillary density of 3,000–4,000 mm^2, which is substantially higher than the 500–2,000 capillaries/mm^2 found in skeletal muscle [45]. Anemia, for example, which can result from either a reduced hematocrit or reduced hemoglobin concentration within red cells, decreases oxygen delivery to tissues. Therefore, *during exercise* when oxygen demand is increased, and since more oxygen cannot be extracted by the myocardium, *blood flow* is increased in the *coronaries* linearly with *oxygen demand* as *hemoglobin* concentration and oxygen extraction increase only slightly. This is different from *skeletal muscles* which during exercise are able to increase both *oxygen extraction* and *blood flow* [46]. Exercise is the most important physiological stimulus for increased myocardial oxygen demand. The approximately sixfold increase in oxygen demands of the *left ventricle* during heavy exercise is met principally by augmenting coronary blood flow, as hemoglobin concentration and oxygen extraction which is already almost 80% at rest increase only modestly in most species. In contrast, in the *right ventricle*, oxygen extraction is lower at rest and increases substantially during exercise, similar to skeletal muscle, suggesting fundamental differences in blood flow regulation between these two cardiac chambers. The increase in heart rate also increases the relative time spent in systole, thereby increasing the net extravascular compressive forces acting on the microvasculature within the wall of the left ventricle, in particular in its subendocardial layers. Hence, appropriate adjustment of coronary vascular resistance is critical for the cardiac response to exercise [19].

During exercise, myocardial VO_2 may increase 200–300%. Exercise is associated with neurohumoral and hemodynamic alterations that improve the response of coronary circulation. For example, activation of the sympathetic nervous system during exercise acts to limit the increase in *coronary blood flow* by opposing metabolic vasodilatation. However, *coronary vasodilatation* counters that effect. Consequently, adequate control of coronary vascular resistance is critical. Coronary resistance vessel tone is the result of a myriad of vasodilator and vasoconstrictor influences, which are exerted by the myocardium, endothelium, and neurohumoral status [42]. Maintenance of α-adrenergic and β-adrenergic tone in the presence of lower circulating catecholamine levels appears to be due to increased receptor responsiveness to adrenergic stimulation. Exercise training also alters local control of coronary resistance vessels. Thus, arterioles exhibit increased myogenic tone, likely due to a calcium-dependent protein kinase C signaling-mediated alteration in voltage-gated calcium channel activity in response to stretch [19].

Inward remodeling of coronary microvessels distal to a stenosis is accompanied by exaggerated vasoconstrictor responses to endothelin-1. These structural and functional alterations may aggravate flow abnormalities distal to a chronic coronary artery stenosis. However, in contrast to the school of thought that myocardial ischemia produced by a coronary artery stenosis causes maximal microvascular dilation, studies have shown that the coronary microvessels retain some degree of vasodilator reserve during ischemia and remain responsive to vasoconstrictor stimuli [47]. On the other hand, exercise training is associated with adaptations in the coronary microvasculature including increased arteriolar densities and/or diameters, which provide a morphometric basis for the observed increase in peak coronary blood flow rates in exercise-trained animals. In larger animals trained by treadmill exercise, the formation of new capillaries maintains capillary density at a level commensurate with the degree of exercise-induced physiological myocardial hypertrophy. Nevertheless, training alters the distribution of coronary vascular resistance so that more capillaries are recruited, resulting in an increase in the permeability-surface area product without a change in capillary numerical density.

Hemodynamic alterations that accompany exercise can augment the ability to increase coronary blood flow during exercise. Failure of coronary blood flow to increase adequately during exercise could limit myocardial oxygen availability, thereby impairing cardiac performance (Fig. 4.7). Coronary blood flow is determined by hemodynamic factors such as perfusion pressure and vascular resistance. The latter is determined by vascular anatomy and structure, as well as by changes in diameter of the vascular lumen resulting from contraction and relaxation of vascular smooth muscle (local regulation of blood flow).

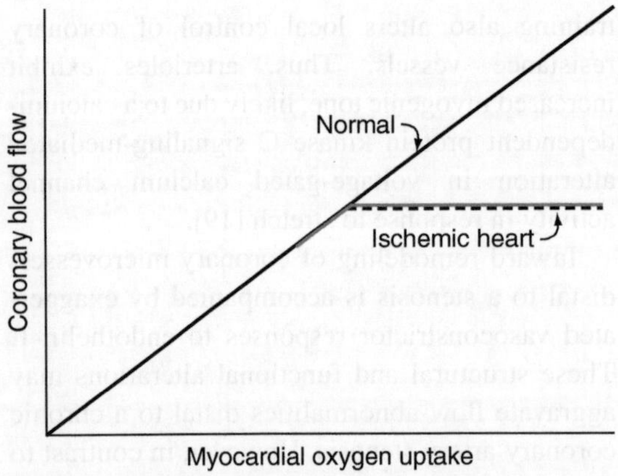

Fig. 4.7 Since myocardium's (a-v)O_2 is almost 70% at rest, it is necessary during exercise to increase coronary blood flow with increased myocardial oxygen demand. Therefore, the relationship between coronary blood flow and myocardial oxygen demand is linear. In the event that blood flow does not keep up with oxygen demand as in coronary artery disease patients, ischemia is reached

However, studies of myocardium isolated from failing ventricles have demonstrated reductions of energy expenditure that might result in decreased myocardial oxygen demands during exercise.

Blood flow in the coronaries occurs during *diastole*, since during systole the coronaries are occluded mechanically. Thus, *coronary blood flow* is determined by diastolic pressure and length, depending on heart rate. As *heart rate* accelerates, systole shortens, but not nearly as much as diastole. As a result, the heart is forced to do more work with less time for blood flow in the coronaries. It seems that this shortening of *diastole time* may be the most important factor limiting maximal heart rate. In addition, increase in heart frequency will reduce *filling time* which, in turn, will also reduce *stroke volume*, and therefore, the amount of blood reaching the myocardium through the coronaries is reduced. There has been debate about the extent to which the cardiac hypertrophy that accompanies certain exercise training programs confounds coronary flow reserve. In general, *physiological hypertrophy* as a result of exercise training does not lead to the impairment of coronary vasodilator capacity that is seen in pathological hypertrophy. It seems that there is an expansion of resistance vasculature commensurate with physiological hypertrophy through growth in number of smaller arterial vessels, in response to training.

Coronary blood flow is determined also by hemodynamic factors such as perfusion pressure and vascular resistance. The latter is determined by vascular anatomy and structure, as well as by changes in diameter of the vascular lumen resulting from contraction and relaxation of vascular smooth muscle (local regulation of blood flow). The *delivery of oxygen* to the myocardium (*oxygen supply*) is determined by two factors: coronary blood flow and the *oxygen content* (concentration) of the arterial blood (Eq. 4.4).

$$O_2\,\text{delivery} = \text{CBF}\cdot\text{CaO}_2, \tag{4.4}$$

where CBF = coronary blood flow (mL · min^{-1}) and CaO_2 = arterial oxygen content (mLO_2 · mL $blood^{-1}$).

Therefore, the primary determinant of oxygen delivery in the absence of *hypoxemia* is coronary blood flow [48].

In *coronary artery disease patients*, three main factors can reduce coronary blood flow: (a) stenotic lesions cause a narrowing of vessel, particularly the large epicardial coronaries (e.g., left anterior descending or circumflex arteries), (b) diseased coronary vessels are more susceptible to vasospasm, which can lead to a temporary restriction of coronary flow at rest. This can occur *during exercise* in susceptible individuals, and (c) thrombus formation, particularly at the site of a ruptured atherosclerotic plaque.

Myocardial VO_2 is determined by heart rate, the intramyocardial tension and contractile state. Other less important determinants of myocardial VO_2 are external work of the heart, activation energy, basal myocardial metabolism, and increased peripheral resistance or afterload. An elevation in *heart rate*, in addition to its positive inotropic effect on the myocardium, also adds to the metabolic needs for oxygen because of the increased number of beats per minute. In addition, heart rate determines the frequency at which the myocardial wall is stressed. Thus, increased myocardial VO_2 with higher heart beats is caused by an increase in the total tension developed and by an increase in myocardial *contractility*.

Heart rate increases with exercise and, as at rest, correlates well with coronary blood flow. As discussed earlier, between 40% and 90% VO_{2max} further increase in cardiac output is met only by increased heart rate. This means that heart rate increases proportionally to the increase in VO_2 demand. Therefore, it becomes evident that the work of the heart, *cardiac output*, coronary blood flow, and heart rate all increase in a parallel manner and peak together. The increase in *heart rate* also increases the relative time spent in systole, thereby increasing the net extravascular compressive forces acting on the *microvasculature* within the wall of the *left ventricle*, in particular in its subendocardial layers. Hence, appropriate adjustment of coronary vascular resistance is critical for the cardiac response to *exercise*.

Intramyocardial tension or the pressure developed by the ventricular wall is a meaningful determinant of myocardial VO_2. Left ventricular wall tension is defined by *Laplace's law* which states "that the wall tension is equal to the pressure within the cylinder times the radius of the curvature of the wall." The tension is also related to the thickness of the wall and the radius of the ventricle. Therefore, at a fixed pressure and wall thickness, an increase in venous return will increase tension and thus myocardial VO_2.

The *contractile state* of the left ventricular is achieved by an increase in the metabolism of myocardial cells. Metabolism level is influenced by the activity level of the sympathetic nervous system via catecholamine in the blood stream and in the ends of the nerves in the heart. *Preload* and *afterload* also influence *contractility state*, while contractility state determines the velocity of contraction.

The combination of a high heart rate and systolic blood pressure suggest high VO_2 by the heart. In fact, the product of heart rate multiplied by systolic blood pressure (Eq. 4.5) or *double product* or the rate-pressure product (RPP) was suggested in order to estimate myocardial oxygen demand, which turns out to be an excellent predictor of myocardial load.

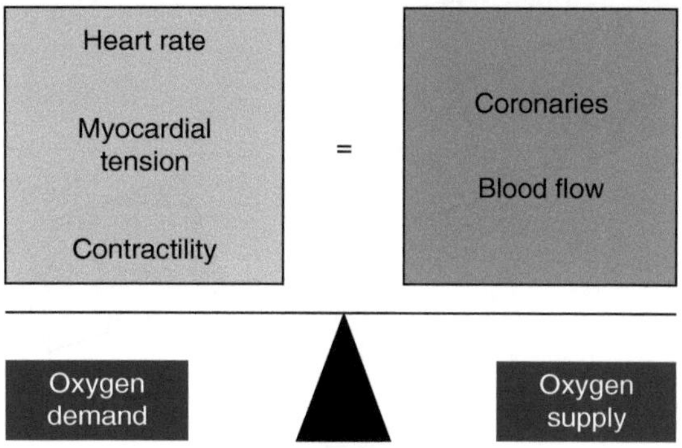

Fig. 4.8 Variables affecting myocardial oxygen demand–supply. Increased heart rate, wall tension, and contractility will increase oxygen demand, which will be balanced by the augmentation of coronaries blood flow

$$(HR \cdot SBP)/100, \qquad (4.5)$$

where HR = heart rate, SBP = systolic blood pressure, and 100 = 100%.

This method measuring myocardial oxygen demand correlates very well in wide range of exercise intensities. The double product is also a good tool to estimate the *angina threshold*, that is, the point in which the imbalance between oxygen supply and demand occurs. This is a very important variable for clinician and cardiac patients.

The *rate-pressure product* (*RPP*) has been used as an indirect measure of myocardial oxygen consumption. The rate-pressure product has been shown to correlate well with myocardial VO_2 under both *isometric effort* and *dynamic exercise* conditions. During *aerobic exercise*, *heart rate* and *systolic blood pressure* increase; the heart has to work harder and will require more oxygen and nutrients to keep going. The response of the heart rate and blood pressure to a fixed level of exercise tends to decrease with regular, *vigorous aerobic exercise*. Therefore, a well-trained person is better able to satisfy the demands of the heart for oxygen and nutrients during exercise than an untrained person [49].

Figure 4.8 summarizes the factors determining myocardial VO_2 and blood flow and reveals that, as long as coronary blood flow is adequate to keep oxygen supply and demand balanced, left ventricular function will function normal.

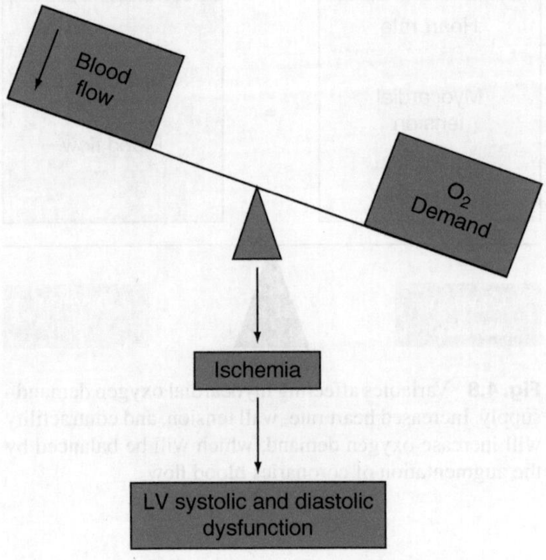

Fig. 4.9 During exercise with increased heart rate, contractility, and end-diastolic volume (wall tension,) oxygen demand is not met due to narrow coronaries that reduce blood flow. Consequently, an imbalance between oxygen demand (increased) and supply (blood flow decrease) is reached, and ischemia

However, coronary abnormalities may impair coronary vasodilation, limiting the ability to increase coronary blood flow to meet increased metabolic demands. With the reduction of blood flow in coronary artery disease, oxygen supply is reduced significantly, bringing about an imbalance in oxygen supply and demand and ischemia (Fig. 4.9).

Cardiac Output Redistribution

The redistribution of the blood is brought about by several mechanisms. *During exercise*, generalized vasodilatation occurs because of the accumulation of *vasodilatory metabolites*. This leads to a decrease in the peripheral resistance, which, in turn, elicits a strong increase in the sympathetic activity through the activation of *baroreceptors*. The distribution of sympathetic input varies among tissues. The blood vessels of the skin and splanchnic bed are strongly innervated by the *sympathetic nervous system*. The blood flow of these tissues is under strong sympathetic regulation. As an example, *skin blood flow* may be reduced to near zero by in cold ambient, thereby reducing heat loss to the environment. So strong is the sympathetically mediated temperature regulation mechanism that blood flow to the skin may be reduced until frostbite occurs. By contrast, the vascular flow of the brain and heart appears to be under near total control of *metabolic regulation*. Skeletal muscle combines both mechanisms. At rest, skeletal muscle arterioles are under strong sympathetic tone. With exercise, metabolic demand increases and blood flow increases by metabolic *autoregulation*, overriding the sympathetic input. At the onset of exercise, stimulation of nerves to the venous capacitance vessels moves large quantities of blood from peripheral veins into the systemic circulation. Blood is redistributed throughout the circulatory system. Local, neural, and hormonal factors determine *blood distribution* throughout the body's vasculature. The body can divert blood and, thus, oxygen where it is most needed. During exercise, these factors redistribute blood in a predictable fashion:

- Increased blood flow to the working musculature. However, blood flow to skeletal muscles varies with level of activity and fiber type. Muscular *autoregulation* occurs almost entirely in response to decreased oxygen concentrations.
- Decreased *visceral blood flow*. The redistribution of blood away from visceral organs allows more blood volume in active circulation.
- Decreased renal blood flow decreases filtration which results in the preservation of blood volume.
- Increasing blood volume, that is, *venous return*. During rest, roughly two thirds of blood volume is present in the venous system. At the onset of exercise, a large volume of blood is ejected from this venous pool into the active circulation. This is due to overall *vasoconstriction* in the venous system along with the activation of the *skeletal muscle pump*.
- Vasoconstriction of the *spleen* – increased blood volume in active circulation.
- *Cerebral blood flow* is tightly regulated to meet neuronal needs, since neurons cannot

tolerate periods of ischemia, and increased blood CO_2 causes marked *vasodilation*.

- Increased blood flow to the *skin*, thus, helps to promote heat loss, maintaining *core temperature*. In the skin, local autoregulatory events control oxygen and nutrient delivery to the cells, while *neural mechanisms* control the core temperature regulation function.
- *Autoregulatory* controls of blood flow to the *lungs* are the opposite of what happens in most tissues: low pulmonary oxygen causes vasoconstriction, while higher oxygen causes vasodilation.
- Movement of blood through the *coronary circulation* of the *heart* is influenced by aortic pressure and the pumping of the *ventricles*.

The redistribution of *cardiac output* during exercise to specific tissues is generally proportional to the metabolic activity of the tissue. Accordingly, the overwhelming majority of cardiac output during exercise is devoted to the *working skeletal muscle*. The *autoregulation mechanism* is responsible for redistributing cardiac output during *dynamic endurance exercise* since blood flow to the exercising muscles is regulated by the metabolic demand [4]. An adult has cardiac output of about 5 L · min^{-1} at rest. With a body weight of 70 kg, this corresponds to an average blood flow of 7.7 mL · min^{-1} · dL^{-1} of tissue with VO_2 of 3.5 mLO_2 · kg · min^{-1}, or 245 mLO_2 · min^{-1}. However, blood flow varies greatly among tissues, as shown in Fig. 4.10. During *dynamic endurance exercise*, VO_2 is increased significantly (20–25 times of resting values), and thus in sedentary young adult, *cardiac output* increases four- to fivefold from resting values, up to 25 L · min^{-1}. This increase in oxygen supply during exercise is achieved due to the differential redistribution of cardiac output to the body's organs (Fig. 4.11).

Figure 4.10 reveals that at *rest* 27% out of the total cardiac output (5 L · min^{-1}) goes to the skeletal muscles and the rest 73% goes to the *liver*, *kidneys*, *digestive track*, *heart*, and *brain*. In addition, the cutaneous blood flow initially decreases, but it later increases during the course of exercise. During *dynamic exercise*, 85% of the total cardiac output (25 L · min^{-1}) goes to the *skeletal muscles* and only15% is devoted to the liver, kidneys, digestive tract, heart, brain, and viscera. The percentage of blood to the brain decreases, but the absolute amount increases. The same percentage of blood as in the brain goes to cardiac muscle, but the absolute amount also increases. In addition, from Fig. 4.11, it can be concluded that during dynamic *endurance exercise*, blood flow to the liver, kidneys, and digestive tract is reduced both absolutely and relatively. The adequacy of this adjustment for brain, exercising skeletal muscle and myocardium, is particularly striking; skeletal muscle will, for example, when arterial oxygen partial pressure is reduced, take blood supply from non-exercising tissues sustaining its own oxygen delivery at normal levels [3]. Blood flow to visceral tissues and inactive skeletal

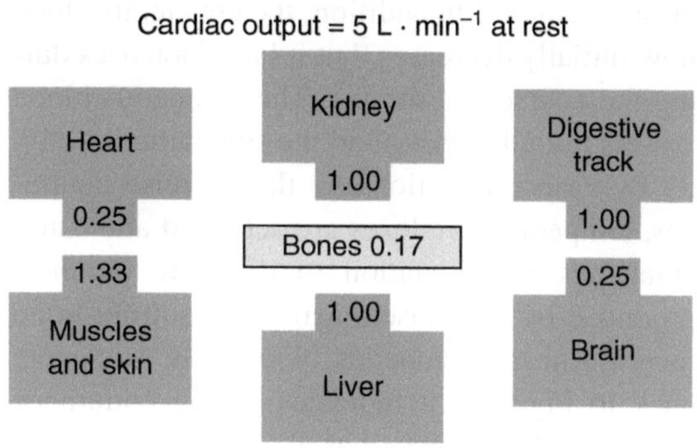

Fig. 4.10 Cardiac output (5 L · min^{-1}) distribution in various body organs at rest. Note that the amount of blood flow to the muscles and skin is almost as that of the liver

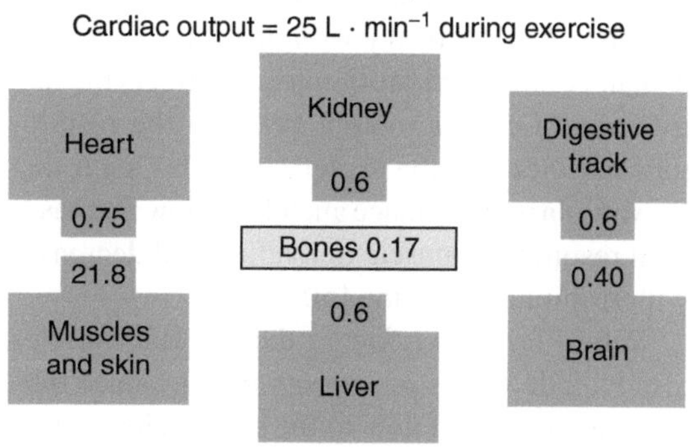

Fig. 4.11 Cardiac output (25 L · min^{-1}) redistribution at rest and during peak dynamic aerobic exercise in absolute liters and relative (percent) values. Muscles and skin blood flow increased relatively and absolutely

muscle reduces. In addition, the cutaneous blood flow initially decreases, but it later increases during the course of exercise. The cutaneous blood vessels initially respond to the sympathetic activity by vasoconstriction. As the exercise continues, temperature reflexes are activated and cause cutaneous vasodilatation to dissipate the heat produced by the muscle activity, resulting in an increase in the cutaneous blood flow. Referring back to Fig. 4.4, it indicates during endurance exercise which organ has the influence of the sympathetic nervous system, which has the autoregulation, and which has both.

It is worth to note that evidence shows that the *respiratory muscles* demand a significant portion of the *cardiac output* and VO_2 during maximal exercise. During heavy exercise, this metabolic demand of the respiratory muscles affects the distribution of cardiac output between the respiratory muscles and the skeletal muscles such that leg vascular conductance and blood flow increases with respiratory muscle unloading and decreases with respiratory loading [50].

Values for *blood flow* to the skeletal muscles also include values of *skin blood flow*, since during exercise, blood flow to the skin is closely tied to *body core temperature* regulation, which is dependent on exercise intensity and ambient temperature.

The cutaneous blood vessels initially respond to the sympathetic activity by vasoconstriction. As the exercise continues, temperature reflexes are activated and cause cutaneous vasodilatation to dissipate the heat produced by the muscle activity, resulting in an increase in the cutaneous blood flow.

As mentioned above, regulation of blood flow and vascular tone *during endurance exercise* in humans is complex due to the different types of *skin* in various regions of the body and the vast array of *nerves* involved in regulation of blood flow. At the beginning of exercise, the demand of blood flow to muscles results in *cutaneous vasoconstriction* by the sympathetic nervous system which innervates the resistance vessels (i.e., the arterioles). The *neurotransmitter released* is *norepinephrine* which acts on both *α-receptor* and *β-receptor*. As *body core temperature* rises, the *thermoregulatory reflex* processes predominate and the *skin blood vessels* dilate, increasing blood flow and heat conduction to the skin. The increase in *skin blood flow* with increase in body core temperature represents the combination of withdrawal of vasoconstrictor activity and elevation of active vasodilator activity.

Respiratory Muscle Work

The respiratory system has sufficient capacity responding to the demand for maximal oxygen and CO_2 elimination in healthy subjects exercising at sea level. This, however, may change at *peak strenuous exercise*. But in the case of respiratory muscle fatigue, the major consequence will be an increased sympathetic vasoconstrictor outflow to working skeletal muscle through a respiratory muscle metaboreflex, thereby reducing working muscles blood flow and increasing the severity of exercise-induced anaerobiosis and working muscle fatigue [50]. The energy expenditure required by the *respiratory muscles* during exercise is a function of their work rate, *cost of breathing*, and efficiency. During exercise, *ventilatory requirement* increases further worsen the potential imbalance between inspiratory muscle load and capacity. Up to 75% of VO_{2max} respiratory mechanical loading and unloading affects total VO_2 and cardiac output. However, it does not change the needed amount of blood flow to working skeletal muscles. Above 75% of VO_{2max}, the work of breathing required during maximal exercise compromises blood flow to working skeletal muscles and reduces exercise performance because of sympathetically mediated vasoconstriction. *Cardiovascular disease patients* and *sedentary subjects* have a reduced cardiac function and increased work of breathing, due to the low V_T and high f and, thus, pulmonary insufficiency. This in turn will increase the demand for oxygen by the diaphragm and expiratory abdominal muscles. Increased skeletal working muscle blood flow demand on one hand and the increased demand for oxygen by the diaphragm and expiratory abdominal muscles on the other hand may result in competition between the

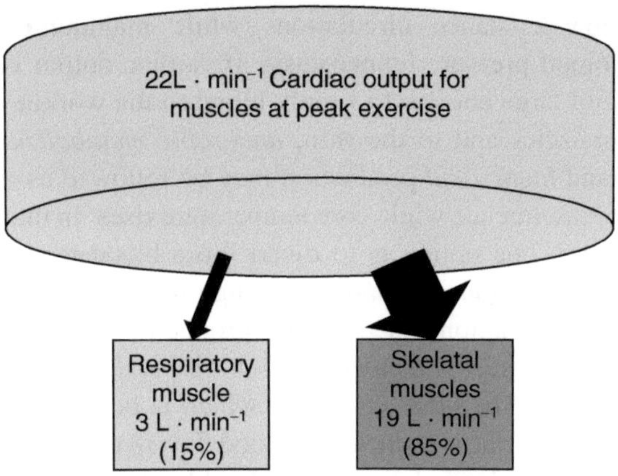

Fig. 4.12 At maximal aerobic exercise of the total blood flow to the working skeletal muscles, 14–16% of the cardiac output is directed to the respiratory muscles

diaphragm and expiratory abdominal muscles on one hand and skeletal working muscle vascular beds on the other hand. Thus, *peripheral fatigue* of *working skeletal muscles* resulting from high-intensity sustained exercise is, in part, due to the increased demand for oxygen by the diaphragm and expiratory abdominal muscles.

The respiratory muscle work normally expends during maximal exercise [51]. The diaphragm has multiple sources of blood supply and a distinctive high aerobic enzymatic capacity that make it the most fatigue-resistant of all the skeletal muscles. In addition, a unique resistance to vasoconstrictor influences on vascular diameter and therefore a substantial fatigue resistance [52]. In most of the cases, the diaphragm has no reduction in force output or velocity of shortening. This has two significant effects on the cardiovascular system: First, of the total blood flow to the skeletal muscles, 14–16% of the *cardiac output* is directed to the respiratory muscles (Fig. 4.12); and secondly, local reflex vasoconstriction significantly compromises blood flow to working muscles [53].

High level of exercise intensity in conjunction with contracting respiratory muscles is the reason for *respiratory muscle fatigue* in healthy subjects. The fatigue appears to be due to elevated levels of respiratory muscle work combined with an increased competition for *blood flow* with skeletal working muscles. These suggest that respiratory muscle fatigue may be involved in limiting exercise tolerance or that other factors including alterations in the sensation of dyspnea or mechanical load may be important. This places a large demand on the myocardium muscle even in well-trained subjects because of the ventilation required by strenuous sustained exercise. This is a significant limitation to exercise performance by reducing blood flow to skeletal working muscle.

Cardiac Output in Warm Environments

The combined metabolic and thermoregulatory demands of *exercise* in the heat place an exceptional burden on the circulation, more than can be met through *cardiac output* and blood flow *redistribution*. Blood flow to muscle is not reduced by heat stress in *exercise*, and *cardiac output* is insufficient to meet competing demands from skin and muscle [54]. *During exercise*, *heat production* can be increased from 4 KJ · min^{-1} at rest and increases up to 2,000 KJ · min^{-1} at peak exercise, or from 80 W to several hundred watts. Under these conditions, the controlling mechanism (the temperature regulation system) must act in order to avoid tissue damage. In hot, compared to cool, environments, exercise capacity is reduced. Because cardiac output to the exercising muscles is reduced, this could be a major contributor to the reduced performance in hot conditions. However, heat acclimation lowers heart rate [55] and increases plasma volume and stroke volume and, thus, maximal cardiac output in hot conditions [56]. The mechanism for the increased plasma volume may be an isosmotic volume expansion caused by influx of protein to the vascular compartment and a sodium retention induced by a significant increase in aldosterone [57]. Environmental heat stress can challenge the limits of human cardiovascular and temperature regulation, body fluid balance, and thus aerobic performance. Hyperthermia reduces VO_{2max} [58, 59], which leads to higher relative exercise intensity and an exponential decline in aerobic performance at any given exercise workload. That local hyperthermia also induces vasodilatation of the skeletal muscle microvasculature, thereby contributing to heat stress and *exercise* hyperemia. The increased muscle vasodilatation in the face of elevated muscle sympathetic vasoconstrictor activity is closely related to the rise in arterial plasma ATP and local tissue temperature [60].

It has been proposed that performance may be impaired by the development of hyperthermia and concomitant rise in cardiovascular strain, increasing relative *exercise* intensity. A *thermoregulatory*-mediated rise in cardiovascular strain is associated with reductions in sustainable power *output*, VO_{2peak}, and maximal power output during prolonged *exercise* in the heat [61]. Other possible cause for the reduced physical performance is a decrease in hemoglobin concentration from the vascular volume. This in turn will increase relatively exercise intensity which increase cardiovascular strain, and as a consequence, an earlier fatigue ensues [62]. Severe heat stress has been shown to markedly suppress VO_{2max} and work capacity without altering the initial rate of rise in whole-body VO_2 [63]. These results can be reversed following heat acclimatization.

Heat stress increases muscle blood flow and cardiac output in humans, presumably in sole response to an augmented thermoregulatory demand of the skin circulation. In ambient temperatures of 20–28°C, VO_2 is linearly with cardiac output and can increase blood flow to the working muscles. However, in temperatures above 22°C, cardiac output is not increased in a linear way with VO_2.

During dynamic exercise, the amount of blood flow to myocardium and active muscle is required to meet the aerobic energetic demands for muscular activity, while blood flow to skin is required to meet the demands of temperature regulation. These two demands for blood flow can result in *blood flow redistribution* due to the competition for the available *cardiac output*. Consequently, *dynamic exercise* in a warm environment creates a competition between *skin* (cutaneous vasodilatation) and active muscle for the available cardiac output [64]. The *blood flow competition* between skin and active muscle for the available cardiac output can be solved by having an integrated cardiovascular response to perfuse these two low-resistance circulations while maintaining blood pressure homeostasis. If cardiac output is not large enough to supply blood to the working muscles and to the skin, *anaerobic metabolism* and *lactic acid* production may be followed as a consequence while core temperature rises. In that case, one option is to divert more blood to the working muscles and not enough for the skin. In this situation, lactic acid production is low. However, *core temperature* will rise to dangerous levels. The other condition which is better than the first one is reducing in blood flow to the working muscles and diverts a higher blood flow to the skin. At this condition, lactic acid production will increase, and thus, an imbalance in acid–base is reached bringing to a halt in exercising before core temperature reaches high and dangerous levels [65].

This suggests that the combined *metabolic* and *thermoregulatory* demands of *exercise* in the heat place an exceptional burden on the circulation, more than can be met through *cardiac output* and *blood flow redistribution*. Under these conditions, vasoconstriction decreases blood flow to the kidneys, liver, pancreas, spleen, and digestive track. In thermally stressful environments, renal and splanchnic flows are further reduced, with this additional fraction of the available cardiac output redirected to the skin to facilitate heat dissipation [66]. Blood flow to muscle is not reduced by heat stress in *exercise*, and *cardiac output* is insufficient to meet competing demands from skin and muscle. Endurance exercise causes a cutaneous vasoconstriction at *exercise* onset through increased vasoconstrictor activity. As *exercise* continues, internal temperature reaches a threshold for increased active vasodilator activity that is elevated by *exercise*. This vasodilator function compromises temperature regulation [54]. It is unclear at present how these two mechanisms that lead to augmented skin blood flow, that is, increased cardiac output and visceral vasoconstriction, are affected by individual subject characteristics such as VO_{2max}. Additional blood flow to skin is not a concern. Instead, circulatory control elements prevent muscle vascular conductance from reaching such high levels. Otherwise, blood pressure could be severely

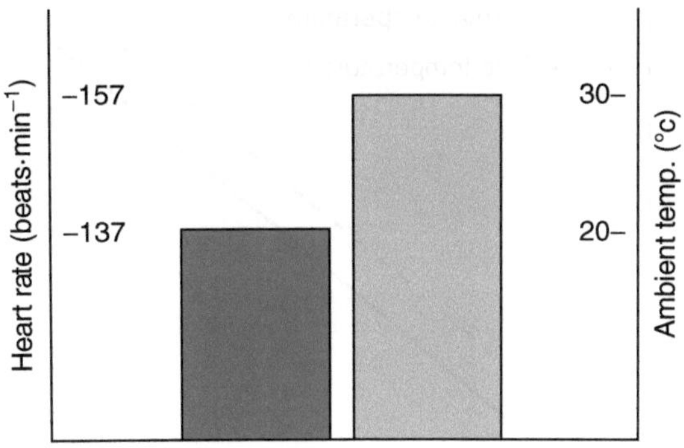

Fig. 4.13 At the same absolute workload, heart rate will be significantly higher at ambient of 30°C compared to environment temperature of 20°C

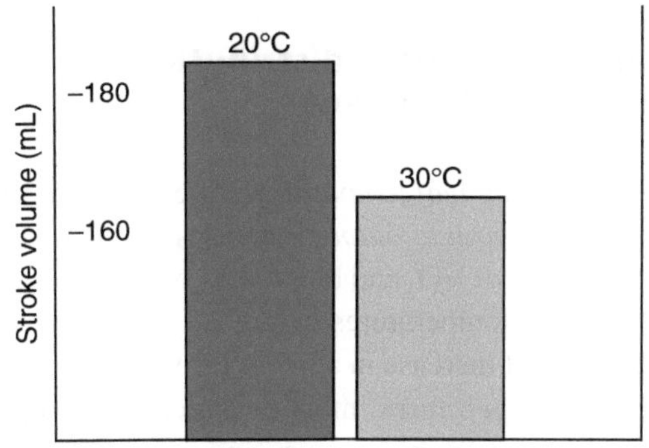

Fig. 4.14 At the same absolute workload, stroke volume will be significantly higher at ambient of 20°C compared to environment temperature of 30°C

threatened. Such a compromised blood pressure regulation is, in fact, seen in conditions wherein sympathetic vasoconstrictor function is compromised [67].

The heat transfer to the skin by the circulation during exercise is possible following the opening of closed blood vessels in the skin. In warm environment compared to normal ambient temperatures, during submaximal dynamic exercise at the same absolute load, *heart rate* will be higher (Fig. 4.13), while *stroke volume* is lower (Fig. 4.14). *Core temperature* has been shown to increase heart rate and reduce stroke volume when skin blood flow, blood volume, and *cardiac output* are constant [68].

It is worth to point out that the $(a\text{-}v)O_2$ and *cardiac output* are not influenced by *ambient temperatures* below 28°C. In any case, at any given ambient temperature, cardiac output will increase. As an example, during running at a speed of 12 km · h^{-1} in an ambient temperature of 35°C, heart rate value will reach 170 beats · min^{-1}, compared to 130 at an ambient temperature of 10°C. The increased 40 beats · min^{-1} is the result of the need to augment cardiac output in order to add blood flow to the skin for heat dissipation.

Additional factor that will further reduce cardiac output during dynamic exercise in warm environment is dehydration. It reduces substantially plasma volume that develops during exercise, thus reducing venous return and stroke volume. These effects are exacerbated when the exercise is performed in a hot environment. Mild hypohydration exacerbated cardiovascular and thermoregulatory strain and tended to impair endurance performance, but aerobic fitness attenuated the physiological effects. Yet, athletes that often dehydrate in exercise are hypervolemic and have less cardiovascular sensitivity to acute hypervolemia. This, however, may have negative consequences in coronary artery disease patients exercising in hot environment. Dehydration reduces aerobic endurance performance and results in increased body temperature, heart rate, perceived exertion, and possibly increased reliance on anaerobic metabolic pathway as an energy source [69]. *Cardiac output* will be the same in different ambient temperatures; however, in hot environments, cardiac output is insufficient to deliver oxygen and to dissipate body's heat. Even though, the internal organs have a significant reduction in blood flow. The dehydration coupled with the relatively reduced cardiac output may bring to decrease in sweating rate and increase in *core temperature* and hence stopping exercise. During prolonged exercise, there is an additional reduction in cardiac output due to a further decrease in *stroke volume* due to reduction in *venous return*. Under normal conditions, the movement of water between compartments helps to maintain reasonable level of sweating in the hot environment without influence on cardiac output. However, the loss of water through sweat interferes with the movement of water

Table 4.1 Summary of hemodynamic responses in different environment temperatures during dynamic aerobic exercise

Variable	At 22°C	At 40°C
Heart rate	Increase	Increase more
Stroke volume	Maximal	Reduced
Cardiac output	Increase	Increase
Skin flow	Increase	Increase more
Plasma volume	Normal	Reduced
Oxygen uptake	Increase	Increase more
Minute ventilation	Normal	Reduced

from the extracellular compartment to the cardiovascular compartment and, thus, reduces venous return.

In ambient temperatures of 22–28°C (mild stress) or in ambient temperatures of 32–40°C (stressful), any loss of water of 3–4% body weight will bring to a significant decrease in *cardiac output*. At that stage, *heart rate* cannot be further increased, that is, the reduction in *stroke volume* is so significant that any increase in heart rate cannot compensate for the cardiac output reduction. *Acclimatization* to warm environment and the benefits of aerobic training improve physical performance in trained and untrained persons. In trained, the improvement is greater than that of the untrained. This is due to the larger amount of body water in the trained following training. This in turn facilitates temperature regulation by keeping *core temperature* low in the warm ambient. Cardiac output is reduced less under the same environment condition following acclimatization. The reduction in *venous return* is attenuated, so stroke volume is reduced not as much as before acclimatization.

The influence of the acclimatization on cardiac output is still controversial. One approach holds that acclimatization period should be 12 weeks, while the second thought is that 6-week training is sufficient. Table 4.1 compares physiological responses to endurance exercise in different ambient temperatures.

Under high extremely ambient temperatures, VO_{2max} in untrained is lower than that achieved by them in normal temperatures (20–22°C). However, in few well-trained athletes, there is no difference in VO_{2max} in both temperatures.

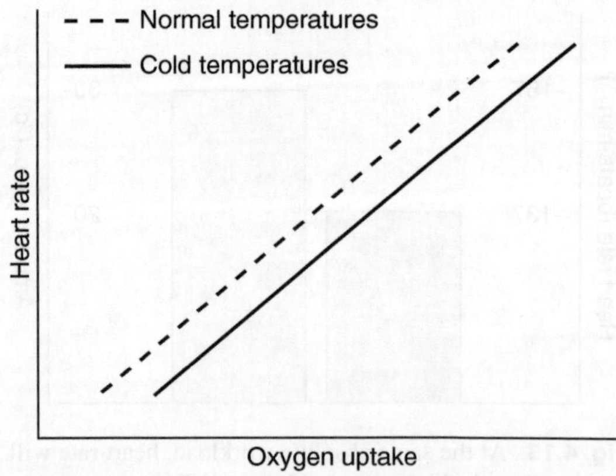

Fig. 4.15 Differences in heart rate responses for the same workload in normal ambient compared to cold environments

Cardiac Output Redistribution in Cold Environment

When the *ambient temperatures* are between 2°C and 22°C, *cardiac output* increases linearly with the increase of VO_2 and blood flow to the muscles. In ambient temperatures below 2°C, cardiac output does not increase in a linear fashion with VO_2. In *cold temperatures*, most of the cardiac output goes to the working muscles and not to the skin. These will increase moderately blood flow to the internal organs. The decrease in heat transfer to the skin, during endurance exercise, in the cold environment (water and air alike) is possible from the vasoconstriction of blood vessels. This increases blood volume in the chest and, therefore, *venous return* is increased as well as *stroke volume*. As a result, during submaximal dynamic endurance exercise in a cold surrounding *heart rate* will be lower and stroke volume larger compared to the same workload at normal temperature (Fig. 4.15). During efforts between 40% and 85% VO_{2max}, there is no linear relationship between heart rate and VO_2 as in normal ambient temperatures. Therefore, the submaximal PWC170 cycle test is not valid in these cold temperatures.

Cardiac Output at Altitude

At 2,300 m and above, cardiac output, heart rate, *stroke volume*, blood volume, and *blood pressure* respond to *hypoxia* by increasing function to

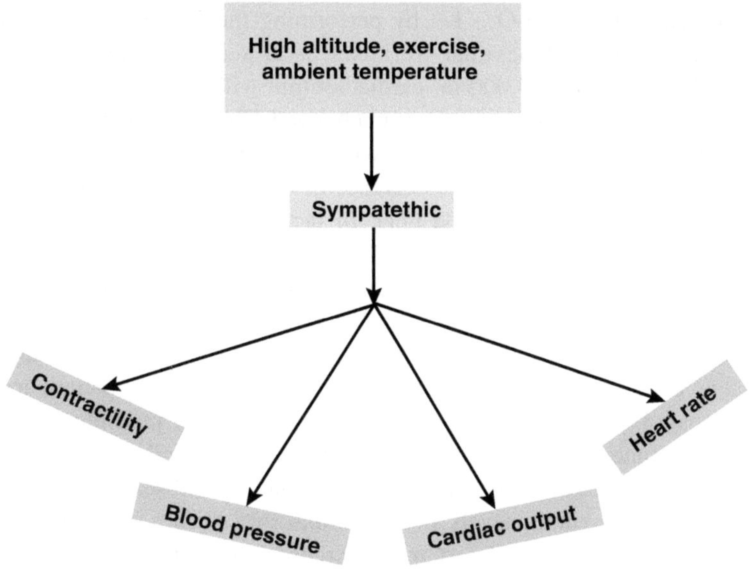

Fig. 4.16 Effect of hypoxia (high altitude), exercise, and ambient temperature on the systemic circulation response at high altitude. High altitude, exercise, and ambient temperature are factors affecting the sympathetic nervous system at high altitude, and as a result, cardiac output, contractility, blood pressure, and heart rate are increased in order to deliver more oxygen

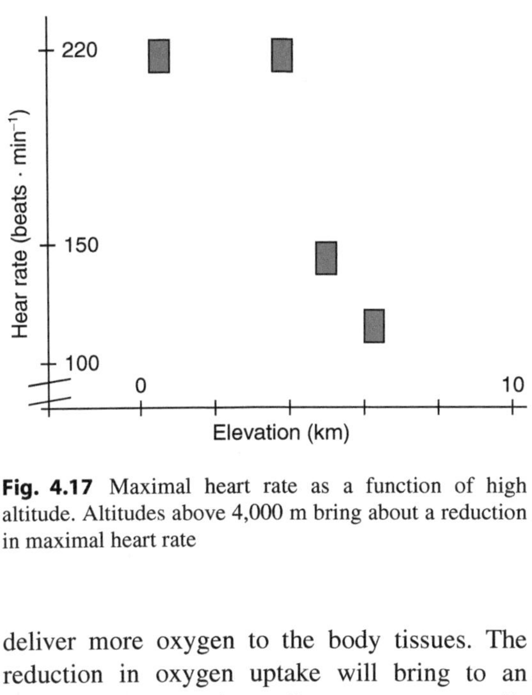

Fig. 4.17 Maximal heart rate as a function of high altitude. Altitudes above 4,000 m bring about a reduction in maximal heart rate

deliver more oxygen to the body tissues. The reduction in oxygen uptake will bring to an immediate increase in *cardiac output*, contractility, and blood pressure (Fig. 4.16).

Maximal heart rate up to 4,000 m does not change in its response compared to sea level. However, above 4,000 m, maximal heart rate is 145 beats · min^{-1}, and at 6,000 m, maximal heart rate decreases to 125 beats · min^{-1} (Fig. 4.17).

Heart rate variability during exercise effort at *high altitude* is difficult to explain due to subject's fitness level, hormonal changes, changes in the sympathetic and parasympathetic nervous systems, ambient temperature, wind, and humidity.

Plasma volume decreases by up to 25% within the first few hours of exposure to altitude and does not plateau until after a few weeks. This is partially a deliberate response by the body as reducing the watery part of blood in effect increases the density of red blood cells. However, *heart rate* increases enough to compensate for this and to actually slightly raise cardiac output. While no extra red blood cells have been produced in this acute phase, the amount of hemoglobin per unit of blood (called hematocrit) is now increased resulting in greater oxygen transport for a given *cardiac output* [70]. *Stroke volume* is reduced within 1 h from arrival to heights of 2,300 m and above. This decrement in stroke volume lasts for 1 week which thereafter it stabilizes. The reduced stroke volume is due to the fast body's fluid losing. As a result, heart rate is increased for maintaining an appropriate cardiac output to deliver the needed *oxygen demand*. The increase in heart rate is related to increased sympathetic activity and vagal withdrawal. With the decrease in plasma volume, the hematocrit concentration is increased, which in turn increases myocardium's work especially during left ventricular ejection.

At sea level, during submaximal aerobic exercise when cardiac output is 11 L · min^{-1}, $(a\text{-}v)O_2$

may equal to 99 $mLO_2 \cdot L^{-1}$ by performing the same absolute submaximal workload as at sea level; at altitude of 4,000 m, cardiac output will be 12.8 $L \cdot min^{-1}$ while $(a\text{-}v)O_2$ is unchanged. The acute increase in cardiac output with the exposure to altitude is due to the decrease in oxygen content in the arterial blood [71]. In fact, after 10 days of acclimatization to altitude results in a lower cardiac output at any given submaximal exercise intensity compared to sea level. Cardiac output returns to its values at sea level when oxygen extraction by the working muscles is increased (Fick equation), that is, oxygen extraction becomes more efficient reducing the need to increase cardiac output [71]. During exhaustive exercise at maximum levels, both maximal *stroke volume* and maximal *heart rate* decrease with altitude [72]. This obviously combines to have a significant effect on maximal cardiac output. In combination with the reduced diffusion gradient to drive oxygen from the blood to working tissues, VO_{2max} and endurance performance is held up. With acclimatization, *cardiac output* falls at rest and during exercise in association with a decrease in left ventricular work but an increase in right ventricular work.

In normal subjects, altitude exposure is associated with an increase in cardiac output with tachycardia and no change in stroke volume, whereas *blood* pressure may temporarily be slightly increased. The relationships between workload, cardiac output, and VO_2 are preserved in all circumstances, but there is a decrease in VO_{2max}, which is accompanied by a decrease in maximal cardiac output. The decrease in maximal cardiac output is minimal in acute *hypoxia* but becomes more pronounced with *acclimatization* [73]. The major factor increasing cardiac stress is hypoxia. Thus, risk assessment regarding *high-altitude* exposure of coronary artery disease patients is of increasing interest. With acute exposure to hypoxia, epicardial coronary arteries dilate. An increase in resting myocardial blood flow compensates for the reduced oxygen content of the blood and contributes to the maintenance of myocardium function [74], whereas exercise-induced coronary flow reserve is preserved at least to 4,500 m. After a few days of acclimatization, cardiac output returns to normal, but heart rate remains increased, so that stroke volume is decreased.

At rest and for a given external workload, myocardial oxygen demand is increased at altitude, particularly in non-acclimatized individuals, and there is some evidence that blood flow reserve is reduced in *coronary artery disease patients*. Even though left ventricular function is preserved at the start of exercise, indices of systolic function are slightly reduced, while diastolic filling pattern are altered later [73]. Regardless of a possible imbalance between oxygen demand and oxygen delivery, selected coronary artery disease patients with stable angina, high *double product*, and sufficient work capacity have shown that exposure and exercise at altitudes of 3,000–3,500 m is generally safe [75]. During the first days at altitude, patients with *stable angina* may develop symptoms of *myocardial ischemia* at slightly lower double products. However, it is recommended to train at sea level before going to altitude, and the altitude-related decrease in exercise capacity should be considered. Coronary artery disease patients should avoid traveling to elevations above 4,500 m owing to severe hypoxia at these altitudes.

References

1. Kim HJ, Jansen KE, Taylor CA. Incorporating autoregulatory mechanisms of the cardiovascular system in three-dimensional finite element models of arterial blood flow. Ann Biomed Eng. 2010;38:2314–30.
2. Timothy W. Theoretical models for regulation of blood flow. Microcirculation. 2008;15:765–75.
3. Wolff CB. Normal cardiac output, oxygen delivery and oxygen extraction. Adv Exp Med Biol. 2007;599:169–82.
4. Murrant CL, Sarelius IH. Local and remote arteriolar dilations initiated by skeletal muscle contraction. Am J Physiol Heart Circ Physiol. 2000;279:H2285–94.
5. Sun D, Huang A, Koller A, Kaley G. Flow-dependent dilation and myogenic constriction interact to establish the resistance of skeletal muscle arterioles. Microcirculation. 1995;2:289–95.
6. Sagiv M, Goldhammer E, Ben-Sira D, Sagiv M, Amir R. Adolescents' left ventricular response to peak Wingate anaerobic test. Pediatric Exercise Science. 2006;17:22–9.
7. Sagiv M, Ben-Sira D, Goldhammer E. Direct vs. indirect blood pressure measurement at peak anaerobic exercise. Int J Sports Med. 1999;20:275–8.

8. Sagiv M, Ben-Sira D, Goldhammer E, Soudry M. Left ventricular contractility and function at peak aerobic and anaerobic exercises. Med Sci Sports Exerc. 2000; 32:1197–201.
9. Nicosia RF, Villaschi S. Auto-regulation of angiogenesis by cells of the vessel wall. Int Rev Cytol. 1999; 185:1–43.
10. Walley KR. Heterogeneity of oxygen delivery impairs oxygen extraction by peripheral tissues: theory. J Appl Physiol. 1996;81:885–94.
11. McDonough P, Behnke BJ, Padilla DJ, Musch TI, Poole DC. Control of microvascular oxygen pressures in rat muscles comprised of different fibre types. J Physiol. 2005;563:903–13.
12. Chakkalakal JV, Stocksley MA, Harrison MA, et al. Expression of utrophin A mRNA correlates with the oxidative capacity of skeletal muscle fiber types and is regulated by calcineurin/NFAT signaling. Proc Natl Acad Sci USA. 2003;100:7791–6.
13. Harms CA. Effect of skeletal muscle demand on cardiovascular function. Med Sci Sports Exerc. 2000; 32:94–9.
14. Sun D, Huang A, Koller A, Kaley G. Adaptation of flow-induced dilation of arterioles to daily exercise. Microvasc Res. 1998;56:54–61.
15. Green DJ, O'Driscoll G, Blanksby BA, Taylor RR. Control of skeletal muscle blood flow during dynamic exercise: contribution of endothelium-derived nitric oxide. Sports Med. 1996;21:119–46.
16. Liao JC, Kuo L. Interaction between adenosine and flow-induced dilation in coronary microvascular network. Am J Physiol Heart Circ Physiol. 1997;272:H1571–81.
17. Jackson WF. Arteriolar oxygen reactivity: where is the sensor? Am J Physiol. 1987;253:H1120–6.
18. Fraser SJ, Newby DE, Uren NG. Regulation of coronary perfusion. Heart Metab. 2004;22:37–41.
19. Duncker DJ, Bache RJ. Regulation of coronary blood flow during exercise. Physiol Rev. 2008;88:1009–86.
20. Carlson BE, Arciero JC, Secomb TW. Theoretical model of blood flow auto-regulation: roles of myogenic, shear-dependent, and metabolic responses. Am J Physiol Heart Circ Physiol. 2008;295:H1572–9.
21. Delp MD, Laughlin MH. Time course of enhanced endothelium-mediated dilation in aorta of trained rats. Med Sci Sports Exerc. 1997;29:1454–61.
22. Jones CJ, DeFily DV, Patterson JL, Chilian WM. Endothelium-dependent relaxation competes with alpha-1 and alpha-2 adrenergic constriction in the canine epicardial coronary microcirculation. Circulation. 1993;87:1264–74.
23. Kuvin JT, Karas RH. Clinical utility of endothelial function testing: ready for prime time? Circulation. 2003;107:3243–7.
24. Bönner G. Kinin-related effects of angiotensin-converting enzyme inhibition. Clin Physiol Biochem. 1990;8 Suppl 1:6–15.
25. Mombouli JV, Vanhoutte PM. Kinins and endothelial control of vascular smooth muscle. Annu Rev Pharmacol Toxicol. 1995;35:679–705.
26. Rush JW, Aultman CD. Vascular biology of angiotensin and the impact of physical activity. Appl Physiol Nutr Metab. 2008;33:162–72.
27. Coates D. The angiotensin converting enzyme. Int J Biochem Cell Biol. 2003;35:769–73.
28. Jones A, Woods DR. Skeletal muscle RAS and exercise performance. Int J Biochem Cell Biol. 2003; 35:855–66.
29. Gordon S, Davis BS, Carlson CJ, et al. Ang II is required for optimal overload-induced skeletal muscle hypertrophy. Am J Physiol Endocrinol Metab. 2001;280: E150–9.
30. Guyton AC, Hall JE, editors. Textbook of medical physiology. 9th ed. Philadelphia: WB Saunders; 2000. p. 227–30.
31. Amir O, Amir R, Yamin C, et al. The ACE deletion allele is associated with Israeli elite endurance athletes. Exp Physiol. 2007;92:881–5.
32. Baudin B. New aspects on angiotensin-converting enzyme: from gene to disease. Clin Chem Lab Med. 2002;40:256–65.
33. Danser AH, Schalekamp MADH, Bax WA, et al. Angiotensin-converting enzyme in the human heart. Effect of the deletion/insertion polymorphism. Circulation. 1995;92:1387–8.
34. Rigat B, Hubert C, Alhenc-Gelas F, et al. An insertion/deletion polymorphism in the angiotensin I-converting enzyme gene accounting for half the variance of serum enzyme levels. J Clin Invest. 1990;86:1343–6.
35. Williams AG, Dhamrait SS, Wootton PT, et al. Bradykinin receptor gene variant and human physical performance. J Appl Physiol. 2004;96:938–42.
36. Van Geel PP, Pinto YM, Voors AA, et al. Angiotensin II type 1 receptor A1166C gene polymorphism is associated with an increased response to angiotensin II in human arteries. Hypertension. 2000;35: 717–21.
37. Tang DD, Anfinogenova Y. Physiologic properties and regulation of the actin cytoskeleton in vascular smooth muscle. J Cardiovasc Pharmacol Ther. 2008; 13:130–40.
38. Cassis L, Helton M, English V, et al. Angiotensin II regulates oxygen consumption. Am J Physiol Regul Integr Comp Physiol. 2002;282:R445–53.
39. Krejci V, Hiltebrand L, Banic A, Erni D, Wheatley AM, Sigurdsson GH. Continuous measurements of microcirculatory blood flow in gastrointestinal organs during acute haemorrhage. Br J Anaesth. 2000;84:468–75.
40. Shier D. Hole's human anatomy and physiology. New York: McGraw-Hill; 2002.
41. Ramanathan T, Skinner H. Coronary blood flow. Contin Educ Anaesth Crit Care Pain. 2005;5:61–4.
42. Duncker DJ, Merkus D. Regulation of coronary blood flow. Effect of coronary artery stenosis. Arch Mal Coeur Vaiss. 2004;97:1244–50.
43. Opie LH, Lopaschuk GD. Fuels: aerobic and anaerobic metabolism. In: Weinberg RW, Bersin J, Aversa F, editors. Heart physiology, from cell to circulation. Philadelphia: Lippincot Williams & Wilkins; 2004. p. 306–54.

44. Tune JD, Gorman MW, Feigl EO. Matching coronary blood flow to myocardial oxygen consumption. J Appl Physiol. 2004;97:404–15.
45. Gute D, Fraga C, Laughlin MH, Amann JF. Regional changes in capillary supply in skeletal muscle of high-intensity endurance-trained rats. J Appl Physiol. 1996; 81:619–26.
46. Laughlin MH, Korthuis RJ, Duncker DJ, Bache RJ. Regulation of blood flow to cardiac and skeletal muscle during exercise. In: Handbook of physiology. Exercise: regulation and integration of multiple systems. Bethesda: American Physiological Society; 1996. p. 705–69.
47. Sorop O, Merkus D, de Beer VJ, et al. Functional and structural adaptations of coronary microvessels distal to a chronic coronary artery stenosis. Circ Res. 2008;102:795–803.
48. Segal SS. Regulation of blood flow in the microcirculation. Microcirculation. 2005;12:33–45.
49. Forjaz CL, Matsudaira Y, Rodrigues FB, Nunes N, Negrão CE. Post-exercise changes in blood pressure, heart rate and rate pressure product at different exercise intensities in normotensive humans. Braz J Med Biol Res. 1998;31:1247–55.
50. Romer LM, Polkey MI. Exercise-induced respiratory muscle fatigue: implications for performance. J Appl Physiol. 2008;104:879–88.
51. Olson TP, Joyner MJ, Dietz MM, Eisenach JH, Curry TB, Johnson BD. Effects of respiratory muscle work on blood flow distribution during exercise in heart failure. J Physiol. 2010;588:2487–501.
52. Dempsey JA, Romer L, Rodman J, Miller J, Smith C. Consequences of exercise-induced respiratory muscle work. Respir Physiol Neurobiol. 2006;151:242–50.
53. Harms CA, Wetter TJ, McClaran SR, et al. Effects of respiratory muscle work on cardiac output and its distribution during maximal exercise. J Appl Physiol. 1998;85:609–18.
54. Johnson JM. Exercise in a hot environment: the skin circulation. Scand J Med Sci Sports. 2010;20 Suppl 3:29–39.
55. Nielsen B, Strange S, Christensen NJ, Warberg J, Saltin B. Acute and adaptive responses in humans to exercise in a warm, humid environment. Pflugers Arch. 1997;434:49–56.
56. Lorenzo S, Halliwill JR, Sawka MN, Minson CT. Heat acclimation improves exercise performance. J Appl Physiol. 2010;109:1140–7.
57. Nielsen B, Hales JR, Strange S, Christensen NJ, Warberg J, Saltin B. Human circulatory and thermoregulatory adaptations with heat acclimation and exercise in a hot, dry environment. J Physiol. 1993; 460:4674–85.
58. González-Alonso J, Calbet JA. Reductions in systemic and skeletal muscle blood flow and oxygen delivery limit maximal aerobic capacity in humans. Circulation. 2003;107:824–30.
59. González-Alonso J, Crandall CG, Johnson JM. The cardiovascular challenge of exercising in the heat. J Physiol. 2008;586:45–53.
60. González-Alonso J. Hyperthermia impairs brain, heart and muscle function in exercising humans. Sports Med. 2007;37:371–3.
61. Periard JD, Cramer MN, Chapman PG, Caillaud C, Thompson MW. Cardiovascular strain impairs prolonged self-paced exercise in the heat. Exp Physiol. 2011;96:134–44.
62. Cheuvront SN, Kenefick RW, Montain SJ, Sawka MN. Mechanisms of aerobic performance impairment with heat stress and dehydration. J Appl Physiol. 2010;109:1989–95.
63. Nybo L, Jensen T, Nielsen B, et al. Effects of marked hyperthermia without dehydration on VO_2 kinetics during intense exercise. J Appl Physiol. 2001;90: 1057–64.
64. Lynn BM, Minson CT, Halliwill JR. Fluid replacement and heat stress during exercise alter post-exercise cardiac haemodynamics in endurance exercise-trained men. J Physiol. 2009;587:3605–17.
65. Drust B, Rasmussen P, Mohr M, Nielsen B, Nybo L. Elevations in core and muscle temperature impair repeated sprint performance. Acta Physiol Scand. 2005;183:181–90.
66. Pearson J, Low DA, Stöhr E, Kalsi K, Ali L, Barker H, González-Alonso J. Hemodynamic responses to heat stress in the resting and exercising human leg: insight into the effect of temperature on skeletal muscle blood flow. Am J Physiol Regul Integr Comp Physiol. 2011;300:R663–73.
67. Puvi-Rajasingham S, Smith GD, Akinola A, Mathias CJ. Abnormal regional blood flow responses during and after exercise in human sympathetic denervation. J Physiol. 1997;505:841–9.
68. González-Alonso J, Rodriguez M, Coyle EF. Stroke volume during exercise: interaction of environment and hydration. Am J Physiol Heart Circ Physiol. 2000;278:H321–30.
69. Merry TL, Ainslie PN, Cotter JD. Effects of aerobic fitness on hypohydration-induced physiological strain and exercise impairment. Acta Physiol (Oxf). 2010; 198:179–90.
70. McArdle WD, Katch FL, Katch VL. Essentials of exercise physiology. 2nd ed. Philadelphia: Lippincott Williams & Wilkins; 2000.
71. Mollard P, Woorons X, Letournel M, Cornolo J, Lamberto C, Beaudry M, Richalet JP. Role of maximal heart rate and arterial O_2 saturation on the decrement of VO_{2max} in moderate acute hypoxia in trained and untrained men. Int J Sports Med. 2007;28: 186–92.
72. Wilmore JH, Costill DL. Physiology of sport and exercise. 3rd ed. Champaign: Human Kinetics; 2005. Human Rate of Reaction.

73. Naeije R. Physiological adaptation of the cardiovascular system to high altitude. Prog Cardiovasc Dis. 2010;52:456–66.
74. Koepfli P, Wyss CA, Namdar M, Siegrist PT, Luscher TF, Camici PG, Kaufmann PA. Beta-adrenergic blockade and myocardial perfusion in coronary artery disease: differential effects in stenotic versus remote myocardial segments. J Nucl Med. 2004;45:1626–31.
75. Dehnert C, Bärtsch P. Can patients with coronary heart disease go to high altitude? High Alt Med Biol. 2010;11:183–8.

Left Ventricular Function

5

Left Ventricular Function Measurements

Many of the substitute endpoints used in clinical research on heart disease are parameters obtained using imaging techniques. The most frequently used endpoint is left ventricular ejection fraction (LVEF). At rest and at peak aerobic exercise, left ventricular contractility measurements can be obtained in a clinical setting by noninvasive methods [1], usually employing M-mode echocardiography which is the most frequently used method to evaluate left ventricular function in clinical trials. The ultrasound-derived measurements of left ventricular internal minor axis throughout the cardiac cycle are very frequently estimated visually. There are three important noninvasive variables to evaluate left ventricular function measurements at rest and during exercise: (a) *Systolic blood pressure* over left ventricular *end-systolic volume ratio* (*P*/*V*), which can be obtained by *echocardiography* and radionuclide methods, (b) *Doppler measurements*, and (c) the relationship between *diastolic volume* of the ventricle and its *stroke volume*, that is, *ejection indices*: The relative reduction in cavity size, expressed as ejection fraction or *shortening fraction* which can be obtained by *echocardiography* and *radionuclide* methods. These measurements can provide very important information for prescribing exercise intensity and following exercise training programs in athletes, health subjects, and cardiac patients. These three methods were previously employed in order to detect changes in left ventricular function at rest and during dynamic aerobic, anaerobic, and isometric exercises. In addition, the development of high resolution ultrasonic imaging and *Doppler ultrasound* has made it possible to measure *transmitral* and *aortic flow patterns* – which measure *left ventricular diastolic and systolic function* – noninvasively.

Left ventricular systolic function is generally assessed by measuring the extent and velocity of fiber shortening, ejection fraction, and velocity of circumferential fiber shortening [2, 3]. Meta-analysis studies [4, 5] have shown that in the groups of athletes studied, overall systolic function as judged by fractional fiber shortening or ejection fraction is similar to that of sedentary control subjects. It was suggested that there is no relation between cardiac geometry and left ventricular systolic function in athlete's heart, due to chamber mechanics rather than myocardial mechanics. Studies of myocardial contractile function in hypertrophied left ventricles resulting from hypertension suggest that intrinsic myocardial performance may be depressed, even when left ventricular ejection fraction remains normal. However, the presumed innocent nature of the athlete's heart does not allow more invasive studies to be conducted on athletes. Left ventricular diastolic function is commonly assessed by studying the pattern of ventricular filling through the mitral valve [6]. The diastolic function parameter generally used is the *E*/*A* ratio. Meta-analysis has demonstrated a normal or slightly enhanced diastolic function in athletes compared with sedentary control subjects [5].

M.S. Sagiv, *Exercise Cardiopulmonary Function in Cardiac Patients*,
DOI 10.1007/978-1-4471-2888-5_5, © Springer-Verlag London 2012

Left Ventricular Function During Aerobic Exercise

The normal response through *dynamic exercise* is an increased *left ventricular contractility*, *ejection fraction*, *ejection fraction indices*, *changed volume over time* (d*v*/d*t*), *stroke volume*, *end-diastolic volume* and *cardiac output*, and a decrease in *left ventricular end-systolic volume* without any *wall motion abnormalities*. In normal subjects, left ventricular contractility state and function differ at peak all-out *anaerobic effort* compared with maximal *aerobic effort* [1]. During the *aerobic effort*, left ventricular contractility and function increase likely due to the relatively lower *afterload* opposing the ejection of the left ventricle [7, 8]. The low afterload is known to be mediated through the peripheral *autoregulation mechanism* occurring in the active muscles. Thus left ventricle ejects against *volume overload*. Such lower afterload allows *cardiac output* to increase as a result of increases in *ejection fraction*, stroke volume [9], and *heart rate* [10]. The increase in *stroke volume* during *aerobic exercise* is a result of left ventricular dilation (*end-diastolic volume*), suggesting higher preload and decrease in *end-systolic volume*. Such response may reflect both an increase in *inotropic* and a decrease in total peripheral resistance by the attenuation of the sympathoexcitatory *chemoreceptor reflex* drive by *exercise training* [11].

In *ischemic heart disease*, resting measures of left ventricular function may be normal or minimally reduced. However, with increasing myocardial work, reduction in left ventricular performance indices has been well documented [12]. Most of the studies involve dynamic exercise in supine position. A few reports have shown similar but less impressive changes with isometric dead lift [13]. During upright isometric exercise, *end-diastolic volume* and *end-systolic volume* are decreased in *coronary artery disease patients*, as in normal subjects when utilizing large muscle mass. At rest, at the upright position *ejection fraction* and d*v*/d*t* for coronary artery disease patients are significantly lower than normal subjects. However, during *upright isometric exercise*, there are further declines in ejection fraction and d*v*/d*t* with increasing isometric tension and muscle mass [13]. These suggests that left ventricular function in coronary artery disease patients with moderate work capacity is maintained in the face of higher afterload conditions when total cardiac output requirements are only moderately increased [14].

Regional wall motion abnormality is a term commonly used in echocardiography. It can also be applied to other modalities of imaging the motion of the cardiac structures. Regional wall motion abnormality means that the motion of a region of the heart muscle is abnormal. The presence of qualitative wall motion abnormalities has been demonstrated to be an independent predictor of cardiovascular events in groups of patients with myocardial infarction, unstable angina, typical chest pain, and congestive heart failure [15]. It can be reduced (hypokinesia), absent (akinesia), or increased (hyperkinesia). Occasionally, it can be opposite of what is expected, moving out in systole rather than moving in. This type of abnormal motion seen is termed dyskinesia. The regional wall motion abnormalities give a hint to the coronary arteries which are diseased. For example, if the inferior wall of the left ventricle is hypokinetic, this means that the right coronary artery is involved. If the whole left ventricle is hypokinetic, then it is called global hypokinesia. This occurs in dilated cardiomyopathy. Then it is not a regional wall motion abnormality. *Wall motion abnormalities* occur in part of the *coronary artery disease patients* during the second level of exercise when ST-segment depression is present. During exercise in coronary artery disease patients, abnormalities in left ventricular function frequently develop before angina pectoris and electrocardiographic evidence of myocardial ischemia [16]. The frequency of wall motion abnormalities in coronary artery disease patients increases in proportion to the magnitude of imposed left ventricular afterload associated with increasing muscle mass in isometric exercise [13].

Left Ventricular Function During Anaerobic Exercise

All-out *anaerobic effort* in healthy subjects do not produce the expected increase in the *left ventricular end-diastolic volume*, ejection fraction, stroke volume, and cardiac output, while *left ventricular end-systolic volume* remains unchanged (Fig. 5.1) from resting values [1].

Contractility is increased significantly from resting values during all-out *anaerobic effort*; however, at peak *aerobic exercise*, contractility of the *left ventricle* is further significantly increased compared to values obtained at peak all-out anaerobic effort [1]. This may suggest that the increase in *left ventricular inotropic state* is not adequate to increase left ventricular *end-diastolic volume* and reduce end-systolic volume, and thus *ejection fraction* remains unchanged during all-out anaerobic exercise [17]. It seems that the lower ventricular function at peak anaerobic exercise compared with aerobic-type exercise is due, partially, to the elevated *systolic* and *diastolic blood pressures* and to the smaller reduction in *total peripheral resistance*. The lower reduction in total peripheral resistance is because of the elevated concentrations of *vasoactive substances* due to tissue *hypoxia* and *acidosis*. Thus, the smaller reduction in *total peripheral resistance* and the increase in afterload at peak anaerobic effort may force the ventricle to eject blood against a relatively higher pressure, that is, to eject against modest *pressure overload*. This coupled with lower peak heart rate and a relatively short duration of any anaerobic bout could explain the lower *cardiac output* during all *anaerobic effort* compared to that of maximal aerobic exercise.

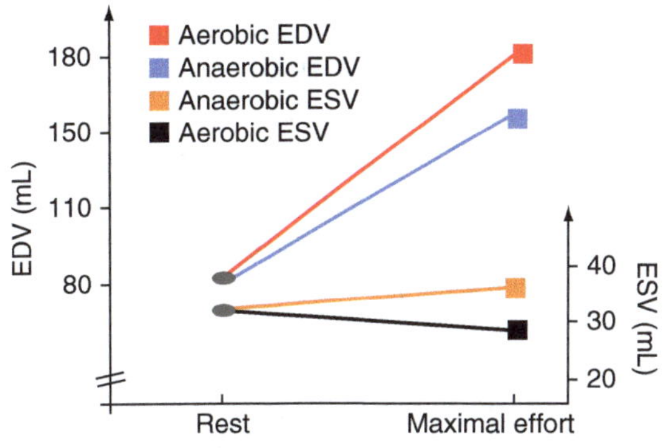

Fig. 5.1 Left ventricular volumes in healthy subjects: Left ventricular end-diastolic volume (*EDV*) and left ventricular end-systolic volume (*ESV*) responses at peak aerobic and anaerobic exercises. At maximal aerobic exercise, compared to the anaerobic bout, value for left ventricular end-diastolic volume is higher and end-systolic volume is lower

Left Ventricular Function During Isometric Exercise

Isometric exercise produces a characteristic *pressor response* increase in blood pressure which may be important in maintaining perfusion of muscle during sustained contraction. During isometric exercise in normal subjects and *cardiac patients* with mild impairment *left ventricular contractility*, *left ventricular function* is normally maintained or improved. *Cardiac patients* with poor left ventricular function may show deterioration during isometric exercise, although this pattern of response is difficult to predict from resting studies [13]. The response is moderate increased left *ventricular contractility* and function, that is, increase or unchanged in *ejection fraction*, *ejection fraction indices*, changed dv/dt, *stroke volume*, *end-diastolic volume*, and *cardiac output*, and a decrease or unchanged in *end-systolic volume* without any *wall motion abnormalities* [18]. During *isometric effort*, although left ventricle ejects against *pressure overload*, it increases moderately contractility and function likely due to increase in the *inotropic state* of the *myocardium* in the face of the increased *afterload* [7, 8]. *Sustained isometric* muscle contraction such as *dead lift* (Fig. 5.2), which involves large muscle mass, produces a characteristic increase in *afterload* [19].

The high afterload during isometric bout is a result of vasoactive substances due to tissue *hypoxia* and *acidosis*. In normal individuals, the increase in *afterload* is mediated by a rise in cardiac output with little or no change in systemic vascular resistance. Therefore, the *autoregulation*

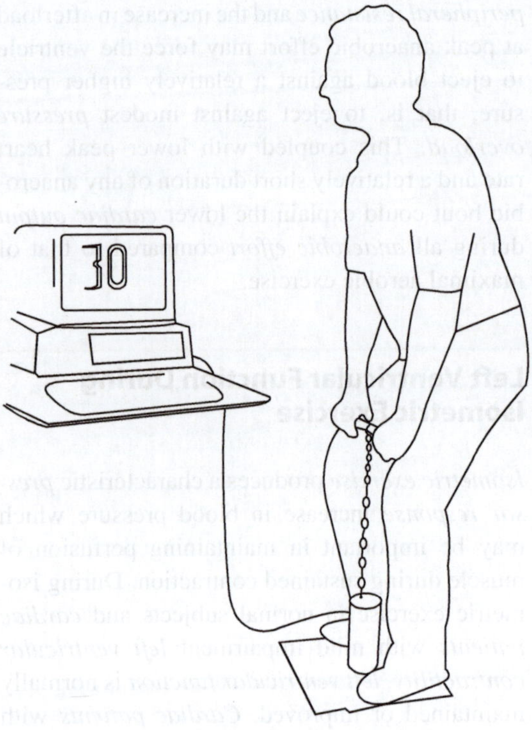

Fig. 5.2 Dead-lift maneuver at 30% maximal voluntary contraction

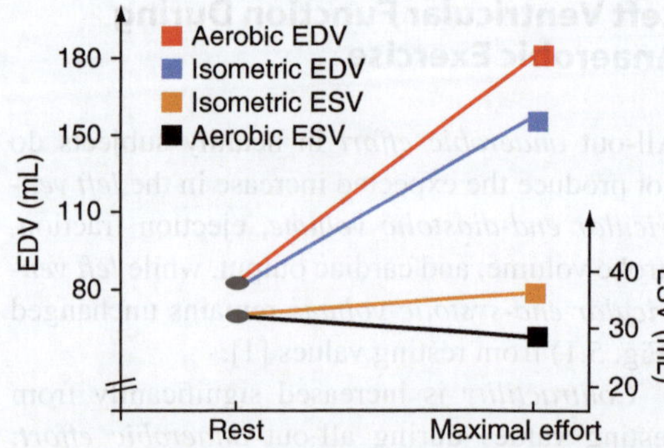

Fig. 5.3 Left ventricular volumes in healthy subjects: Left ventricular end-diastolic volume (*EDV*) and left ventricular end-systolic volume (*ESV*) responses at peak aerobic and isometric exercises. At maximal aerobic exercise, compared to the isometric bout, value for left ventricular end-diastolic volume is higher and end-systolic volume is lower

mechanism does not occur in the active muscles. Such high *afterload* allows a small increase in cardiac output (12 L · min^{-1}) mainly due to increase in *heart rate* [20].

The unchanged *stroke volume* during *isometric exercise* is a result of moderate increase in left ventricular dilation (*end-diastolic volume*), suggesting higher *preload* and unchanged *end-systolic volume*. This response is mediated by combined central and peripheral afferent input to medullary cardiovascular centers [21].

Compared to resting values, isometric effort produce a slight but significant increase in left ventricular *end-diastolic volume* and *cardiac output*, while left ventricular *ejection fraction*, *stroke volume*, *end-systolic volume* (Fig. 5.3) are unchanged [19]. *Contractility* is increased significantly from resting values during *isometric effort*; however, at peak *anaerobic* and *aerobic exercises*, contractility of the left ventricle is significantly higher compared to values obtained at peak *isometric effort* [1, 21]. This may suggest that the increase in left ventricle is adequate to increase left ventricular end-diastolic volume, and *inotropic state* is not adequate to reduce end-systolic volume, and thus *ejection fraction* remains unchanged.

It seems that the lower ventricular function during isometric maneuver compared with the aerobic-type exercise is due, partially, to the unchanged or increased *total peripheral resistance* from resting values [22]. The lower reduction in total peripheral resistance is because of the elevated concentrations of *vasoactive substances* due to tissue *hypoxia* and *acidosis*. Thus, total peripheral resistance response and the increase in afterload during isometric exercise may force the ventricle to eject blood against a relatively higher pressure. This coupled with lower *venous return* compared to aerobic exercise could explain the lower *cardiac output* during *isometric maneuver* compared to that of *maximal aerobic exercise*. Sustained isometric muscle contraction such as *dead lift* (Fig. 5.2), which involves large muscle mass, produces a characteristic increase in *afterload* [19].

In normal healthy subjects, athletes, and *coronary artery disease patients*, *left ventricular systolic* and *diastolic function* and *contractility* are increased, however, not to the same extent as during aerobic exercise [23]. In addition, the increased *pressor response* [13] has a significant effect on left ventricular global performance [19].

Left Ventricular Systolic Function

Systolic function is the contraction of the ventricle in order to eject blood into the aorta. The extent of myocardial fiber shortening is a reflection of the interaction between the initial fiber stretch: Preload or end-diastolic volume, the load opposing shortening, afterload, and the intrinsic contractile state [24, 25].

Preload is an expression of the length-active tension relationship on which *Starling's law* is based: Force of contraction and/or extent of shortening depend on initial muscle length, which in turn is dependent on muscle length of the myosin and actin myofilament within the sarcomere. Thus, performance of the myocardium is influenced by the length of the sarcomere and therefore, in the intact heart, by *ventricular end-diastolic volume*. The major determinants of ventricular end-diastolic volumes are *venous return*, ventricular compliance, *left ventricular filling time*, and ventricular pressure.

Afterload for any shortening contracting muscles is the total force that opposes shortening minus the stretching force that existed prior to contraction. Thus, for the *myocardium*, afterload is the force against which myocardium fibers must contract during the ejection phase of systole. Afterload may also be defined as the tension, force (per unit of cross-sectional area), or stress in the ventricular wall after the onset of shortening. *Ejection fraction* and maximum rate of change of left ventricular volume (dv/dt_{max}) are the results of the extent of left ventricular fiber shortening during systole, which varies inversely with afterload at any level of diastolic fiber length (preload) and contractility. The overall determinant of left ventricular afterload is aortic impedance which is a composite of resistance, compliance, and inertia.

The strength of left *ventricular contraction* may be influenced in two ways: (a) Through alteration of *preload* as a result of intrinsic regulatory process and (b) by altering the *inotropic contractile state*, which is an extrinsic effect. Factors which alter contractility in vivo are sympathetic nerve activity, circulating catecholamine, exogenous inotropic agents, physiological and pharmacological depressants, loss of contractile mass, and intrinsic myocardial depression. The continuity of cardiac output depends on the beat-by-beat adjustment of ventricular function to input-output coupling with systemic and pulmonary circulation.

Dynamic steady-state aerobic exercise lasting up to 30 min is associated with an increase in *cardiac output* secondary to an increase in *heart rate* and *stroke volume*. The heightened stroke volume is due, in part, to a Frank-Starling-mediated increase in end-diastolic volume, that is, preload reserve, and to enhanced systolic emptying secondary to an increase in myocardial contractility, that is, contractile reserve. During dynamic steady-state exercise lasting above 30 min, stroke volume has been shown to gradually decrease, while cardiac output remains unaltered due to a compensatory elevation in heart rate [26]. The prolonged strenuous exercise mediated decline in stroke volume may be due, in part, to a reduction in preload reserve secondary to the diminished plasma volume associated with dehydration and thermoregulatory peripheral vasodilatation. These findings suggest that the alteration in left ventricular systolic function after prolonged strenuous exercise may result in cardiac drift due, in part, to impairment in myocardial contractility. Several investigators have found that the decline in left ventricular systolic performance associated with prolonged strenuous exercise was independent of changes in left ventricular preload [26] or afterload [27]. However, study by Alshaher et al. examined the impact of prolonged exercise leading to physical exhaustion on left ventricular systolic and diastolic function in untrained healthy subjects, and to examine cardiovascular determinants of exercise performance. It was concluded that prolonged exercise leading to physical exhaustion is not associated with systolic or diastolic dysfunction. Reduced early left ventricular diastolic filling and the relative increase in left atrial contribution seen with prolonged exercise are likely due to preload reduction rather than true diastolic dysfunction [28].

Goodman et al. suggested that in healthy, trained men, no cardiac fatigue is seen after prolonged exercise under controlled conditions; ejection fraction during the postexercise recovery period is similar to the pre-exercise value. These results indicate that prolonged exercise of moderate duration may not induce abnormal left ventricular systolic function following long-lasting mild aerobic exercise [29]. In another study, Goodman's findings were confirmed. In that study, seven, healthy, trained male subjects exercised for 3 h using semi-recumbent ergometer cycling at 70% of VO_{2max}, while preload to the left ventricle was maintained via saline infusion. It resulted in no evidence of a depression in left ventricular systolic function, while left ventricular diastolic function declined postexercise [8]. A widely held belief in exercise physiology is that although alterations in preload reserve may contribute to the decreased stroke volume, however, a previous investigation has found that echocardiographic images obtained after cessation of exercise are not representative of the acute left ventricular changes that occur during exertion [30]. Therefore, the time course of alteration in left ventricular systolic performance during prolonged intense exercise (similar to that observed during a competitive endurance event) is not well known.

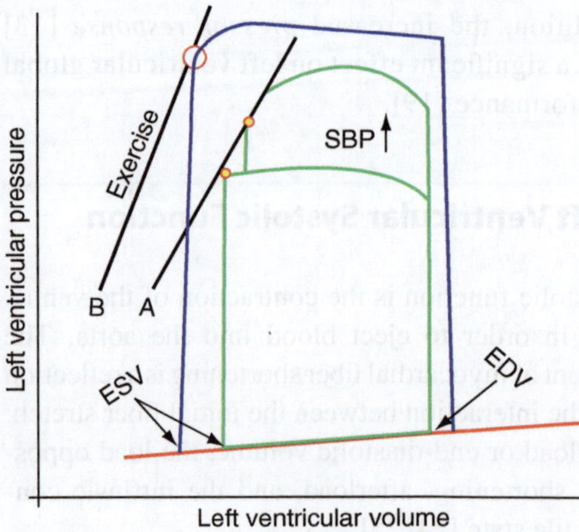

Fig. 5.4 The left ventricular pressure–volume loop from a healthy person at rest (*A*) and exercise (*B*). The pressure–volume ratio is a widely applicable pathophysiological tool. The events that take place during the cardiac cycle are shown as pattern of the instantaneous pressure values (*y axis*) versus those of intraventricular volume (*x axis*), end-diastolic volume (*EDV*), and end-systolic volume (*ESV*). During exercise, end-diastolic volume is increased; there is a shift of the curve to the left due to increase in contractility in the face on increased systolic blood pressure. Thus, end-systolic volume decreases and stroke volume increases

Left Ventricular End-Systolic Pressure–Volume Ratio (*P*/*V*)

The most accurate approach to inherent left ventricular pump properties is based on the analysis of pressure–volume curves [31]. The systolic blood pressure to end-systolic volume ratio is a noninvasive index used to estimate the slope of the end-systolic pressure–volume relationship. This is thought to be a better surrogate of myocardial contractility than *ejection fraction* since it is independent of *preload* and *afterload* and little affected by *heart rate* [32]. However, caution must be taken when using this index of contractility, since it represents only one point within the pressure–volume loop. As such, it is only an estimate of the slope of the end-systolic pressure–volume relationship. It includes the concept of the interrelationship of force, length, velocity, and time [25]. The extent of myocardial fiber shortening is a reflection of the interaction between initial fiber stretch (preload), the load opposing shortening (afterload), and the intrinsic contractile state. Based on this relationship, the left ventricular end-systolic pressure–volume ratio is a measure of left ventricular contractility independent of preload [13, 33]. Therefore, it is a load-insensitive method for evaluating left ventricular contractility. As afterload increases, the extent of systolic fiber shortening decreases. Figure 5.4 describes the mechanics of ventricular contraction which include the concepts of force, length, velocity, and time [25].

The left ventricular end-systolic pressure–volume ratio has shown to be prognostic useful, and it is the only index of cardiac function to emerge as independent predictor of total mortality. These studies [34, 35] have demonstrated that left ventricular *end-systolic pressure–volume ratio*, measured noninvasively, can be prognostic useful. Nevertheless, further studies are needed to confirm the prognostic value of left ventricular end-systolic pressure–volume ratio in cardiovascular disease patients [35].

The *systolic blood pressure over left ventricular end-systolic volume ratio* increases during all kinds of exercise in healthy individuals. During dynamic aerobic exercise, although *systolic blood pressure* increases, contractility is increased, and the heart works against *volume overload* [36]. Consequently, the ratio is increased due to a significant decrease in end-systolic volume values [1].

During isometric exercise, the ventricle works against increased *afterload*, that is, systolic and diastolic blood pressures are elevated significantly, and as a result, end-systolic volume is slightly changed from resting values. Thus, the ratio increases moderately. During dynamic *anaerobic exercise*, *total peripheral resistance* and afterload are not reduced to the level observed at peak dynamic aerobic exercise [1, 37], but they are still lower than those observed during isometric exercise [1]. Such insufficient reduction in total peripheral resistance and afterload is responsible for the lesser augmentation in the ratio compared to dynamic aerobic exercise [1].

Coronary artery disease patient increase left ventricular end-systolic pressure–volume ratio from resting values during aerobic exercise and to the less extent during isometric exercise. This may be a reflection of participation in physical training program. These results were performed with trained coronary artery disease patients with stable exercise capacity of 8–12 METs [13]. Figure 5.5 shows the increase of left ventricular end-systolic pressure–volume ratio in normal subjects during aerobic, anaerobic, and isometric exercise [1], while Fig. 5.6 shows the response of coronary artery disease patients compared to normal subjects during aerobic and dead-lift isometric exercise [13].

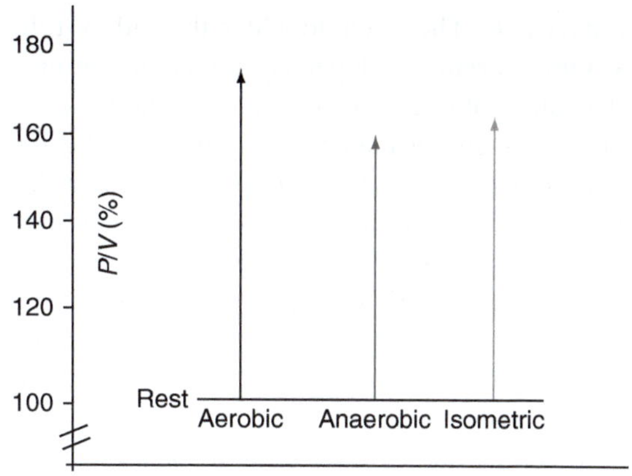

Fig. 5.5 Left ventricular end-systolic pressure–volume ratio (*P*/*V*) changes relatively from resting values (100%) in healthy subjects at peak aerobic, anaerobic, and isometric dead-lift exercises

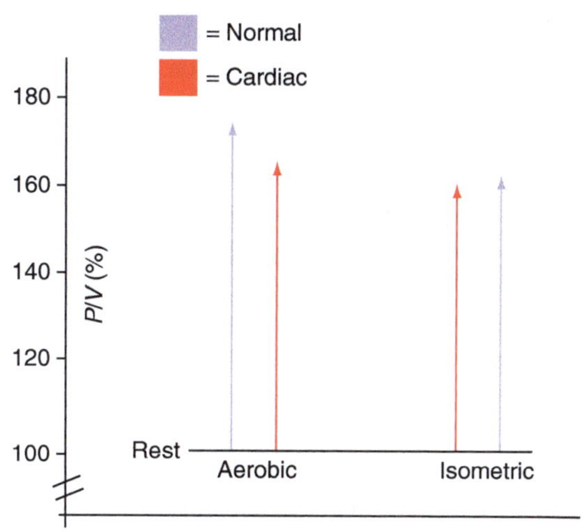

Fig. 5.6 Left ventricular end-systolic pressure–volume ratio (*P*/*V*) changes relatively from resting values (100%) in normal subjects compared to coronary artery disease patients at peak aerobic and isometric dead-lift exercises

Left Ventricular Ejection Fraction

Ejection indices are determined by left ventricular *end-diastolic volume*, left ventricular *end-systolic volume*, and *left ventricular inotropic state*. In normal subjects during dynamic *aerobic exercise*, end-diastolic volume varies according to the body position and the state of exercise training, whereas end-systolic volume is uniformly reduced [1]. The extent to which the end-systolic volume is reduced depends on changes in end-diastolic volume in response to dynamic exercise; it is also a major determinant of the left ventricular *ejection fraction*. It is suggested that the delta end-systolic volume during the circulatory adaptive response to orthostatic and exercise stresses in humans is related to the delta end-diastolic volume, and this relationship modulates the delta ejection fraction in response to these stresses [38].

Ejection fraction is useful in distinguishing normal from abnormal contractile states. It is often useful in determining contractility in the basal state in the presence of chronic heart disease, though the dynamics of left ventricular ejection fraction is a complex function of left ventricular volumes and depends on chamber size and shape, preload, and afterload [39, 40]. Although clear evidence exists on the relationship of left ventricular ejection fraction and ventricular volumes for prognosis in patients who have had acute myocardial infarction [41], left ventricular ejection fraction as a measure of ventricular function during systole assumes that the fraction of blood displaced from the left ventricle is proportional to the force generated. However, there are various pathological situations where left ventricular *ejection fraction* does not correspond to left ventricular function [42]. In addition, it is not reliable for dilated or asymmetrical ventricles where the relationships between their axes are altered. Another limitation is related to alterations in the motion of the interventricular septum, as occurs in the case of complete left branch block, pacemaker rhythm, or right ventricular volume overload. Thus, it is understandable why left ventricular ejection fraction would not detect subtle changes in myocardial contractile state. Therefore, although left ventricular ejection fraction has been demonstrated to predict mortality [43], it presents several constrains in the assessment of cardiac function in cardiovascular disease patients. First, left ventricular ejection fraction is commonly evaluated at rest and shows poor correlation with exercise capacity and symptomatic status of the patients [44]. Second, it does not truly represent a measure of cardiac function because it equates left ventricular end-diastolic dimension. Dilation of the heart is a common consequence of the activation of compensatory mechanisms to maintain *stroke volume* at a cost of increased central venous pressure.

As left ventricular *ejection fraction* is determined by stroke volume and *end-diastolic volume*, such disarrangement could distort the relationship between left ventricular ejection fraction and stroke volume and turn it more reciprocally dependent on left ventricular geometric structural changes. This was illustrated in the study by Bombardini et al. [34], in which 33 out of 99 *cardiac patients* exhibited a considerable disagreement between left ventricular *ejection fraction* and contractile reserve. In their study, left ventricular ejection fraction failed to predict event in 17 cardiac patients, mostly with *left ventricular dilation* and extensive vasodilator therapy, who exhibited positive left ventricular ejection fraction reserve but abnormally flat *pressure–volume relationship*. Third, it may be largely affected by changes in *preload* and *afterload* [34]. Furthermore, even if resting, left ventricular ejection fraction could give a complete picture of *left ventricular systolic function* during exercise, it would not simultaneously quantify *left ventricular diastolic function* in heart failure [45]. Ejection fraction can be calculated as follows (Eqs. 5.1 and 5.2):

$$EF(\%) = [(EDV - ESV)/EDV]\cdot 100 \quad (5.1)$$

or

$$EF(\%) = SV/EDV\cdot 100, \quad (5.2)$$

where EF = ejection fraction, EDV = end-diastolic volume, ESV = end-systolic volume, SV = stroke volume.

Left ventricular ejection fraction values in healthy young adults *at rest* range from 50% to 65%. *Ejection fraction* values during dynamic *aerobic exercise* measured at VO_{2max} can reach 80–90% in top aerobic athletes and 75% in untrained subjects (Fig. 5.7). During *isometric exercise*, ejection fraction can increase up to 65% (Fig. 5.8), decrease, and sometimes remains unchanged [1]. During

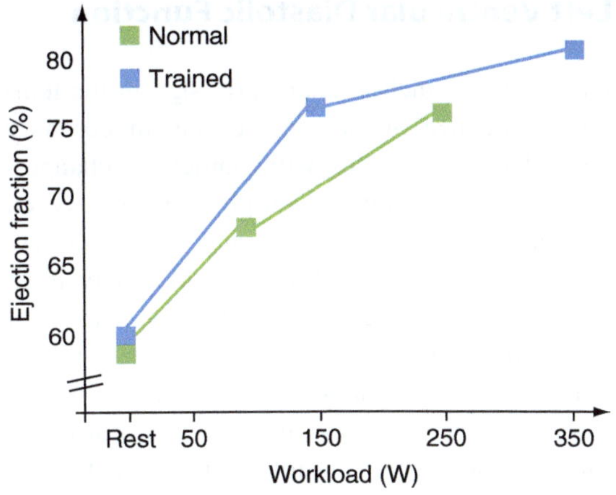

Fig. 5.7 Ejection fraction increases during incremental aerobic exercise in healthy young trained and healthy young sedentary subjects

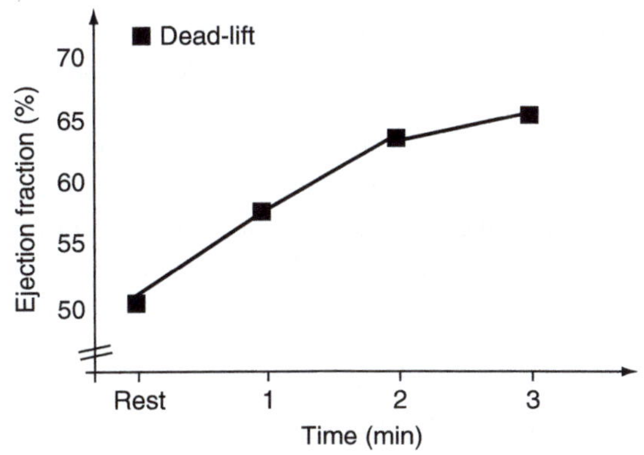

Fig. 5.8 Ejection fraction increases during isometric dead lift in healthy young subjects

anaerobic exercise, *ejection fraction* remains unchanged or slightly increases [37].

Left Ventricular Function in Coronary Artery Disease

In ischemic *heart disease*, resting measures of left ventricular function may be normal or only minimally reduced. However, during aerobic exercise with increase in myocardial work, reduction in left ventricular performance indices has been well documented [12, 46]. Previous studies have suggested that a few patients with *coronary artery disease* increase their ejection fraction during *supine exercise*, whereas in many, the ejection fraction does not change or fall during exercise. During submaximal upright dynamic aerobic exercise in coronary artery disease patients, ejection fraction either decreases, increases, or remains unchanged; *end-diastolic volume* and *end-systolic volume* increase significantly from resting values, thus *stroke volume* remains unchanged or decreases. The discrepancy in the results of *ejection fraction* may be due to different cohorts and protocols used in the different studies. In age-matched normal subjects during submaximal aerobic exercise, global ejection fraction is increased. The difference of ejection fraction response to exercise between the coronary artery disease patients and normal subjects may be due to pronounced increases in relative end-diastolic and especially end-systolic volumes in coronary artery disease patients. Relative stroke volume differs also between patients and controls only at peak exercise.

At maximal exercise effort, control subjects progressively increase ejection fraction from rest to intermediate and maximum levels of exercise. *Coronary artery disease patients*, on the other hand, demonstrate a decrease in ejection fraction from rest to their maximal level of exercise. However, the coronary artery disease patient's responses to intermediate exercise range from a decrease or no change to an increase in ejection fraction. Thus, exercise at maximal intensity is necessary to induce the *left ventricular dysfunction* that is diagnostic of coronary artery disease.

Doppler Indices During Systole

Doppler-derived parameters of aortic flow constitute a reliable index of left ventricular systolic function. Their normal ranges, age, gender variations, and responses to exercise in untrained and athletic populations have been reported previously [47]. Doppler-derived parameters are a method to measure aortic diameter and continuous-wave Doppler ultrasound to obtain aortic blood velocity. Patients with aortic stenosis, aortic insufficiency, or a prosthetic valve are not suitable to be measured by this method due to conditions likely to violate the assumptions upon which the calculation of absolute cardiac output is based.

Doppler indices during systole from rest to peak exercise have been shown to be reproducible and can be used to reflect changes in left ventricular systolic function [48]. The velocity and acceleration of blood flow in the ascending aorta have been used to describe left ventricular systolic function in health and disease [49]. During *dynamic aerobic exercise*, the normal responses of Doppler indices during systole from *rest* to *peak exercise* are an increase *in peak velocity* of blood flow through the aortic valve, 1 and 1.3 m · s^{-1}, respectively, and in *flow velocity integral* which is the length of wave movement in the aorta following ejection, 20 and 30 cm, respectively. Decreased values from rest to peak exercise were seen in: flow period, 0.3 and 0.2 s; *acceleration time*, 0.07 and 0.06 s; and *deceleration time*, 0.2 and 0.1 s respectively. During *isometric exercise*, Doppler indices values are *peak velocity* 1.1 m · s^{-1}, *flow velocity integral* 21 cm, flow period 0.3 s, *acceleration time* 0.08 s, and deceleration time 0.2 s. During *dynamic anaerobic exercise*, *Doppler indices* values are closely similar to those obtained during dynamic aerobic exercise. These results indicate that accurate *cardiac output* can be measured by noninvasive ultrasound in most patients. The technique may be useful for extended cardiac output monitoring in acute care patients and for cardiac output assessment in many other types of patients undergoing diagnostic studies and therapeutic interventions, as well as during exercise[50].

During *isometric exercise*, *Doppler indices* values are significantly lower in normal subjects and *coronary artery disease* patients compared to aerobic exercise values [50]. During dynamic *anaerobic exercise*, in healthy subjects, Doppler indices values are closely similar to those obtained during *dynamic aerobic* exercise [51].

Left Ventricular Diastolic Function

Diastolic dysfunction is an early sign in the temporal sequence of ischemic events in coronary heart disease. In cases with borderline changes, exercise stress testing which provokes an oxygen demand-supply imbalance and consecutively impairs early diastolic filling could clarify if an underlying heart disease is present. It is established that *cardiac output* is related to *ventricular filling*, which is strongly influenced by *ventricular diastolic properties*. At rest, most of left ventricular filling occurs early in diastole. This left ventricular filling occurs in response to the pressure gradient produced as left ventricular pressure falls below left atrial pressure. Left ventricular diastolic phases start with the onset of *isovolumic relaxation* and ends with the cessation of inflow to the ventricle. Because mitral valve flow occurs in response to a left atrial to left ventricular pressure gradient, augmented diastolic mitral valve flow during exercise may be due to an increased mitral valve pressure gradient, resulting from a rise in left atrial pressure and/or a fall in left ventricular early diastolic pressure. From the physical point of view, *left ventricular diastolic inflow* is determined by *venous return*, the impedance of the mitral valve, left ventricular interior pressure, and thus the *atrial-ventricular pressure gradient* [52, 53].

Left ventricular filling fraction and peak filling rate are assessed during the first third of diastole, as indices of left ventricular diastolic performance at rest and following *upright bicycle exercise* in normal individuals and patients with *coronary artery disease*. Additionally, left ventricular filling must be accomplished at relatively low filling pressures, otherwise pulmonary vascular congestion may occur [54]. There are several important links between *aerobic exercise* performance and the diastolic phase of the cardiac cycle. During acute exercise, *diastolic function* must be augmented in order for left ventricular filling to match increased *left ventricular output*, that is, cardiac output. This challenges the myocardium because the shortened duration of diastole during exercise may compromise left ventricular filling, thereby limiting the *stroke volume*.

In healthy subjects, exercise training can enhance diastolic function and exercise capacity and prevent deterioration of *diastolic function* in the course of aging. This can be in patients with diastolic dysfunction, in which exercise capacity can be enhanced by exercise training and pharmacological treatment, whereas improvement of diastolic function can only be observed in few patients.

Despite similar resting heart rates, the mean filling fraction remains unchanged from rest to exercise in *normal individuals*, while normal ejection fraction in coronary artery disease patients at rest demonstrates a significant low filling fraction. Presence of symptoms of congestive heart failure in the setting of a normal systolic function is referred to as heart failure with normal ejection fraction or, if evidence of an impaired diastolic function is observed, as diastolic heart failure [55].

In addition, although *coronary artery disease patients* have similar resting heart rates as normal individuals, they demonstrate significant lower peak filling rate during the first third of diastole compared to the normal once. Left ventricular diastolic function may be impaired in the elderly and/or in individuals with ischemic coronary syndromes. Regular aerobic exercise training appears to enhance left ventricular diastolic function and may benefit patients with clinically relevant diastolic dysfunction. These data suggest that (a) indices of diastolic performance can be noninvasively assessed at rest and during exercise using first-pass radionuclide angiocardiography, (b) abnormalities in early diastolic performance are often present at rest in patients with coronary artery disease despite normal systolic performance, and (c) exercise-induced ischemia results in increased early diastolic dysfunction in patients with coronary disease. Diastolic dysfunction is frequent in elderly subjects and in patients with left ventricular hypertrophy, vascular disease, and diabetes mellitus. Patients with diastolic dysfunction demonstrate a reduced exercise capacity and might suffer from congestive heart failure [55]. Reduced exercise capacity in diastolic dysfunction results from a number of pathophysiological alterations such as slowed myocardial relaxation, reduced myocardial distensibility, elevated filling pressures, and reduced ventricular suction forces. These alterations limit the increase of ventricular diastolic filling and cardiac output during exercise and lead to pulmonary congestion.

Doppler-derived left ventricular diastolic indices have been shown to correlate with *exercise capacity* in patients with *heart diseases* [56] as well as in healthy individuals [57]. Left ventricular diastolic indices measurements have been advocated in health and disease because left ventricular systolic function do not often predict exercise capacity [56, 58]. However, it is not clear whether left ventricular *diastolic function* is the strongest predictor of *exercise capacity*. If one would compare left ventricular diastolic indices with more accurate left ventricular systolic indices, the importance of left ventricular systolic function to exercise capacity would likely be emphasized [59].

Left Ventricular Diastolic Indices

Opening of the mitral valve and filling of the left ventricle in diastole is contingent on a pressure gradient, between the left atrium and left ventricle. At rest, such filling occurs in two diastolic phases. The *early* or rapid-*filling* phase occurs when left ventricular pressure falls below that of left atrial pressure at the onset of diastole, causing the mitral valve to open and blood to flow into the ventricle, what is called *mitral peak early diastole* (*E*). During the middle portion of diastole, left ventricular pressure rises, the gradient is eliminated, the valve floats shut, and flow ceases (diastasis), which is shortened at rapid heart rates. Toward the end of diastole, *atrial contraction* (*atrial systole*) again creates a left atrial-left ventricular gradient with flow across the mitral valve or *presystole maximal velocity* (*A*). The two phases of left ventricular filling can be observed using Doppler echocardiography as an initial tall *E* wave (flow from the gradient created by decreasing left ventricular pressure) and a smaller *A* wave which is the effect of an increased gradient by pressure created by left atrial contraction.

During *mitral peak early diastole*, the ventricle is filled with blood flowing from the atria into the ventricle without any energy consumption. At a heart rate greater than 80 beats · min^{-1}, the interval of slow filling shortens almost to nonexistence, and atrial contraction begins at or before the end point of rapid filling. Atria contraction occurring at the time of peak filling in the early diastolic rapid-filling phase (i.e., heart rate, 120 beats · min^{-1}) may not augment mitral flow and chamber filling. *Ventricular filling* in the rapid-filling phase may become more significant for adequate global filling as *heart rate* increases during *physical exercise*. *Heart rate* may increase to exceedingly high values during exercise, especially in athletes who perform strenuously. Therefore, augmented early diastolic filling may suggest the presence of mechanisms to compensate for the decrease in the *diastolic period* during high intensity exercise.

At the end of mitral peak early diastole, 80% of the ventricle is filled. Presystole maximal velocity atrial contraction adds 20% to the ventricle volume. However, atrial action requires ATP.

At rest, filling rate during mitral peak early diastole is 65–70 and 40–50 cm · s^{-1} for presystole maximal velocity. During dynamic aerobic exercise, filling rate obtained in mitral peak early diastole is approximately 60–65 cm · s^{-1}, while for presystole maximal velocity, it is below 40 cm · s^{-1} and sometimes unchanged compared to rest. During isometric exercise, presystole maximal velocity values can increase up to 60 cm · s^{-1}, while during mitral peak, early diastole values are unchanged from rest. During dynamic anaerobic exercise, mitral peak early diastole values can increase to 75–80 cm · s^{-1}, and reach 40–45 cm · s^{-1} during presystole maximal velocity.

Factors contributing to diastolic disturbances can be differentiated into intrinsic and extrinsic left ventricular abnormalities. Intrinsic mechanisms include (a) impaired left ventricular relaxation, (b) increased overall chamber stiffness, (c) increased myocardial stiffness, and (d) increased left ventricular asynchrony. All these factors are part of pathological left ventricular hypertrophy. Factors extrinsic to the left ventricle causing diastolic disorders include (a) increased central blood volume, which will increase left ventricular pressure without altering the left ventricular pressure–volume relation, and (b) ventricular interaction mediated by pericardial restraint, which may cause a parallel upward shift of the diastolic left ventricular pressure–volume curve. Improved understanding of left ventricular relaxation and filling helps to differentiate pathological and physiological myocardial hypertrophy.

The Ratio of Peak Early Diastole/Presystole Maximal Velocity

Patients with similar grade diastolic dysfunction at rest may have a spectrum of alterations in *left ventricular diastolic function* during exercise. Despite similar mitral flow and annular velocities at rest, different responses to exercise are seen in patients with abnormal left ventricular relaxation at rest. Lower left ventricular diastolic functional reserve was associated with higher ventricular elastance during exercise and reduced exercise capacity. The mitral *peak early diastole/presystole maximal velocity ratio* (*E/A*) is an important variable measuring left ventricular diastolic function. Figure 5.9 shows values for the ratio in healthy

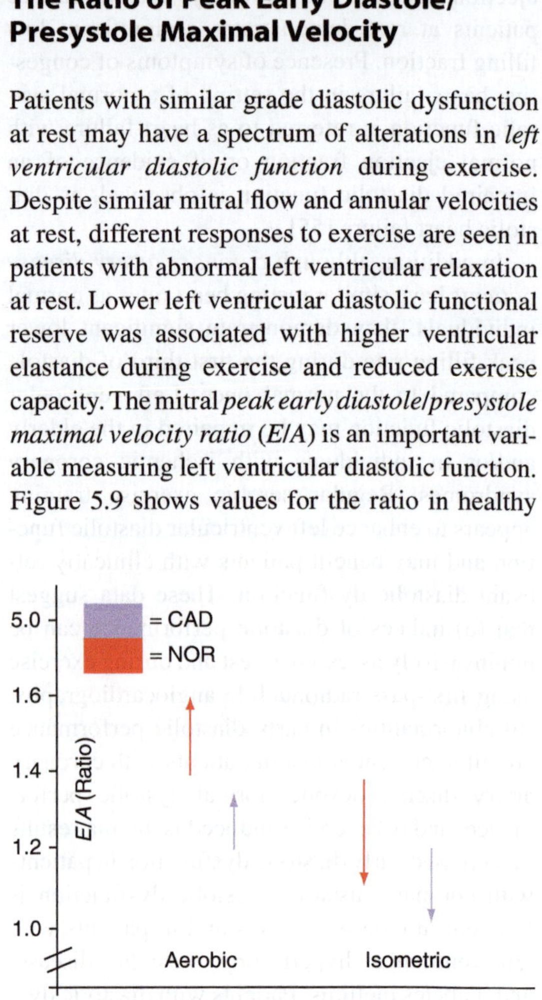

Fig. 5.9 Peak early diastole/presystole maximal velocity ratio (*E/A*) changes from resting values in normal subjects (*NOR*) compared to coronary artery disease patients (*CAD*) at peak aerobic and isometric exercises. During aerobic exercise, both groups increased the ratio, while during the isometric bout, both groups reduced the ratio

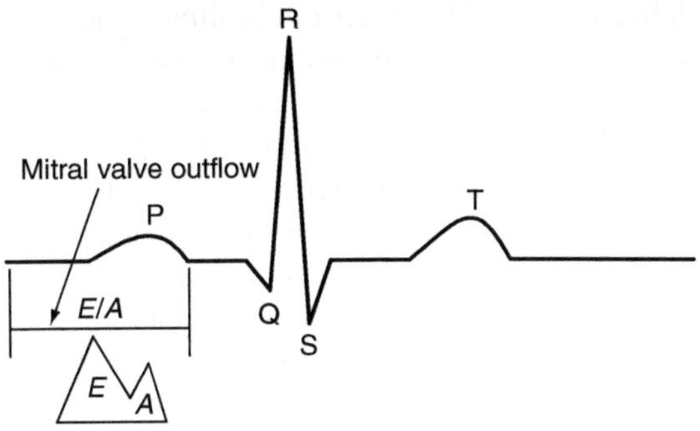

Fig. 5.10 Peak early diastole/presystole maximal velocity ratio (*E/A*) at rest in healthy individuals. The filling of the ventricular starts from mid *PQ* segment and ends up before ejection (*QS* segment)

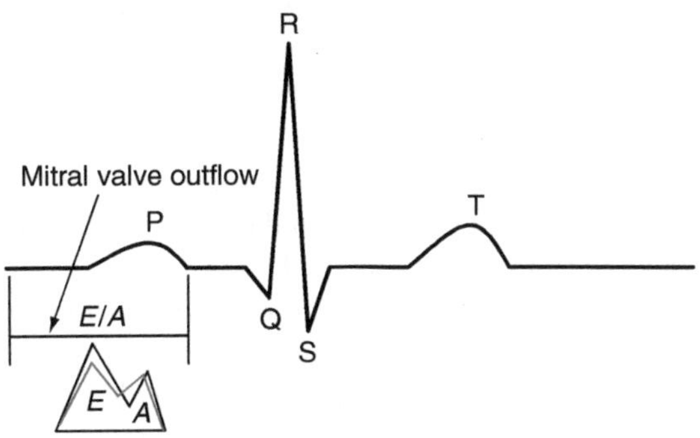

Fig. 5.11 Peak early diastole/presystole maximal velocity ratio (*E/A*) at peak aerobic exercise in coronary artery disease patients. The filling of the ventricular starts from end of the *T*-wave segment and ends up by the *Q* wave (isovolumic stage) before ejection

and *coronary artery disease patients*. In healthy subjects, at rest, the ratio is 1.4, and it increases during dynamic *aerobic exercise* to 1.5 or 1.6 [60]. Coronary artery disease patients increase their ratio modestly from 1.2 to 1.3. Figure 5.10 reveals the relationship between *E* and *A* in normal subjects, while Fig. 5.11 shows the changed ratio *E/A* in coronary artery disease patients.

Conversely, in healthy subjects and coronary artery disease patients, *isometric handgrip exercise* produced evidence of reduced *early filling* including decreased *early diastolic* and *mean acceleration rate* and slightly increased *isovolumic relaxation time*. Thus the response of left ventricular filling dynamics recorded by Doppler differs for *isotonic* exercise and *isometric exertion utilizing large muscle mass* and likely reflects the variable pressure and flow alterations induced by these two forms of exertion.

During *isometric exercise* utilizing large muscle mass, *mitral peak early diastole/presystole maximal velocity ratio* decreases in healthy subjects from 1.4 to 1.1 since values of mitral peak early diastole and presystole maximal velocity are similar [60].

Coronary artery disease and *hypertensive patients* show significant lower values compared to normal individuals at *rest* and *during aerobic* and *isometric effort.*

Atrial Filling Fraction

As mitral flow velocities depend on *preload* and heart rate, the correct interpretation of these values should consider changes in loading conditions within the ventricle [52, 61].

At rest, *filling rate* during *mitral peak early diastole* (*E*) is 65–70 and 40–50 cm · s^{-1} for *presystole maximal velocity* (*A*) *in young subjects* [23, 60], and 60 and 61 cm · s^{-1} in *older subjects.* During dynamic *aerobic exercise*, filling rate obtained in mitral peak early diastole is approximately 60–65 cm · s^{-1}, while for presystole maximal velocity, it is below 40 cm · s^{-1} and sometimes unchanged compared to rest. During *isometric exercise*, presystole maximal velocity values can increase up to 60 cm · s^{-1} in young subjects and up to 70 cm · s^{-1} in older subjects, while during mitral peak early diastole values are unchanged from rest [60] or may even decrease in older subjects. *Cardiac* and *hypertensive patients* show significant lower values at *rest* and *during aerobic* and *isometric effort* compared to normal subjects. During dynamic anaerobic exercise in normal subjects, mitral peak early diastole values can increase to 75–80 cm · s^{-1}, and reach 40–45 cm · s^{-1} during presystole maximal velocity.

Atrial filling fraction measures the percentage of blood volume filled by mitral peak early diastole and the percentage filled by presystole maximal velocity. At *rest*, value of normal subject is 20% and 25% in *coronary artery disease patients*. In healthy individuals, it is reduced to

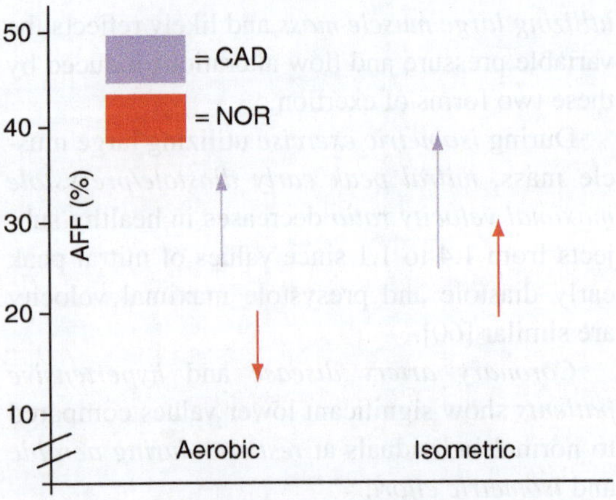

Fig. 5.12 Atrial filling fraction (*AFF%*) changes from resting values in normal subjects (*NOR*) compared to coronary artery disease patients (*CAD*) at peak aerobic and isometric exercises. Coronary artery disease patients increase significantly atrial filling fraction during both modes of exercise while normal subjects reduce it during aerobic exercise and increased it slightly during isometric exercise

15–18% during *aerobic effort* and increased to 25–30% during *isometric exercise*. *Coronary artery disease patients* increase atrial filling fraction during aerobic exercise up to 35% while *hypertensive patients* reaches 40 and sometimes 50%. During isometric exercise, atrial filling fraction in coronary artery disease patients is increased to 40% (Fig. 5.12) and 50% in hypertensive patients.

Exercise Mode and Left Ventricular Hypertrophy

Adaptation of the heart to strength training with a slight increase in left ventricular internal diameter and a large increase in left ventricular wall thickness can be explained on the basis of *blood pressure* response (*pressor response*) and low *cardiac output* during weight lifting [19]. *Endurance training* improves maximal work capacity, as evidenced by higher VO_{2max}, *stroke volume*, *cardiac output*, and by lower *heart rate* and blood pressure [62].

Hypertrophy is a physiological adaptation by which the heart compensates for an increased workload. At some point, this process can be defined as an *athletic heart* in healthy subjects or as *pathological heart* in cardiac patients. Improve in understanding of left ventricular relaxation and filling helps to differentiate pathological and physiological myocardial hypertrophy. *Physiological hypertrophy* is accompanied by a normal or augmented contractile, in which myosin hydrolyzes ATP, and the maximum velocity of muscle shortening is either normal or elevated [63]. *Pathological hypertrophy*, on the other hand, is associated with depressed contractility not necessarily accompanied by concomitant heart failure, in which case the rate of myosin ATPase activity and the velocity of muscle shortening are decreased [63]. To differentiate between physiological and pathological myocardial changes, the relationship between heart size and ergometric performance, as well as the echocardiographically measured ratio between left ventricular myocardial thickness and volume is useful; the latter remains unchanged, on the whole, in endurance- and strength-trained athletes.

Adaptation of the heart to *endurance training* with an increase in both diameter and *wall thickness* is useful if *heart rate* and *blood pressure* responses during intense exercise are taken into account. Endurance training is associated with a *left ventricular eccentric hypertrophy* form, where ventricular wall thickness and cavity size are increased, as a consequence of the volume overload produced during exercise. The cardiac output of trained endurance athletes may increase from 5 to 6 $L \cdot min^{-1}$ at rest up to 40 $L \cdot min^{-1}$ during maximal exercise, with left ventricular end-diastolic diameter of 66–70 mm. [64]. The heart adapts to this *volume overload* with an increase in *internal diameter*. *Blood pressure* also increases during endurance exercise, although to a lesser extent than during strength training [1, 19].

In contrast, *strength training* is supposedly associated with a *left ventricular concentric hypertrophy* form where increased ventricular wall thickness, with no change in cavity size, underpins the elevated *left ventricular mass* as a consequence of the pressure overload produced during strenuous resistive exercise [65]. Pathological left ventricular concentric hypertrophy can be induced by additional factors which play an important role factors such as hypertension, aortic stenosis, cardiomyopathy, or anabolic steroid use can play an important role. D'Andrea et al. [66] evaluated in 263 competitive athletes possible correlations between changes induced by different sport activities in left ventricular structure and cardiac response during maximal physical effort, in 160 top-level endurance athletes. D'Andrea et al. concluded that left ventricular structural changes in competitive athletes represent adaptation to hemodynamic overload induced by training and are consistent with different kinds of sport activity. Work capacity during exercise is positively influenced by preload increase in endurance athletes, while increased afterload due to isometric training in endurance athletes determines higher systemic resistance during physical effort.

Rowing and *cycling* represent typical combined *strength* and *endurance sports*, sometimes exercise last up to 6 h. In healthy individuals, *systolic blood pressure* and *mean arterial blood pressure* are increased during cycling; systolic blood pressure readings of >200 mmHg can be found during maximal exercise testing on the bicycle ergometer [67, 68]. During rowing, *heart rate* increases to near-maximal values of ≈190 beats · min^{-1}, with peak systolic blood pressure waves of ≈200 mmHg [69]. The combination of both extreme volume overload (endurance) and extreme pressure overload (strength) may explain why the largest increases in left ventricular internal dimension and left ventricular wall thickness are found in cyclists and rowers.

Genome and Left Ventricular Mass

Exercise ventricular *systolic pressure or volume overload* leads to increased *wall tension* per sarcomere and greater stretch of myocardium fibers, thus, resulting in augmentation of *end-diastolic sarcomere length*. This in turn activates the genetic apparatus of myocardial cells, resulting in enhanced *nucleic acid*, *protein* and *myosin synthesis*, and possible induction of new genetic expression such as *myosin isozymes*.

Although the heart possesses a relatively high *ribonucleic-to-deoxyribonucleic acid ratio*, following *exercise*, there is an altered base composition in *ribonucleic acids* (*RNA*) in *hypertrophied hearts*.

Humans have about 35,000–65,000 genes with around 1–2 million transcription factors. The basic mechanism by which *exercise* activates *genes* involves a stimulus signal to *deoxyribonucleic acid* (*DNA*), then transcription via *messenger ribonucleic acid* (*mRNA*), and finally, translation into protein [70]. However, if the genetic predisposition is set for lower level range, changes due to physical activity can be trained up to a certain degree. The complex interplay of different physiological responses to exercise with genetic polymorphism can be found in the origins of left ventricular mass in physiological and pathological hypertrophies. It is assumed that *resistive exercise* can be very demanding due to the *pressor response* [68], which might have a significant effect on global performance and mass [71, 72]. Though, in healthy subjects, the effects of successful adaptation on the pressure overload training are still controversial, as *pressure overload* per se does not always produce intrinsic depression of the myocardial *inotropic state*. However, this is not the case in patients with *heart disease* and *hypertension* in which the adaptation to pressure overload is pathologically increased in *left ventricular mass* [71].

Endurance training, on the other hand, improves maximal work capacity, as evidenced by higher VO_{2max}, *stroke volume*, *cardiac output*, and lower *heart rate* and blood pressure [73]. *Left ventricular hypertrophy* is a *physiological* (*eccentric*) adaptation by which the heart compensates for an increased workload. At some point in healthy subjects, this process can be defined as an *athletic heart*, or as *pathological* (*concentric*) in *weightlifters* or *cardiac patients*. An important problem is determining when left ventricular hypertrophy ceases to be physiological and begins to be pathological or when it induces the heart to augment or depress its mechanical function.

Pathological and physiological states of left ventricular hypertrophy have been described primarily using criteria focusing on normal chamber performance and oxygen delivery as well as the reversibility of the hypertrophy once the overload is removed. Both states are also defined by the nature of the imposed load and the resulting myocardial adaptations [74].

The *pathological hypertrophy* undergoes a complex series of changes in both myocyte and non-myocyte elements. In an attempt to compensate for the reduction in left ventricular function, the sympathetic nervous (SNS), renin-angiotensin-aldosterone systems (RAAS), and other neurohumoral mechanisms are activated. The altered signal transduction in pathological hypertrophy initiates changes in *gene expression* that produce myocyte hypertrophy [75]. Figure 5.13 emphasizes the differences in end-diastolic volume between normal, physiological hypertrophy (eccentric) and pathological hypertrophy (concentric). Figure 5.14 shows that following contraction at peak aerobic exercise change from end-diastolic volume to end-systolic volume during aerobic exercise in normal physiological hypertrophy (eccentric) and pathological hypertrophy (concentric). End-systolic volume value is the smallest in the athletic heart while no significant differences are seen between normal subjects and weightlifters.

In the two modes of exercise, isometric exercise, pressure overload and aerobic exercise, volume overload may result in ventricular hypertrophy. Yet, ventricular physiological measurements discriminate poorly between high-level athletes and cardiac patients. As a result, much research has been directed at elucidating the role of submaximal exercise, cardiovascular responses, and skeletal muscle factors in trying to differentiate better between levels of physiological performance among *athletes* and *cardiac patients* [76].

Family studies were the only possible option before 1990 because studying DNA was laborious and costly. It has shown in a heritability study that many aspects of physical capacity have substantial genetic component. A more recent approach has been to measure genetic markers and other important determinants of left ventricular mass. Such studies center on renin-angiotensin system and the identification of a candidate gene.

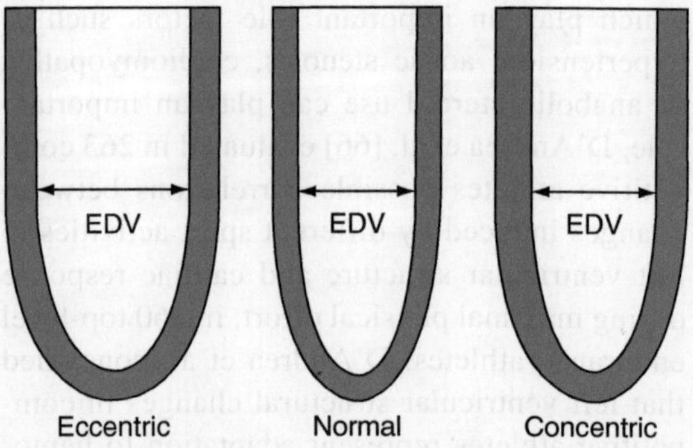

Fig. 5.13 Comparisons of end-diastolic volume (*EDV*) pre-contraction between left ventricular physiological hypertrophy (eccentric), normal left ventricular, and weightlifter left ventricular hypertrophy (concentric)

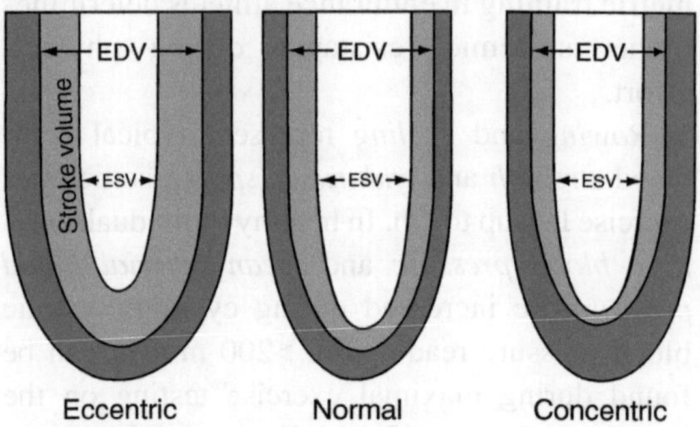

Fig. 5.14 Left ventricular volumes end-diastolic (*EDV*), end-systolic volume (*ESV*), and stroke volume (*SV*) and changes at peak aerobic exercise in endurance athletes (eccentric), normal subjects, and weightlifters (concentric)

Data show that different molecular mechanisms are responsible for different types of left ventricular mass increase seen in athletes and *cardiac patients*.

In Fatini et al.'s [77] study, the association of ACE I/D polymorphism with changes in *left ventricular mass* in response to physical training has been observed, but no association has been found with AT1R A1166C polymorphism. Twenty-eight soccer players and 155 healthy untrained male subjects genotyped for angiotensin-converting enzyme I/D underwent 7 months army training. Pretraining left ventricular mass was significantly higher in players compared to the controls. Training-induced left ventricular mass increase in

22 of 28 players and in all the controls. The percentage of soccer players in whom an increase of left ventricular mass was found after training was statistically different in relation to the angiotensin-converting enzyme D allele. Fatini et al. concluded that soccer play does not select athletes on genotype basis. Training-induced left ventricular mass changes in male elite athletes are significantly associated with the presence of ACE D allele, but not of AT1R C allele. Montgomery et al. found that the absence of the D allele from the 287 base pair marker in the angiotensin-converting enzyme gene resulted in a higher than normal angiotensin-converting enzyme level. Following a 10-week physical training period in male military recruits, echocardiographic measurements of left ventricular mass revealed that persons with D allele in the 287 base pair marker in the angiotensin-converting enzyme had a mixed cardiac response to military basic training, with both eccentric and concentric left ventricular hypertrophy, while individuals with angiotensin-converting enzyme of 11 genotype did not have a cardiac morphology response to training. These two last studies [78] may have implications for which exercise mode will best serve athletes or cardiac patients in terms of modulating cardiovascular function during exercise training. These two last studies by Fatini et al. [77] and Montgomery et al. [78] may have implications for which exercise mode will best serve athletes or cardiac patients in terms of modulating cardiovascular function during exercise training.

Although a few studies have analyzed the association of angiotensin-converting enzyme polymorphism and left ventricular hypertrophy in isotonic exercise-trained subjects who developed eccentric cardiac hypertrophy, there has been no research done in power athletes who developed concentric cardiac hypertrophy. It was hypothesized that angiotensin-converting enzyme genotypic modulation characteristics may affect left ventricular mass in power athletes [79].

Kasikcioglu et al. [80] studied 29 elite Caucasian wrestlers (mean age, 22.6 years) and 51 age-matched sedentary subjects. According to the absence or presence of the insertion segment in the polymerase chain reaction product, the subjects were classified as homozygous deletion-deletion (DD), insertion-insertion (II), or heterozygous insertion-deletion (ID). The association of left ventricular hypertrophy with angiotensin-converting enzyme gene insertion/deletion (I/D) polymorphism was analyzed. Angiotensin-converting enzyme genotyping was performed on peripheral leukocytes using the polymerase chain reaction technique. It was found that left ventricular hypertrophy was more apparent in the athletes than in the controls. Angiotensin-converting enzyme's genotype II frequency was 17.2% in the athletes, 17.6% in the controls; ID frequency was 51.7% in the athletes, 56.8% in the controls; and the DD frequency was 31% in the athletes and 25.4% in the controls. Left ventricular mass and mass index were found to be higher in genotype DD (126.2 ± 2.9 g · m^2) than genotype II (85.5 ± 4.0 g · m^2) or genotype ID (110.1 ± 2.3 g · m^2) in the athletes. Furthermore, VO_{2max} in genotype DD was found to be higher than in II and ID. Kasikcioglu et al. concluded that an association exists between angiotensin-converting enzyme gene I/D polymorphism and left ventricular hypertrophy in strength-trained athletes.

It has been assumed that resistive exercise can be very demanding due to the pressor response [81] which might have a significant effect on left ventricular global performance and mass [82]. However, in healthy subjects, the effects of successful adaptation to the pressure of overload training are still controversial, as pressure overload per se does not always produce intrinsic depression of the myocardial inotropic state. However, this is not the case with coronary artery disease patients and hypertension patients in which the adaptation to pressure overloads is a pathological increase in left ventricular mass.

Exercise and "Athlete's Heart"

Cardiovascular adaptations to exercise have been systematically defined and differ according to type of conditioning: Endurance training such as long-distance running and swimming; and strength training such as wrestling, weightlifting, or throwing heavy objects. Long-term cardiovascular adaptation to dynamic training produces increased VO_{2max} due to increased cardiac output and (a-v) O_2. Strength exercise results in little or no increase in VO_2. Thus, the predominant effect of endurance exercise is to produce volume overload on the left ventricle, while strength exercise causes a pressure overload for the most part. Sports such as cycling and rowing are examples of *isodynamic exercise*. Most athletic disciplines combine endurance and strength modes of physical conditioning to some extent, and training-related physiological alterations represent a complex set of central and peripheral mechanisms operating at structural, metabolic, and regulatory levels [67]. Performing vigorous physical activity entails multiorgan system engagement, but the cardiovascular system plays a critical role. In order to provide enough oxygen to activate muscles during repeated physical activity of high intensity, the heart undergoes profound morphological, functional, and electrophysiological alterations, which have been identified as "*athlete's heart syndrome*" and are generally regarded as a benign increase in cardiac mass, with specific circulatory and cardiac morphological alterations, representing a physiological adaptation to systematic training [83].

Physical exercise is associated with hemodynamic changes which alter the loading conditions of the heart. In *dynamic exercise*, the emphasis is on movement with no or minimal development of force. The main hemodynamic features are increases in *heart rate* and *stroke volume*, the two components of *cardiac output*. *Total peripheral resistance* drops, but the net result is a slight-to-moderate rise in blood pressure. The load on the heart is predominantly that of volume.

During *static exercise*, force is developed with no or minimal movement. The hemodynamic consequences involve a slight elevation of cardiac output, caused by the increase of heart rate, and a more pronounced rise of blood pressure, resulting in a pressure load on the heart. From a theoretical point of view, the hemodynamic alterations and the ventricular loading conditions during exercise could, in the long run, lead to left ventricular hypertrophy. Volume overload would lead to enlargement of the left ventricular internal diameter and a proportional increase of wall thickness, eccentric left ventricular hypertrophy. The pressure overload would induce thickening of the ventricular wall with unchanged internal dimension or concentric left ventricular hypertrophy. It was suggested that these cardiac adaptations serve to normalize wall stress [84].

Athlete's heart is a constellation of morphological cardiac changes, including increased left ventricular volume, increased left ventricular mass, increased left atrial volume, and right ventricular structural changes as physiological responses to exercise training. These structural changes fall within the normal reference ranges of appropriately matched control subjects for most trained individuals. However, there are significant numbers of athletes who have "abnormal" measurements. The ability to distinguish between physiological changes associated with athlete's heart and structural abnormalities that may represent underlying cardiac disease is of paramount importance [85]. These cardiac changes leading to athlete's heart in highly trained athletes are the consequence of several determinants, including type of sport, gender, and possibly, inherited genetic factors. The extent of physiological cardiac remodeling may occasionally be substantial in highly trained athletes and may elicit a differential diagnosis with structural cardiac disease, such as cardiomyopathies [86].

Athlete's heart is a complex but not precisely defined concept, anatomically and functionally and in relation to health and disease. It refers to whole heart enlargement and/or hypertrophy of the cardiac muscle, as well as increasing economy of cardiac performance at rest and during physical activity with higher maximal functional capacities, in adaptive response to vigorous physical activity. *Left ventricular hypertrophy* in athletes is associated with normal systolic and diastolic functions and resting cardiac energy metabolism, supporting its benign nature [87]. In addition, athletes demonstrate a spectrum of alterations in the 12-lead electrocardiogram (ECG) pattern, including marked increase in precordial R-wave or S-wave voltages, ST-segment or T-wave changes, and deep Q-waves, suggestive of left ventricular hypertrophy, which may raise the possibility of a pathologic heart condition, but have also been viewed as a consequence of *morphological cardiac remodeling* induced by athletic conditioning.

Pellicia and Maron [88] postulated that two different morphological forms of athlete's heart can be distinguished: a *strength-trained heart* and an *endurance-trained heart*. There is overwhelming evidence, particularly from echocardiography, that the heart of competitive athletes may differ from that of nonathletes matched for age, gender, and body size. A larger *left ventricular mass* has been shown in athletes performing predominantly *dynamic aerobic exercises* and *anaerobic sports*, in athletes engaged in static training, and in players of ball sports. Enlargement of the *left ventricular internal diameter* was most pronounced and reached about 10% in athletes performing predominantly dynamic sports, while athletes who focused mainly on *strength training* had a lesser increase of internal dimensions, which was limited to 2.5% [66]. Furthermore, the *left ventricular wall* appeared to be thickened in all types of athletes as compared with controls. Even though the morphology of athlete's heart and the impact of different sports on cardiac structure have been investigated previously by several authors [89], they have not been able to satisfactorily resolve the question of whether two types of athlete's heart exist.

Concentric Hypertrophy

Concentric hypertrophy develops in the case of chronic *pressure overload* as through *isometric exercise*, which increases resistance to blood flow by compressing arteries, the chamber radius may not change; however, the wall thickness greatly increases as new sarcomeres are added in parallel to existing sarcomeres [65]. This type of ventricle is capable of generating greater forces and higher pressures, while the increased wall thickness maintains normal wall stress. *Strength exercise* results in little or no increase in VO_2. Thus, the predominant effect of *aerobic exercise* is to produce *volume overload* on the left ventricle, while *strength exercise* causes a *pressure overload* for the most part. Physical activities such as load carriage, cycling, and rowing are examples of *combined endurance* and *strength exercise* (isodynamic). Most athletic disciplines combine endurance and strength modes of physical conditioning to some extent, and training-related physiological alterations represent a complex set of *central* and *peripheral mechanisms* operating at structural, metabolic, and regulatory levels [67].

Rowers, cyclists, and cross-country skiers tend to have the largest hearts, with an average left ventricular wall thickness of 1.3 cm, compared to 1 cm in normal adults. A left ventricular myocardial thickness of 13 mm is seldom exceeded even in the highly endurance-trained or anabolic drug-free strength-trained athletes under physiological conditions. The upper normal value of left ventricular muscle mass is 170 g $\cdot$ m^{-2} for a physiological heart enlargement. *Left ventricular hypertrophy* in athletes is associated with normal systolic and diastolic functions and resting cardiac energy metabolism, supporting its benign nature [87]. The alterations in the 12-lead electrocardiogram pattern in athletes include changes seen in coronary artery disease patients changes such aspre cordial R-wave or S-wave voltages, ST-segment or T-wave changes, and deep Q-waves, suggestive of *left ventricular hypertrophy*; this may raise the possibility of a *pathologic heart* condition, but have also been viewed as a consequence of morphological cardiac remodeling induced by athletic conditioning.

Pathological Left Ventricular Hypertrophy

Unhealthy Cardiac Hypertrophy: Pathological hypertrophy is the response to stress or disease such as hypertension, heart muscle injury (*myocardial infarction*), or neurohormones. *Valvular heart disease* is another cause of pathological hypertrophy.

Left ventricular hypertrophy resulting from *cardiovascular disease* and/or *hypertension* is accompanied by significant morbidity and mortality and in advanced stages may be irreversible.

Pathological left ventricular hypertrophy also leads to an increase in myocardium mass, but the myocardium does not increase its pumping ability, and instead, accumulates myocardial scarring (collagen). In pathological left ventricular hypertrophy, the heart can increase its mass by up to 150%. Cardiac and/or hypertensive patients have a markedly lower average rapid *left ventricular filling rate*. Thus, in those patients with *left ventricular hypertrophy*, abnormal *left ventricular diastolic filling rate* is more closely related to impaired myocardial contractility than to left ventricular chamber *ejection fraction* [90]. Though, abnormal left ventricular diastolic filling is more closely related to impaired *myocardial contractility* than to left ventricular chamber ejection fraction. *Coronary artery disease patients* and/or *hypertensive patients* with reduced ejection fraction and left ventricular filling pattern have higher *left ventricular mass*, eccentric left ventricular geometry (with thin left ventricular wall thickness), or concentric with wall thickness of 12–18 mm, prolonged left ventricular isovolumic relaxation time, atrial filling fraction, and heart rate compared to those patients with normal ejection fraction [91].

Left Ventricular Adaptations

Aerobic exercise training improves *left ventricular contractility* and function; however, anaerobic and isometric exercises do not improve left ventricular function. *Isometric exercise* has the effect on left ventricular dimensions (*concentric hypertrophy*) opposite to that of aerobic effect (*eccentric hypertrophy*) due to different afterload responses. No changes in left ventricular volumes and hemodynamic responses were obtained following *anaerobic dynamic exercise* were noted.

Aerobic exercise training improves left ventricular contractility and function because (a) the better ability of the left ventricle to develop force, (b) increase in myocardial adrenal receptors' sensitivity, (c) increase in body's blood volume will thus increase venous return.

Table 5.1 Changes in cardiovascular variables following different modes of exercise training programs at rest

	Modes of exercise		
Variable	Aerobic	Anaerobic	Isometric
Heart rate	⇩	⇩	⇨
Stroke volume	⇧	⇨	⇨
Cardiac output	⇨	⇨	⇨
Left ventricular hypertrophy	⇧	⇨	⇧
Ejection fraction	⇨	⇨	⇨
End-diastolic volume	⇧	⇨	⇧
End-systolic volume	⇨	⇨	⇨
Total peripheral resistance	⇩	⇨	⇨
Systolic blood pressure	⇩	⇨	⇨
Diastolic blood pressure	⇩	⇨	⇨

Increased blood volume helps to take advantage of the increased filling capacity of the heart, facilitates increase in *stroke volume* through the *Frank-Starling mechanism*, and (d) reduces total peripheral resistance. This adaptation at rest and at peak exercise occurs fairly rapidly with training (Tables 5.1 and 5.2), but is also the first adaptation lost if stopped training for week or two.

Anatomical changes of the left ventricle that induce 5% increase in myocytes length and wall thicknesses are physiological adaptations: Left ventricular eccentric following aerobic dynamic exercise and concentric after isometric exercise training programs are presented in Figure 5.15.

Change in the myocardium resulting from exercise is an increased heart weight without changes in cardiac respiratory enzymes. Left ventricular hypertrophy is related to increases

Table 5.2 Changes in cardiovascular variables following submaximal efforts during aerobic and isometric exercise programs

	Mode of exercise	
Variable	Aerobic	Isometric
Heart rate	↓	→
Stroke volume	↑	→
Cardiac output	→	→
Left ventricular hypertrophy	↑	↑
Ejection fraction	→	→
End-diastolic volume	↑	→
End-systolic volume	→	→
Total peripheral resistance	↓	→
Systolic blood pressure	↓	→
Diastolic blood pressure	↓	→

Table 5.3 Changes in cardiovascular at peak efforts following dynamic aerobic, anaerobic, and isometric exercise programs

	Mode of exercise		
Variable	Aerobic	Anaerobic	Isometric
Heart rate	↓	→	→
Stroke volume	Slightly ↑	→	↓
Cardiac output	↑	→	→
Ejection fraction	↑	→	→
End-diastolic volume	↑	→	→
End-systolic volume	↓	→	→
Total peripheral resistance	↓	→	↑
Systolic blood pressure	↓	→	↑
Diastolic blood pressure	↓	→	↑

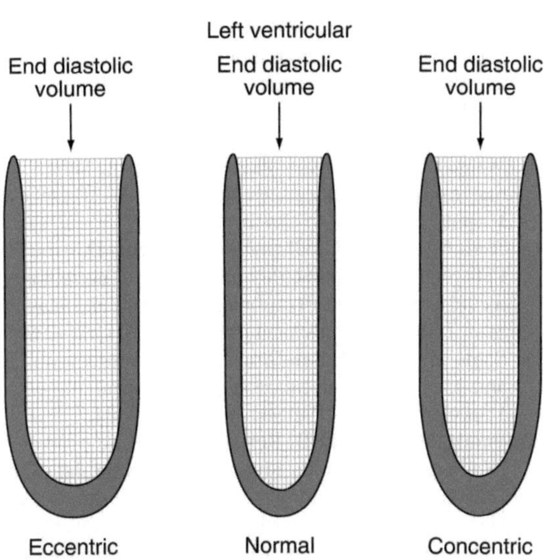

Fig. 5.15 Changes in end-diastolic volume and wall thickness at rest and following dynamic aerobic exercise (eccentric) and isometric exercise (concentric) training programs

in either chamber size or wall dimensions (Table 5.3), increasing *left ventricular end-diastolic volume*, *ejection fraction*, and *left ventricular internal axis* and *decreasing left ventricular end-systolic volume* and *end-diastolic pressure*.

Following dynamic aerobic exercise, *cardiac output* remains unchanged at rest and during submaximal exercise because cardiac output during submaximal exercise is linear with VO_2.

Although an improvement in exercise capacity after exercise training seems to be mainly related to peripheral adaptations, studies have suggested a favorable effect on myocardial adaptations as well as on the outcome of exercise-induced coronary vessel adaptations. *Left ventricular contractility* is increased following aerobic dynamic exercise especially at peak exercise, due to changes in ventricular morphology which is related to left ventricular capacity. The majority of studies, however, have shown minimal or no changes in *ejection fraction* [92]. Factors affecting contractility include an increase in the number of myocardial mitochondria, structural changes in myosin and activity of ATPase enzyme which reduces ATP cleavage time, an increase in venous return, and an increase in calcium released from the sarcoplasmic reticulum, therefore increasing relaxation filling pattern.

Aerobic training brings about enlargement of blood vessel diameter especially in the arterioles thus *systolic*, *diastolic*, and *mean arterial* blood pressures decrease and hence, reducing total peripheral resistance. The decrement in blood pressure is obtained at rest, during submaximal and maximal exercise.

References

1. Sagiv M, Ben-Sira D, Goldhammer E, Soudry M. Left ventricular contractility and function at peak aerobic and anaerobic exercises. Med Sci Sports Exerc. 2000;32:1197–201.
2. Shimizu G, Hirota Y, Kita Y, Kawamura K, Saito T, Gaasch WH. Left ventricular midwall mechanics in systemic arterial hypertension. Circulation. 1991;83: 1676–84.
3. Vinch CS, Aurigemma GP, Simon HU, Hill JC, Tighe DA, Meyer TE. Analysis of left ventricular systolic function using midwall mechanics in patients >60 years of age with hypertensive heart disease and heart failure. Am J Cardiol. 2005;96:1299–303.
4. Barbier J, Ville N, Kervio G, Walther G, Carré F. Sports-specific features of athlete's heart and their relation to echocardiographic parameters. Herz. 2006;31: 531–43.
5. Pluim BM, Zwinderman AH, van der Laarse A, van der Wall EE. The athlete's heart a meta-analysis of cardiac structure and function. Circulation. 2000;101:336–44.
6. Gibbons R, Balady G, Timothybricker J, et al. ACC/AHA 2002 guideline update for exercise testing: summary article a report of the American College of Cardiology/ American Heart Association Task Force on practice guidelines. J Am Coll Cardiol. 2002;40:1531–40.
7. Calabrò R, Pisacane C, Pacileo G, Russo MG. Hemodynamic effects of a single oral dose of enalapril among children with asymptomatic chronic mitral regurgitation. Am Heart J. 1999;138:955–61.
8. Dawson EA, Shave R, Whyte G, et al. Preload maintenance and the left ventricular response to prolonged exercise in men. Exp Physiol. 2007;92:383–90.
9. Sullivan MJ, Cobb FR, Higginbotham MB. Stroke volume increases by similar mechanisms during upright exercise in normal men and women. Am J Cardiol. 1991;67(16):1405–12.
10. Foster C, Gal RA, Port SC, Schmidt DH. Left ventricular ejection fraction during incremental and steady state exercise. Med Sci Sports Exerc. 1995;27: 1602–6.
11. Izdebska E, Izdebski J, Cybulska I, Makowiecka-Ciesla M, Trzebski A. Moderate exercise training reduces arterial chemoreceptor reflex drive in mild hypertension. J Physiol Pharmacol. 2006;57 Suppl 11:93–102.
12. Ding HJ, Lin CC, Wang JJ, Ho ST, Kao A. Correlation of abnormal response of left ventricular ejection fraction after exercise and left ventricular cavity-to-myocardium count ratio of technetium-99m-tetrofosmin single photon emission computed tomography in patients with coronary artery disease. Jpn Heart J. 2002;4:505–14.
13. Sagiv M, Hanson P, Besozzi M, Nagle F. Left ventricular responses to upright isometric handgrip and dead-lift in men with coronary artery disease. Am J Cardiol. 1985;55:1298–302.
14. Digenio AG, Noakes TD, Joughin H, Daly L. Effect of myocardial ischaemia on left ventricular function and adaptability to exercise training. Med Sci Sports Exerc. 1999;3:1094–101.
15. Cicala S, de Simone G, Roman MJ, et al. Prevalence and prognostic significance of wall-motion abnormalities in adults without clinically recognized cardiovascular disease: the Strong Heart Study. Circulation. 2007;116:143–50.
16. Chizyński K, Płachcińska A, Kuśmierek J. Assessment of left ventricular ejection fraction and wall motion in patients after myocardial infarction with and without persistent electrocardiographic ST-segment elevation–using gated radionuclide angiography. Wiad Lek. 2003;56:515–9.
17. Poole DC, Gaesser GA, Hogan MC, Knight DR, Wanger PD. Pulmonary and leg VO_2 during submaximal exercise: implications for muscular efficiency. J Appl Physiol. 1992;72:805–10.
18. Sagiv M, Amir O, Goldhammer E, Ben-Sira D, Amir R. Left ventricular contractility in response to upright isometric exercise in heart transplant recipients and healthy men. J Cardiopulm Rehabil Prev. 2008;28(1):17–23.
19. Sagiv M, Sagiv M, Ben-Sira D. Weight lifting training and left ventricular function in adolescent subjects. J Sports Med Phys Fitness. 2007;47:329–34.
20. Smith DL, Fernhall B. Resistance exercise produces cardiovascular benefits advanced cardiovascular exercise physiology. Champaign: Human Kinetics; 2011.
21. Hanson P, Nagle F. Isometric exercise: cardiovascular responses in normal and cardiac populations. Cardiol Clin. 1987;5:157–70.
22. Van Hook JW, Gill P, Easterling TR, Schmucker B, Carlson K, Benedetti TJ. The hemodynamic effects of isometric exercise during late normal pregnancy. Am J Obstet Gynecol. 1993;169:870–3.

23. Sagiv M, Soudry M, Sagiv A, Rudoy J, Ben-Gal S. Doppler evaluation of left ventricular systolic and diastolic function during isometric exercise in marathon runners. Int J Sports Cardiol. 1995;4:125–30.
24. Hess O, Carroll J. Clinical assessment of heart failure. In: Brauwald E, Libby P, Bonow R, Man D, Zipes D, editors. Braunwald's heart disease: a textbook of cardiovascular medicine. 8th ed. Philadelphia: Saunders; 2007. p. 569–72.
25. Weber KT, Janicki JS. The dynamics of ventricular contraction: force, length, and shortening. Fed Proc. 1980;39:188–95.
26. Haykowsky M, Welsh R, Humen D, Warburton D, Taylor D. Impaired left ventricular systolic function after a half-ironman race. Can J Cardiol. 2001;17: 687–90.
27. Douglas PS, O'Toole ML, Hiller WD, Hackney K, Reichek N. Cardiac fatigue after prolonged exercise. Circulation. 1987;76:1206–13.
28. Alshaher M, El-Mallakh R, Dawn B, Siddiqui T, Longaker RA, Stoddard MF. Cardiac manifestations of exhaustive exercise in nonathletic adults: does cardiac fatigue occur? Echocardiography. 2007;24: 237–42.
29. Goodman JM, McLaughlin PR, Liu PP. Left ventricular performance during prolonged exercise: absence of systolic dysfunction. Clin Sci (Lond). 2001; 100:529–37.
30. Vanoverschelde JL, Younis LT, Melin JA, et al. Prolonged exercise induces left ventricular dysfunction in healthy subjects. J Appl Physiol. 1991; 70:1356–63.
31. Burkhoff D, Mirsky I, Suga H. Assessment of systolic and diastolic ventricular properties via pressure-volume analysis: a guide for clinical, translational, and basic researchers. Am J Physiol Heart Circ Physiol. 2005;289:H501–12.
32. Warburton DE, Haykowsky MJ, Quinney HA, Blackmore D, Teo KK, Humen DP. Myocardial response to incremental exercise in endurance-trained athletes: influence of heart rate, contractility and the Frank-Starling effect. Exp Physiol. 2002;87:613–22.
33. Thompson RB, van den Bos EJ, Esposito DJ, Owen CH, Glower DD. The effects of acute afterload change on systolic ventricular function in conscious dogs with normal vs. failing hearts. Eur J Heart Fail. 2003;5:741–9.
34. Bombardini T, Galderisi M, Agricola E, Coppola V, Mottola G, Picano E. Negative stress echo: further prognostic stratification with assessment of pressure-volume relation. Int J Cardiol. 2008;126:258–67.
35. Grosu A, Bombardini T, Senni M, Duino V, Gori M, Picano E. End-systolic pressure/volume relationship during dobutamine stress echo: a prognostically useful non-invasive index of left ventricular contractility. Eur Heart J. 2005;26:2404–12.
36. Palmieri V, Palmieri EA, Arezzi E, et al. Peak exercise oxygen uptake and left ventricular systolic and diastolic function and arterial mechanics in healthy young men. Eur J Appl Physiol. 2004;9:664–8.
37. Sagiv M, Ben-Sira D, Sagiv M, Goldhammer E. Left ventricular function at peak all-out anaerobic exercise in older men. Gerontology. 2005;51:122–5.
38. Renlund DG, Gerstenblith G, Fleg JL, Becker LC, Lakatta EG. Interaction between left ventricular end-diastolic and end-systolic volumes in normal humans. Am J Physiol. 1990;258:H473–81.
39. Carabello BA, Nolan SP, McGuire LB. Assessment of preoperative left ventricular function in patients with mitral regurgitation: value of the end-systolic wall stress-end-systolic volume ratio. Circulation. 1981;64:1212–7.
40. Carabello BA. Evolution of the study of left ventricular function: everything old is new again. Circulation. 2002;105:2701–3.
41. San Roman JA, Candell-Riera J, Arnold R, et al. Quantitative analysis of left ventricular function as a tool in clinical research. Theoretical basis and methodology. Rev Esp Cardiol. 2009;62:535–51.
42. Dittoe N, Stultz D, Schwartz BP, Hahn HS. Quantitative left ventricular systolic function: from chamber to myocardium. Crit Care Med. 2007;35 Suppl 8:330–95.
43. Parameshwar J, Keegan J, Sparrow J, Sutton GC, Poole-Wilson PA. Predictors of prognosis in severe chronic heart failure. Am Heart J. 1992;123:421–6.
44. Clark AL. Origin of symptoms in chronic heart failure. Heart. 2006;92:12–6.
45. Francis DP, Davies LC, Coats AJ. Diagnostic exercise physiology in chronic heart failure. Heart. 2001; 86:17–20.
46. Bestetti A, Di Leo C, Alessi A, Triulzi A, Tagliabue L, Tarolo GL. Post-stress end-systolic left ventricular dilation: a marker of endocardial post-ischemic stunning. Nucl Med Commun. 2000;22:685–93.
47. Fisman EZ, Pelliccia A, Motro M, Auerbach I, Frank AG, Tenenbaum A. Effect of intensive resistance training on isotonic exercise Doppler indexes of left ventricular systolic function. Am J Cardiol. 2002; 89:887–91.
48. Hadjis T, Jobin J, Bourbeau J, Desagagnés P, Juneau L, Sampalis J. Aortic flow velocity indices during upright exercise: reliability and relationship to cardiac output. Can J Cardiol. 1995;11:100–4.
49. Sagiv M, Ben-Gal S, Ben-Sira D. Effects of gradient and load carried on human haemodynamic responses during treadmill walking. Eur J Appl Physiol. 2000;83:47–50.
50. Sagiv M, Sagiv A, Ben-Sira D, Ben-Gal S, Soudry M. Effects of chronic overload training and aging on left ventricular systolic function. Gerontology. 1997;43:307–15.
51. Ben-Sira D, Sagiv M. The effect of gender on left ventricular function immediately after the wingate test. Eur J Appl Physiol Occup Physiol. 1997;75:549–53.
52. Zile MR, Brutsaert DL. New concepts in diastolic dysfunction and diastolic heart failure: part I: diagnosis, prognosis, and measurements of diastolic function. Circulation. 2002;105:1387–93.
53. Zile MR, Brutsaert DL. New concepts in diastolic dysfunction and diastolic heart failure: part II: causal mechanisms and treatment. Circulation. 2002;105:1503–8.

54. Libonati JR. Myocardial diastolic function and exercise. Med Sci Sports Exerc. 1999;31:1741–7.
55. Barmeyer A, Müllerleile K, Mortensen K, Meinertz T. Diastolic dysfunction in exercise and its role for exercise capacity. Heart Fail Rev. 2009;14:125–34.
56. Eriksson SV, Caidahl K, de Faire U, Lindvall K, Rehnqvist N, Hamsten A. Diastolic and systolic function as predictors of exercise capacity after myocardial infarction in young men. Cardiology. 1998;90: 8–12.
57. Vinereanu D, Florescu N, Sculthorpe N, Tweddel AC, Stephens MR, Fraser AG. Left ventricular long-axis diastolic function is augmented in the hearts of endurance-trained compared with strength-trained athletes. Clin Sci (Lond). 2002;103:249–57.
58. Grewal J, McCully RB, Kane GC, Lam C, Pellikka PA. Left ventricular function and exercise capacity. JAMA. 2009;301:286–94.
59. Witte KK, Nikitin NP, De Silva R, Cleland JG, Clark AL. Exercise capacity and cardiac function assessed by tissue Doppler imaging in chronic heart failure. Heart. 2004;90:1144–50.
60. Abinader EG, Sharif D, Sagiv M, Goldhammer E. The effects of isometric stress on left ventricular filling in athletes with isometric or isotonic training compared to hypertensive and normal controls. Eur Heart J. 1996;17:457–61.
61. Stoddard MF, Pearson AC, Kern MJ, Ratcliff J, Mrosek DG, Labovitz AJ. Influence of alteration in preload on the pattern of left ventricular diastolic filling as assessed by Doppler echocardiography in humans. Circulation. 1989;79:1226–36.
62. González-Alonso J, Mortensen SP, Jeppesen TD, et al. Haemodynamic responses to exercise, ATP infusion and thigh compression in humans: insight into the role of muscle mechanisms on cardiovascular function. J Physiol. 2008;586:2405–17.
63. Randhawa AK, Singal PK. Pressure overload-induced cardiac hypertrophy with and without dilation. J Am Coll Cardiol. 1992;20:1569–75.
64. Wilmore JH, Costill DL. Physiology of sport and exercise. 3rd ed. Champaign: Human Kinetics; 2005.
65. Naylor LH, George K, O'Driscoll G, Green DJ. The athlete's heart: a contemporary appraisal of the 'morganroth hypothesis'. Sports Med. 2008;38:69–90.
66. D'Andrea A, Limongelli G, Caso P, et al. Association between left ventricular structure and cardiac performance during effort in two morphological forms of athlete's heart. Int J Cardiol. 2002;86:177–84.
67. Mitchell JH, Haskel W, Snel P, Van Camp SP. Task force 8: classification of sports. In: Maron BJ, Zfpes DP, editors. 36th Bethesda conference: eligibility recommendations for competitive athletes with cardiovascular abnormalities. J Am Colle Cardiol. 2005;45: 1364–7.
68. Vitcenda M, Hanson P, Folts J, Besozzi M. Impairment of left ventricular function during maximal isometric dead lifting. J Appl Physiol. 1990;69:2062–6.
69. Clifford PS, Hanel B, Secher NH. Arterial blood pressure response to rowing. Med Sci Sports Exerc. 1994;26:715–9.
70. Briton SL, Koch LG. Animal genetic models for complex traits of physical capacity. Exerc Sport Sci Rev. 2001;1:7–14.
71. Breisblatt WM, Wolf CJ, McElhinny B, Salerni R, Smith VE. Comparison of ambulatory left ventricular ejection fraction and blood pressure in systemic hypertension in patients with and without increased left ventricular mass. Am J Cardiol. 1991;67: 597–603.
72. Storto G, Nicolai E, Petretta M, et al. Cardiac performance during exercise in hypertensive patients without ventricular hypertrophy. Eur J Clin Invest. 2009;39: 664–70.
73. Sagiv M. Genome and left ventricular mass response to various exercise modes in health and disease. Med Sport. 2001;54:277–9.
74. Richey PA, Brown SP. Pathological versus physiological left ventricular hypertrophy: a review. J Sports Sci. 1998;16:129–41.
75. Tomaselli GF, Marbán E. Electrophysiological remodeling in hypertrophy and heart failure. Cardiovasc Res. 1999;42:270–83.
76. Bouchard C, Rankinen T, Simoneau JA, et al. Genomic scan for maximal oxygen uptake and its response to training in the heritage family study. J Appl Physiol. 2000;88:551–9.
77. Fatini C, Guazzelli R, Manetti P, et al. RAS genes influence exercise-induced left ventricular hypertrophy: an elite athletes study. Med Sci Sports Exerc. 2000;32:1868–72.
78. Montgomery HE, Clarkson P, Dollery CM, et al. Association of angiotensin-converting enzyme gene I/D polymorphism with change in left ventricular mass in response to physical training. Circulation. 1997;96:741–7.
79. Dursunoglu D, Evrengül H, Tanriverdi H, Turgut G, Genç O, Kaftan HA. Angiotensin-converting enzyme polymorphism in healthy young subjects: relationship to left ventricular mass and functions. Acta Cardiol. 2005;60:153–8.
80. Kasikcioglu E, Kayserilioglu A, Ciloglu F, Akhan H, Oflaz H, Yildiz S, et al. Angiotensin-converting enzyme gene polymorphism, left ventricular remodeling, and exercise capacity in strength-trained athletes. Heart Vessels. 2004;19:287–93.
81. Sagiv M, Shapiro Y, Ben-Sira D, Shapira H. Effect of isometric vs. running training on left ventricular and hemodynamic alterations at rest on healthy adolescent girls. Int J Cardiol. 1986;1:30–4.
82. Miller DD, Ruddy TD, Zusman CM, Okada RD, Strauss HW, Kanarek W, et al. Left ventricular ejection fraction responses during exercise in asymptomatic systemic hypertension. Am J Cardiol. 1987;59:409–13.
83. Maron BJ, Pelliccia A. The heart of trained athletes: cardiac remodeling and the risks of sports, including sudden death. Circulation. 2006;114:1633–44.

84. Fagard F. Athlete's heart. Heart. 2003;89:1455–61.
85. Atchley Jr AE, Douglas PS. Left ventricular hypertrophy in athletes: morphologic features and clinical correlates. Cardiol Clin. 2007;25:371–82.
86. Pelliccia A, Di Paolo FM, Maron BJ. The athlete's heart: remodeling, electrocardiogram and preparticipation screening. Cardiol Rev. 2002;10:85–90.
87. Perseghin G, De Cobelli F, Esposito A, et al. Effect of the sporting discipline on the right and left ventricular morphology and function of elite male track runners: a magnetic resonance imaging and phosphorus 31 spectroscopy study. Am Heart J. 2007;154:937–94.
88. Pelliccia A, Maron BJ. Outer limits of the athlete's heart, the effect of gender, and relevance to the differential diagnosis with primary cardiac diseases. Cardiol Clin. 1997;15:381–96.
89. Spirito P, Pellicia A, Proschan MA, et al. Morphology of the "athlete's heart" assessed by echocardiography in 947 elite athletes representing 27 sports. Am J Cardiol. 1994:74:802–6. Fagard RH. Impact of different sports and training on cardiac structure and function. Cardiol Clin. 1997;15:397–412.
90. Palmieri V, Bella JN, DeQuattro V, et al. Relations of diastolic left ventricular filling to systolic chamber and myocardial contractility in hypertensive patients with left ventricular hypertrophy (the PRESERVE study). Am J Cardiol. 1999;84:558–62.
91. Wachtell K, Papademetriou V, Smith G, et al. Relation of impaired left ventricular filling to systolic midwall mechanics in hypertensive patients with normal left ventricular systolic chamber function: the Losartan Intervention for Endpoint Reduction in Hypertension (LIFE) study. Am Heart J. 2004;148:538–44.
92. Belardinelli R, Georgiou D, Purcaro A. Low dose dobutamine echocardiography predicts improvement in functional capacity after exercise training in patients with ischemic cardiomyopathy: prognostic implication. J Am Coll Cardiol. 1998;31:1027–34.

Blood Pressure and Hypertension

6

Introduction

Physical inactivity increases the risk of many chronic disorders. Numerous studies have convincingly demonstrated that undertaking and maintaining moderate levels of physical activity (e.g., brisk walking 3 h a week) greatly reduces the blood pressure. Constant and adequate pressure in the arterial system is required to drive blood into all of the organs. Abnormally low blood pressure results in inadequate perfusion of organs, while abnormally high blood pressure can cause heart disease, vascular disease, and stroke. Exercise may affect the risk of developing clinically manifested *coronary artery disease* through two mechanisms. One is a direct effect on the heart and circulation, such as increasing blood flow through collateral blood vessels or improving cardiac output. The other is an indirect impact through the effect of exercise on risk factors such as obesity, blood pressure, or blood concentration of lipoprotein fractions [1, 2].

Cardiovascular disease patients with cardiovascular risk factors may be characterized by function and structural vascular abnormalities. Vascular *endothelium* plays a fundamental role in modulating vascular tone and structure. The physiological production of the relaxing factors including *nitric oxide*, prostacyclin, and hyperpolarizing relaxing factors protects the vessel wall by antagonizing the first pathogenetic steps of atherosclerosis and thrombosis. With *atherosclerosis*, arteries are thickened and narrowed by fatty material and calcium. Narrowed arteries reduce blood flow and increase risks for heart attack, stroke, and other diseases. Endothelial cells may also produce endothelium-derived contracting factors [3]. Irregular endothelial function is largely related to hypertension. The endothelium-dependent vasodilation index has been consistently used in studies as an indicator of the endothelial function. This index seems to be capable of identifying high-risk patients. Endothelial damage and dysfunction (Fig. 6.1) is considered to be a major underlying mechanism for the elevated cardiovascular risk associated with increased adiposity [4].

Alterations in endothelial cells and stem/endothelial progenitor cell function associated with overweight and obesity predispose to

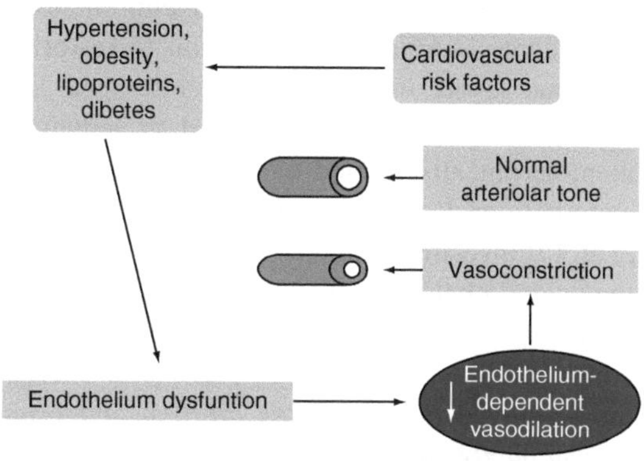

Fig. 6.1 Endothelium dysfunction resulting in an arterial vasoconstriction due to the presence of cardiovascular risk factors

M.S. Sagiv, *Exercise Cardiopulmonary Function in Cardiac Patients*,
DOI 10.1007/978-1-4471-2888-5_6, © Springer-Verlag London 2012

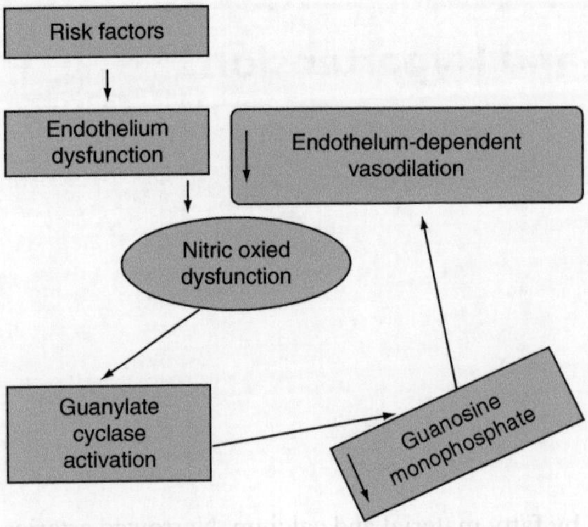

Fig. 6.2 Cardiovascular risk factors influence on endothelium-dependent vasodilation

atherosclerosis and thrombosis. *Endothelium* dysfunction is associated with smoking, excessive alcohol intake, *physical inactivity*, abdominal obesity, diabetes, hypertension, and decreased antioxidant defenses, all of which reduce nitric oxide production. Thus, guanylate cyclase activation by *nitric oxide* is impaired in individuals with *endothelial dysfunction*. For this reason, accumulation of cyclic guanosine monophosphate in the endothelium fails to occur, and consequently, the endothelium-dependent vasodilation is affected (Fig. 6.2).

Studies have verified that regular *aerobic exercise* may prevent the loss of endothelium-dependent vasodilation, in addition to restoring previous levels in sedentary middle-aged and elderly men [5]. When compared to sedentary men, aerobically trained men show a preserved endothelium-dependent vasodilation [6]. Luk et al. [7] investigated the effect of exercise training on endothelial function and exercise capacity in *coronary artery disease patients* compared to controls. Luk et al. suggested that exercise training improved *flow-mediated dilation* and *exercise capacity* in stable coronary artery disease patients independent of the changes in inflammation, oxidative stress, or endothelial progenitor cells. The beneficial effects of *exercise training* on flow-mediated dilation and exercise capacity are interrelated, and more pronounced in those with baseline impaired exercise capacity. Clarkson et al. [5] found positive results of a 10-week aerobic and *anaerobic exercise* training program in healthy military recruits. Training increased *endothelium-dependent vasodilation* in these individuals. In coronary artery disease, *aerobic exercise training* is associated with an improvement in endothelial function. In patients with recent acute myocardial infarction, aerobic exercise training is associated with improved endothelial function independently of the type of training, but this effect disappeared after 1 month of detraining [8]. This result suggests that even individuals with a history of a cardiac event may obtain improvement of the endothelial function.

Exercise Effects on Atherosclerosis

Atherosclerosis occurs when fat deposits, or plaque, line the walls of the arteries. It is also recognized as a chronic inflammatory disorder that results from the interactions between modified lipoproteins and various components of the immune system including monocyte-derived macrophages, T-lymphocytes, and a variety of cytokines secreted by these and other cells in the artery wall [9]. Many times, individuals with atherosclerosis do not have any symptoms until an artery is narrowed by 40%. Many factors contribute to the development of atherosclerosis, but the oxidation of the protein and lipid components of low-density lipoprotein particles is believed to be among the most important initiating events [9]. Plaque becomes thick and hard and narrows the course that blood flows in the arteries. Plaque causes arteries to become stiff and inflexible.

Risk factors for atherosclerosis include being male (if female, being past menopause), *hypertension*, high low-density *lipoprotein cholesterol* or *triglycerides* circulating in the blood, *diabetes*, being *overweight*, smoking, a family history of heart disease, sedentary lifestyle, and diets high in saturated fat and trans fatty acids. The exact cause of atherosclerosis is unknown, although it is believed that atherosclerosis begins with an injury in the endothelium. Although regular *physical activity* is recommended for prevention of cardiovascular diseases, no data are available on its antiatherosclerotic effects in the general population. Physical exercise is a deterrent of cardiovascular disease and atherogenesis in animal models [10]. Regular exercise is recommended for prevention of heart disease, but surprisingly, little long-term data document the effects of exercise on atherosclerosis progression. However, epidemiological studies suggested that a graded relationship of decreasing coronary artery disease rates with increasing levels of activity, demonstrating beneficial effects of exercise on atherosclerotic risk factors [11]. Moreover, there is an inverse association between intensity of physical activity and the risk of coronary heart disease events [12].

The accumulated data suggest that regular aerobic exercise imparts cardiovascular benefits and may even reduce the risk of coronary events [13]. However, it is also well recognized that physical exercise increase the metabolic rate of working muscles, which in turn leads to increase whole body VO2 associated with an increased production of reactive oxygen species [14]. The pathogenesis of atherosclerosis has been linked to oxidative damage [15]. Thus, the paradox of exercise reflects the balance between the cardiovascular benefits attributable to exercise and the potential risk of causing tissue injury and atherosclerosis. However, Wilund [16] suggested that engaging in regular physical activity reduces the risk of developing cardiovascular disease, but it is not certain to what degree this may be due to the anti-inflammatory effects of exercise. Following acute exercise, there is a transient increase in circulating levels of anti-inflammatory cytokines, whereas chronic exercise reduces basal levels of proinflammatory cytokines. Exercise training also induces the expression of antioxidant and anti-inflammatory mediators in the vascular wall that may directly inhibit the development of atherosclerosis. Beneficial effects of aerobic and resistive training on the immune system in elderly subjects were seen in elderly subjects exercising aerobically at 60–70% of their work capacity gain a statistically significant higher lymphocyte T cell function as compared with their resistive counterparts [17].

Rauramaa et al. found that aerobic physical exercise do not attenuate progression of atherosclerosis, except in a subgroup of men not taking statins [18]. One possible mechanism that helps to overcome the narrowing of the arteries is through moderate intensity aerobic exercise generating almost 1,000 kcal · week^{-1} that enhances endothelium-dependent vasodilation in humans and attenuates exercise-induced peroxidation and cardiovascular mortality in the elderly [19].

The magnitude of the exercise effect is influenced by characteristics of the exercise intervention, individual variation, and whether exercise produces concomitant reductions in body weight. Second possible mechanism is the increase in the diameter of large arterioles, small arteries, and conduit arteries following exercise training. In addition, another important aspect of exercise-induced changes in capillarity is the onset and persistence of exercise-induced arteriogenesis. The induction of arteriogenesis is an important vascular adaptation, since arteriogenesis leads to the formation of large conductance arteries capable of compensating for the loss of function of occluded arteries [20]. Exercise along with dietary changes may prevent atherosclerosis from developing. According to the National Heart Lung and Blood Institute, lifestyle changes might be the only atherosclerosis treatment that is needed. *Physical activity* prevents many established atherosclerotic risk factors, such as elevated *blood pressure*, *insulin resistance* and *glucose intolerance*, elevated *triglyceride* concentrations, low high-density *lipoprotein cholesterol* concentrations, and obesity [21]. In addition to all the benefits of exercise, regular physical activity also helps to increase production of *nitric oxide* in cells lining the arteries, and thus improve circulation, which is impaired by atherosclerosis. Exercise might also stimulate the creation of new cells that line arteries, replacing aging cells and repairing damaged arteries. Additionally, exercise reduces the risk of developing heart disease if atherosclerosis exists already. The physical activity effect on atherosclerotic risk factors can be large in some individuals and obviate the need for other interventions. In general, the effect of exercise on atherosclerotic risk factors is substantially less than that achieved by pharmacological therapies, although the exercise effect can be significantly magnified by other lifestyle changes such as changes in dietary composition and weight loss.

Blood Pressure During Aerobic Exercise

Blood pressure is the force that drives blood through the circulatory system and is influenced by *blood volume*, *cardiac output*, and *total peripheral resistance* (*TPR*). Pressure in the arterial system fluctuates with the cardiac cycle. Blood pressure reaches a peak in systole and is lowest in diastole. Therefore, blood flow between two points is directly proportion to the driving force (pressure) between them. Any changes in cardiac output or total peripheral resistance to blood flow and blood volume influences blood pressure as well as blood flow. Blood pressure is noted as two separate values: systolic and diastolic blood pressures. The *systolic blood pressure* represents the amount of pressure exerted against the aortic wall following the *left ventricular ejection*. The diastolic blood pressure value represents the amount of pressure exerted against the aortic wall before the left ventricular ejects. It is a very important physiological variable since it is the pressure that the left ventricular has to develop in order to eject against the pressure existing in the aorta. Therefore, low diastolic blood pressure means less pressure opposing left ventricular ejection. At rest, most of the blood resides in the venous system. With the onset of *aerobic exercise*, there is constriction of the *venous system* which increases blood return to the heart and in turn increases *stroke volume* as explained by the Frank-Starling principle. This is facilitated by both *sympathetic* and *catecholamine* hormonal stimulation which increases *heart rate* and left ventricular contractility.

During upright *aerobic exercise*, the increase in exercise *systolic blood pressure* varies between individuals [22], the normal blood pressure response is to observe a progressive and steadily increase in *systolic blood pressure*. In healthy males, it increases from about 112–120 mmHg at rest [23] to 180–190 mmHg or more during *maximal exercise*. It follows the same general trend as heart rate. *Maximum systolic pressure* in a normal person may be as little as 150 and no more than 220 mmHg. Therefore, it is essential that blood pressure be maintained within a narrow range of values that is consistent with the needs of the tissues. A failure of the systolic blood pressure to rise with an increase in intensity, called exertional hypotension, is considered abnormal and may occur in patients with number of cardiovascular problems. Following exercise, systolic blood pressure progressively declines during an active recovery. With a passive and seated recovery, systolic blood pressure may drop abruptly due to the pooling of blood in the peripheral areas of the body.

Diastolic blood pressure changes little during dynamic *aerobic exercise* in normal subjects. Normally, there is either no change or a slight decrease of less than 10 mmHg during exercise or may increase by 10–20 mmHg, presumably from the occlusion of blood flow caused by the forceful contractions of the exercising muscle [24]. The slight decrease in *diastolic blood pressure* is due primarily to the vasodilation of the arteries from the exercise bout. Thus, the expansion in artery diameter may lower blood pressure during the diastolic phase. An increase in diastolic blood pressure of more than 10 mmHg during or after *aerobic exercise* represents an unstable form of hypertension, and may be associated with *coronary artery disease*.

Following exercise, *blood pressure* rapidly returns to normal, caused by a pooling of blood in the dilated, previously exercised muscle beds. This pressure decrement is more pronounced following *intense exercise*. The baroreceptors work to counter the circulating vasodilatory substances to initially return homeostasis within 10 min following exercise. However, there may also be a drop in diastolic blood pressure called post-exercise hypotension during the *recovery phase* of exercise due to the *vasodilation*.

Post-exercise Hypotension

Post-exercise hypotension is a phenomenon of a prolonged decrease in resting *blood pressure* in the minutes and up to 7–12 h following acute exercise. However, its occurrence in *normotensive* humans is inconsistent. Although post-exercise hypotension can be detected in normotensive individuals [25], it was found to be much less consistent and of lesser magnitude than in hypertensive individuals.

This may be due to other compensatory mechanisms, such as the *baroreflex*, that are activated in normotensive subjects, and prevent the degree of *post-exercise hypotension* from affecting orthostatic tolerance [26]. Although the mechanisms of the vasodilation underlying post-exercise hypotension are poorly understood, the sympathetic nervous system [27], baroreflex resetting [27], nitric oxide [28], and an unknown vasodilator have all been implicated [29].

Several mechanisms have been proposed to account for this post-exercise hypotension including the release of vasodilator metabolites from the exercising muscle, resetting of the baroreflex control of sympathetic tone and inhibition of muscle *sympathetic nervous activity*. A further possibility relates to the need to dissipate heat accumulated during the exercise period [30]. The amount of pressure reduction appears to be dependent on the *intensity of the exercise* performed, the *mode of exercise*, *duration*, and the recovery *posture* of the individual. The greater the exercise intensity performed, the lower the blood pressure value following exercise. Furthermore, *cycling* and *heavy resistance training* with the quadriceps, probably due to the very large increase in muscle blood flow to the legs, is associated with a greater hypotensive effect than is seen following running. However, the largest reductions in pressure are observed in those individuals who have stopped exercise and stood motionless in an *upright position*. Another explanation for the *hypotensive* effect following exercise is the changes in *plasma volume*. As exercise begins, the increase in blood pressure forces water to leave the cardiovascular system to the extracellular compartment which in turn increases *albuminous concentration* of the blood. At the cessation of exercise, water returns to the cardiovascular system due to *osmotic pressure*.

Although there are reports of *gender* differences in *blood pressure* and sympathetic nerve activity, post-exercise hypotension appears to be unaffected by gender, since gender-specific and mixed-gender studies have found similar degrees of *hypotension*. It also occurs independent of *age*, having been observed in young middle-aged and older adults [26]. After a single bout of dynamic exercise, there are profound changes in the mechanisms that regulate and determine arterial pressure, resulting in a post-exercise hypotension that lasts nearly 2 h in sedentary but otherwise healthy individuals [29]. In sedentary individuals, post-exercise hypotension after a single bout of aerobic exercise is due to a peripheral vasodilation. Endurance exercise training has the potential to modify this response and perhaps reduce the degree of post-exercise hypotension. The magnitude of post-exercise hypotension is similar in sedentary and endurance-trained men and women but that endurance-trained men and women achieve this fall in pressure via different mechanisms. In sedentary men and women, hypotension was the result of vasodilation, while in endurance-trained men, hypotension was the result of a reduced cardiac output [31].

Resistive exercise elicits more pronounced increments in both systolic and diastolic blood pressure. *Systolic* and *diastolic* blood pressures rise rapidly to extremely high values during the *concentric contraction* phase for each lift and decline with the *eccentric contraction*. The greatest peak pressures occur during the *double-leg press* where the mean value is 320/250 mmHg, with pressures in one subject exceeding 480/350 mmHg. Peak pressures with the *single-arm curl* exercise reached a mean group value of 255/190 mmHg when repetitions were continued to failure. A portion of the observed increase in *blood pressure* was caused by a *Valsalva maneuver*. Thus, the mechanical compression of blood vessels during weight-lifting exercises combined with a potent *pressor response* and a *Valsalva response* produces extreme elevations in blood pressure. Pressures are extreme even when exercise is performed with a relatively small *muscle mass* [26, 32].

Narloch and Brandstater have suggested that during *heavy weight lifting*, the extreme pressure values seen with Valsalva are dramatically reduced when the exercise is performed without Valsalva maneuver [33]. The changes in blood pressure during *resistance exercise* are oscillatory and related to the phase of the lift. Blood pressure increases to maximal values as determined by the resistance encountered during the lifting phase. Pressure then declines, often to below resting values at the completion of the lift, and then increases again during the lowering phase of the exercise [34]. The restoration of baseline blood pressure is similar to that of *endurance exercise*, although the transient pressure is often more pronounced following heavy resistance exercise.

During *anaerobic bouts*, systolic, diastolic, and *mean arterial blood pressures* values are higher than that of *aerobic exercise* and lower than during *weight lifting* [35].

From the above values, it can be concluded that the type of exercise influences blood pressure responses. Activities such as dynamic aerobic which are rhythmic in nature cause less increase in blood pressure than activities that are static or involve slow muscular movements such as weight lifting. By contracting the muscles, there is a temporarily slower or even stop in blood flow through the tissues until relaxation occurs. This temporarily increases blood resistance and pressure. When performing aerobic exercise, muscles alternately contract and relax; it is during the relaxation phase in which muscle blood flow is restored and resistance decreased. However, an individual performing a heavy, *isometric contraction* will have a greater rise in *blood pressure* due to the higher *resistance* to *blood flow* by the contracting muscles.

Post-exercise hypotension has been consistently seen in hypertension and pre-hypertension but has been inconsistently observed in normal individuals. There are many reasons why exercise may work as a treatment for hypertensive patients. Post-exercise hypotension is a prolonged decrease in blood pressure following acute exercise during which total peripheral resistance is reduced and it remains reduced post-exercise. This can be a main factor influencing post-exercise hypotension [26]. The short-term reduction in blood pressure after exercise can be seen even in elderly hypertensive patients. This decrease is associated with a decrease in stroke volume and left ventricular end-diastolic volume. The 22-h post-exercise reduction in blood pressure demonstrates the clinical relevance of aerobic type exercise in elderly hypertensive patients [36]. The diagnostic value of the post-exercise hypotension in evaluating the presence of coronary artery disease was studied on 82 subjects with normal blood pressure and 24 patients with hypertension; all had significant narrow coronary arteries (patients with coronary artery disease). It was concluded that the post-exercise hypotension response is useful for detecting coronary artery disease in patients with and without hypertension and for evaluating the severity of coronary artery disease [37].

Mean Arterial Blood Pressure

Due to the differences of blood pressure (systolic – diastolic), it is important to calculate mean arterial blood pressure (MABP) that represents the average pressure in the arterial system. This value is important because it is the difference between mean arterial pressure and the venous pressure that drives blood through the capillaries of the organs. Because more time is spent in diastole than in systole, mean arterial pressure is not simply the average of the systolic and diastolic pressures. During *aerobic exercise*, *mean arterial blood pressure* increases from about 93 mmHg at rest to about 120 mmHg at *maximal*

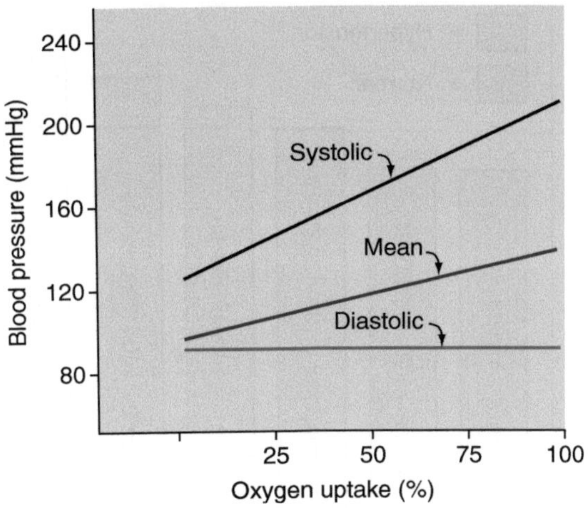

Fig. 6.3 Systolic, diastolic, and mean arterial blood pressure responses during dynamic aerobic exercise in healthy normal subjects

exercise (Fig. 6.3), while during weight lifting, it reaches 293 mmHg and an intra-arterial measurement of 132 mmHg during dynamic anaerobic effort [35].

Mean arterial blood pressure is calculated as follows (Eq. 6.1):

$$\text{MABP} = 1/3(\text{SBP} - \text{DBP}) + \text{DPB} \quad (6.1)$$

where MABP = mean arterial blood pressure, SBP = systolic blood pressure, and DBP = diastolic blood pressure.

The three most important variables effecting mean arterial blood pressure are total peripheral resistance, cardiac output, and blood volume. Therefore (Eq. 6.2):

$$\text{MABP} = Q \cdot \text{TPR} \quad (6.2)$$

where MABP = mean arterial blood pressure, Q = cardiac output, and TPR = total peripheral resistance.

Blood vessels provide resistance to the flow of blood because of friction between moving blood and the wall of the vessel. The *total peripheral resistance* refers to the sum total of vascular resistance to the flow of blood in the systemic circulation. Because of their small radius, arterioles provide the greatest resistance to blood flow in the arterial system. Adjustment in the radius of arterioles has a significant effect on total peripheral resistance, which in turn has a significant effect on *mean arterial blood pressure*. *Resistance* and *pressure* are directly proportional to each other. If resistance increases, then pressure increases. When the radius of arterioles decrease with vasoconstriction, total peripheral resistance increases, which causes mean arterial blood pressure to increase.

The *cardiac output* is a measure of *blood flow* into the *arterial system*. Blood flow is directly proportional to pressure (Eq. 6.3).

$$\text{Flow} = \text{pressure/resistance} \quad (6.3)$$

Therefore, an increase in flow (*cardiac output*) will cause an increase in mean arterial blood pressure. *Blood volume* is directly related *to blood pressure*. If the blood volume is increased, then *venous return* of blood to the heart will increase. An increase in venous return will, by *Starling's Law*, cause *stroke volume* to increase. As stroke volume goes up, the *cardiac output* goes up and the blood pressure rises. Thus, one way to control blood pressure over the long term is to control blood volume.

Hypertension and Arterial Baroreceptors

Constant and adequate pressure in the *arterial system* is required to drive blood into all of the organs. Abnormally low blood pressure results in inadequate *perfusion* of organs, while abnormally high *blood pressure* can cause heart disease, vascular disease, and stroke. Therefore, it is essential that *blood pressure* be maintained within a narrow range of values that is consistent with the needs of the tissues. Therefore, an individual's blood pressure is controlled on a second to second basis by a servo-mechanism known as the arterial *baroreceptors* or *baroreflex*. All forms of exercise result in disturbance of systemic blood pressure and thus of the mechanisms that tend to maintain blood pressure at steady state level. Abnormal changes are in the baroreflex arch in

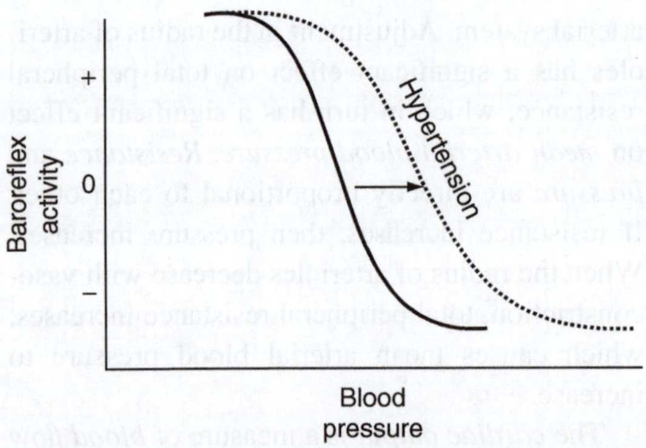

Fig. 6.4 Changes in baroreflex sensitivity and the set point in hypertension (*arrow*). Relationships between the baroreflex arch increase activity (+) and reduced activity (–)

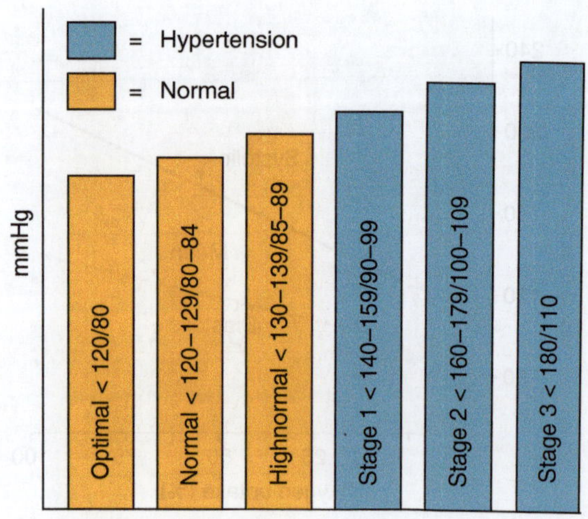

Fig. 6.5 Classification of blood pressure for adults aged 18 years and older with values for normal and abnormal (hypertension) systolic and diastolic blood pressures

hypertensive patients. The first change that the baroreflex causes is the increase levels of blood pressure by changing the set point. Once this point is set, the baroreflex sensitivity for changing the blood pressure is reduced, which thereafter, only significant changes in blood pressures activate it again to increase or reduce blood pressure. The baroreflex controls blood pressure levels mainly through changes in heart rate. For that, heart rate is a variable that expresses baroreflex sensitivity and activity (Fig. 6.4). One of the main mechanisms that bring change in the new baroreflex set point is angiotensin II, via the teorema area since this peptide cannot cross the barrier-blood brain. By changing the set point affects the sympathetic tone to the kidney which in turn activates the rennin and reduces potassium secretion.

Hypertension, when undetected and untreated, may lead to a number of abnormal problems. It is defined as resting systolic and/or diastolic blood pressure greater than 140/90 mmHg. The heart may possibly begin to increase in size, which eventually can cause heart failure. The brain's blood vessels can develop aneurisms, which can lead to a stroke. Finally, *hypertension* may also lead to a stiffening of the arteries. [38]. Figure 6.5 reveals that hypertension patients compared to normal subjects demonstrated different and significantly higher values of systolic and diastolic blood pressure [39].

Arterial baroreceptors play a pivotal role in the rapid reflex adjustments that accompany acute cardiovascular stressors by buffering beat-to-beat fluctuations in *blood pressure* via modulation of autonomic neural activity to the heart and vasculature [40]. *During exercise*, it has been demonstrated that the arterial baroreceptors continues to regulate blood pressure by resetting to operate around the exercise-induced elevation in blood pressure [41]. Moreover, there is convincing evidence that a properly functioning arterial baroreflex is requisite for an appropriate neural cardiovascular response to exercise. The *sympathetic nervous system* plays a critical role in mediating the cardiovascular adjustments necessary for performing and sustaining exercise including increases in *heart rate*, *stroke volume* and arterial blood pressure, and a redistribution of *cardiac output* to active skeletal muscle. Exercise-induced increases in sympathetic nerve activity are mediated by central signals arising from higher brain centers, that is, central command and by peripheral feedback from skeletal muscle, that is, exercise pressor reflex with important modulation provided by the arterial baroreflex.

The *exercise stimuli* exert a powerful drive to elevate *blood pressure* in health and disease.

The *arterial baroreceptors* and the reflexes evoked by activation of those afferent nerve endings in the working *skeletal muscles* are sensitive to metabolic changes (*metaboreflex*) moreover to interact in ways that lead to modulation of the primary cardiovascular reflex responses [42]. This may possibly be facilitated by spinal *sympatho-sympathetic reflexes* arising from the heart and aorta. The role of the *Bainbridge reflex* as a feed-forward mechanism in exercise remains unclear. Other, homeostatic, reflexes may modulate the pressor effects of the exercise stimuli. The balance of evidence strongly suggests that the arterial baroreceptors are still able to restrain disturbances of blood pressure during exercise, even though their control of *heart rate* is modified. *Vagally* innervated cardiopulmonary, and especially *left ventricular*, receptors may also subserve buffer reflexes in exercise, but whether their thresholds are reached has not been determined.

Baroreceptors detect the level of *blood pressure* and pass on information to the cardiovascular control centre in the brain. At the start of *exercise*, the level of required pressure is set to a higher value in the brain's control center. At this time, the *baroreceptors* detect and relay the measured pressure to the brain, but because of the large increase in *muscle blood flow*, this measured pressure is well below the new level required. In order to correct the difference, nerve impulses are sent to the heart to increase *heart rate*, *stroke volume*, and *cardiac output* in order to maintain *blood pressure* at the necessary level.

During submaximal and maximal dynamic exercise, the *baroreflex* remains active in controlling the level of blood pressure. However, *during exercise*, the required pressure is reset to a much greater value than for rest. The level to which blood pressure is reset during exercise is dependent upon the *work intensity* performed and the extent of *arteriole vasodilatation*. *Blood flow* changes remarkably to exercising muscle which, at maximal effort, can increase up to 35-fold. Such a large increase in *blood flow* has severe consequences for blood pressure regulation, as the onset of this large-scale circulation can result in a sudden and substantial drop in pressure. This *vasodilatation* phenomenon forces the heart to increase *cardiac output* significantly and thus considerably raising *systolic blood pressure* in order to maintain appropriate blood pressure and, at the same time, to supply as much blood and oxygen as possible to the working muscles. Therefore, the increase in systolic blood pressure is mainly due to *volume overload*. Thus, the linear increases in heart rate and cardiac output that are observed during dynamic exercise can be explained by the need to maintain blood pressure at a new set point, rather than solely by the need to increase muscle blood flow to allow the delivery of nutrients for metabolism. There is also a small decrease during recovery of less than 4 mmHg (post-exercise hypotension). A significant increase in diastolic pressure (>15 mmHg or above 120 mmHg) is associated with a greater prevalence of *coronary artery disease*. It seems that the *autoregulation mechanism* is responsible for keeping *diastolic blood pressure* values similar and sometimes lower than those measured at rest.

Blood Pressure Adaptations to Resistive Training

Static exercise is associated with a resetting of the operating range and an increase in the reflex gain of the *arterial baroreflex* control of muscle *sympathetic nerve activity* [43]. *During isometric* muscle activity, large increases in *systolic* and *diastolic* blood pressures are noted resulting in increased *mean arterial blood pressure*, which is seemingly inappropriate to the metabolic demand (Fig. 6.6).

This phenomenon, known as a *pressor response*, is characterized by a sustained rise in systolic and diastolic blood pressure to higher levels than during *dynamic exercise* at an equal level of exertion and cardiac output demand. The abrupt and sharp increase in blood pressure occurs in contractions above 20–30% of *maximal voluntary contraction* (*MVC*). This pressor response is a result of the small increase in *cardiac output* (9–12 L · min^{-1}) due to the moderate increase in *heart rate*, and without significant

Fig. 6.6 Systolic, diastolic, and mean arterial blood pressure responses to isometric bout at percentage of maximal voluntary contraction

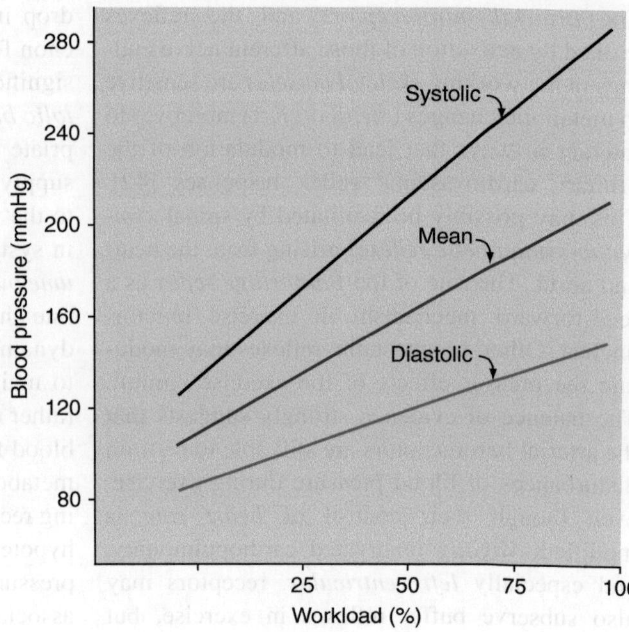

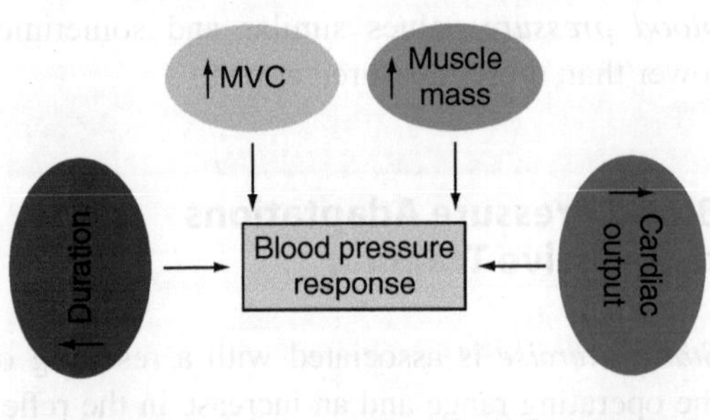

Fig. 6.7 Relations between physiological variables that influence blood pressure response during isometric exercise: muscle mass exercise duration and maximal voluntary contraction (*MVC*)

change in *total peripheral resistance*, and with possible *vasoconstriction* in nonactive muscles due in part to the reflex mechanism originating in active muscles. It has been found that the *pressor response* to *isometric work* increases proportionally to the intensity of contraction, muscle mass involved, and duration along the integrity of the sensor pathway from active muscles [44].

Figure 6.7 summarizes the effects and relationships between cardiac output, *muscle mass*, percentage of maximal voluntary contraction, and exercise duration on *blood pressure* during isometric exercise.

During a resistive exercise bout, systolic and diastolic blood pressures may show dramatic increases, which suggest that caution should be observed in persons with cardiovascular disease, or known risk factors. The extent of the increase in blood pressure is dependent on the time the contraction is held, the intensity of the contraction, and the amount of muscle mass involved in the contraction [44]. More dynamic forms of resistance training, such as circuit training, that involve moderate resistance and high repetitions with short rests are associated with reductions in blood pressure; others have shown decreases in diastolic blood pressure [45], or no change in blood pressure [46], and decreases in systolic blood pressure. The effects of resistance training on blood pressure are varied due largely to differences in study design, which suggests that more research is necessary to clearly understand the role of resistance training in blood pressure management. Thus, even though those studies have shown that resistance training improves blood pressure in people with borderline hypertension [47], many are still concerned that blood pressure may rise to dangerous levels during the workout itself. A study that followed 10 experimental and 16 control subjects through 9 weeks of resistance training found marked increases in strength, but more importantly, the conclusion was that circuit weight training did not exacerbate resting or exercise blood pressure [45].

Anaerobic Bout

During *all out physical activity* (*anaerobic bout*), it is almost impossible to determine *blood pressure* value utilizing the conventional indirect sphygmomanometer. Such an activity is the Wingate anaerobic test, which is characterized by exposing the subjects to an all-out strenuous exercise on a cycle ergometer [48]. Measurements comparing auscultation and intra-arterial values reveal that systolic blood pressure can be measured indirectly at peak anaerobic exercise with satisfactory results. However, at peak all-out anaerobic exercise, the *indirect method* is not valid for the assessment of *diastolic blood pressure* [35].

Although *anaerobic exercise* is dynamic in nature, *blood pressures* responses are similar to those seen during *isometric exercise*, that is, systolic and diastolic blood pressures are increased and thus mean arterial blood pressure (Fig. 6.8). Figure 6.9 summarizes the effects and relationships between *blood volume*, *heart rate*, *stroke volume*, *total peripheral resistance*, and viscosity on blood pressure at rest and during *dynamic aerobic* and *anaerobic exercises*. *Viscosity* or thickness of the fluid gets thicker; the result is an increase in blood pressure. Certain medical conditions can change the viscosity of the blood. For instance, low *red blood cell* concentration, *anemia*, reduces viscosity, whereas increased red blood cell concentration increases viscosity.

In practice, each individual's *autonomic nervous system* responds to and regulates all these interacting factors so that, although the above issues are important, the actual *blood pressure* response of a given individual varies widely because of both split-second and slow-moving responses of the nervous system and end organs. These responses are very effective in changing the variables and resulting blood pressure from moment to moment.

With the *cessation of the dynamic aerobic exercise*, there are rapid and large changes in the return of blood to the heart. This is because once the muscles have stopped contracting, there is no muscle pump action to massage blood back to

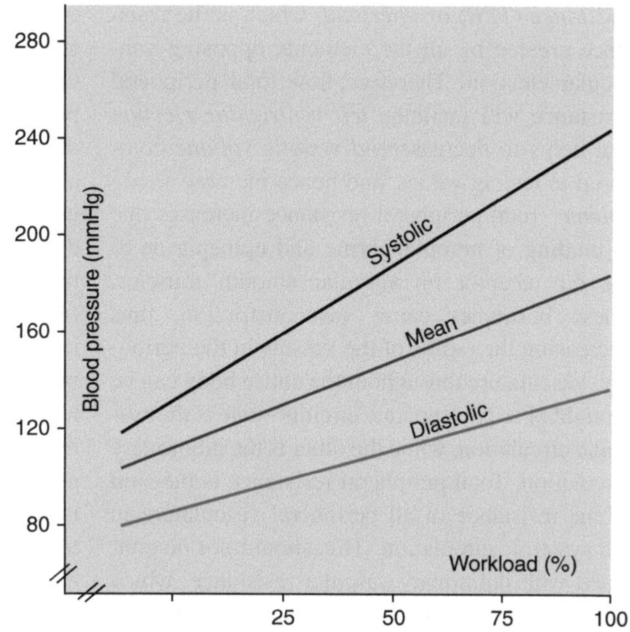

Fig. 6.8 Systolic, diastolic, and mean arterial blood pressure responses to anaerobic bout at percentage of maximal workload

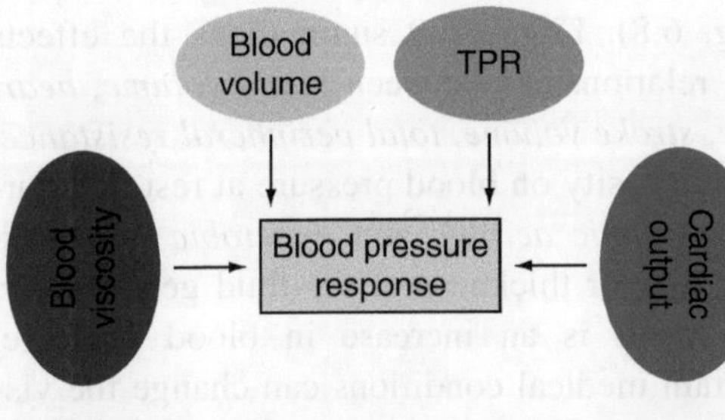

Fig. 6.9 Relations between physiological variables that influence blood pressure response at rest and during aerobic and anaerobic exercises. *TPR* total peripheral resistance

the heart (venous return), and therefore blood remains in the active limbs. If the removal of the muscle pump is combined with an upright posture, the influence of *metabolites* such as *lactic acid*, and elevated body *core temperature*, it will be quite possible that the individual will experience *hypotension* and symptoms of fainting. Values of *post-exercise hypotension* decline between 5 and 20 mmHg compared to pre-exercise values.

Total Peripheral Resistance

The changes in systolic, diastolic, and mean arterial blood pressures influence *total peripheral resistance* (*TPR*) *or afterload*, which is the resistance created by all the elements opposing ventricular ejection. Therefore, low total peripheral resistance will facilitate *left ventricular ejection* that helps to decrease *end-systolic volume* compared to resting values, and hence increase *stroke volume*. Total peripheral resistance increases due to binding of norepinephrine and epinephrine to the $\alpha 1$ receptor on vascular smooth muscles. These hormones cause vasoconstriction, thus decreasing the radius of the vessels in the periphery. Vasculature throughout the entire body can be thought of as two separate circuits – one is the systemic circulation, while the other is the pulmonary circulation. Total peripheral resistance is the sum of the resistance of all peripheral vasculature in the systemic circulation. This should not be confused with pulmonary vascular resistance, which is the resistance in the pulmonary circulation. Total peripheral resistance is represented mathematically by Eqs. 6.4 and 6.5:

$$\mathrm{TPR} = \Delta P / Q. \tag{6.4}$$

or

$$\mathrm{TPR} = (\mathrm{MABP} - \mathrm{MVP})/Q \tag{6.5}$$

Total peripheral resistance can be calculated also as follows (Eq. 6.6):

$$\mathrm{TPR} = (\mathrm{MABP} \cdot 80) / Q \tag{6.6}$$

where TPR = total peripheral resistance, MABP = mean arterial blood pressure, MVP = mean venous pressure, Q = cardiac output; 80 is a constant number.

In young and elderly healthy subjects and coronary artery disease patients (without hypertension), *total peripheral resistance* values at rest is approximately 1,400 dyn · s^{-1} · cm^{-5}. *During aerobic exercise*, values are around 400 dyn · s^{-1} · cm^{-5} [49]. This change occurs because of the tremendous increase in blood flow to working skeletal muscles created by a fivefold increase in cardiac output. Even though systolic blood pressure increases, total peripheral resistance may fall to a one third of the resting values during exercise. Vasoconstriction in nonexercising tissue is not enough to compensate for the vasodilatation in active muscles. The reduced total peripheral resistance during exercise helps to decrease forces opposing left ventricular ejection and end-systolic volume compared to resting values, and hence increase stroke volume. During dynamic *anaerobic bout*, total peripheral resistance values are reduced to 700 dyn · s^{-1} · cm^{-5} [49]. However, this reduction is not similar to the level observed at peak dynamic *aerobic exercise*, but still, during anaerobic exercise, values are lower than that obtained during *isometric exercise* (1,600 dyn · s^{-1} · cm^{-5}). Nevertheless, they are lower than 1,600 dyn · s^{-1} · cm^{-5} seen during isometric exercise [50]. Young and older hypertensive patients did not reduce their total peripheral resistance from resting values 2,049 dyn · s^{-1} · cm^{-5} to cycling bout 2,046 dyn · s^{-1} · cm^{-5} [51].

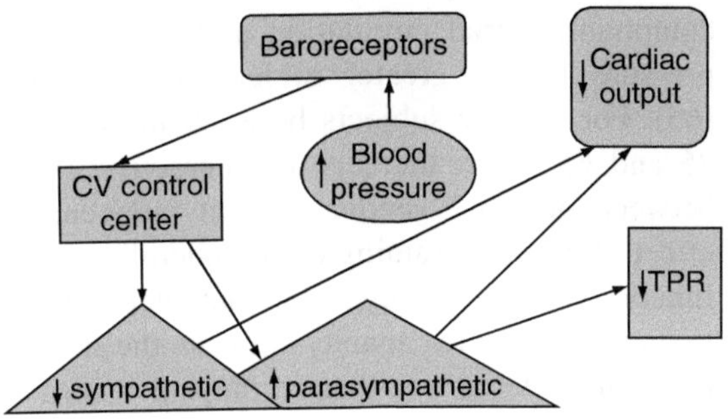

Fig. 6.10 With increased blood pressure, the baroreceptors brings about a reduction in cardiac output and total peripheral resistance (*TPR*) via the autonomic nervous system mainly by reducing heart rate

An increase in blood pressure causes an increase in action potentials sent to the cardiovascular control center.

The cardiovascular control center responds by decreasing sympathetic input and increasing parasympathetic input to the heart. This causes a drop in heart rate and stroke volume, and thus lowers cardiac output. This in turn lowers *mean arterial blood pressure*. The cardiovascular control center also decreases sympathetic input to the blood vessels. This causes *vasodilation*, which lowers resistance and causes blood pressure to drop. Overall, the compensatory mechanisms of the *baroreceptor reflex* act to restore blood pressure back to normal (Fig. 6.10). Conversely, a decrease in *blood pressure* results in a decrease in action potentials sent to the *cardiovascular control center*, which gives rise in *sympathetic input*, which brings about vasoconstriction and increased cardiac output, which causes a rise in blood pressure, thus restoring blood pressure back to normal.

Arterials and Aortic Stiffening

The high prevalence of hypertension imposes a considerable public health problem, and therefore, prevention of hypertension is a major public health objective. Hypertension is a serious health problem that increases the risk of aortic stiffness. These increases in arterial stiffness are thought to contribute to age-related increases in the incidence of cardiovascular disease [52].

Arterial stiffness may predict coronary heart disease beyond classic risk factors. In a longitudinal study, the predictive value of arterial stiffness on coronary heart disease in patients with essential hypertension and without known clinical cardiovascular disease has been assessed [53]. It was found that measurements of arterial stiffness correlate significantly with those of endothelial function, mainly influenced by the relationship of angiotensin-converting enzyme (a key component in the rennin-angiotensin system) and bradykinin. Data show that different molecular mechanisms are responsible for the hypertension and aortic stiffness seen in elderly and in cardiac patients. Moreover, there is growing evidence for a genetic contribution to the pathophysiology of hypertension and aortic stiffness. Genetic studies may help to understand the mechanisms underlying the involvement of the rennin-angiotensin system in arterial regulation. Therefore, *exercise training* has an important role as a primary prevention tool to aortic stiffness. Hypertension may produce *arterial stiffening* by both functional and structural mechanisms. Therefore, the distending or *mean arterial pressure* is an important confounder of measurements of arterial stiffness [54].

Arteries serve a dual role of conducting blood to the peripheral tissues and buffering the pressure pulsations that are a necessary accompaniment of intermittent ventricular pumping. Isolated systolic hypertension may increase arterial stiffness, especially in older subjects, but not peripheral artery stiffness, although the underlying mechanisms are somewhat unclear [55].

Aortic elasticity is an important determinant of *left ventricular performance* and *coronary blood flow*. As a consequence of arterial stiffness, left ventricular workload is increased and so is myocardial oxygen demand, leading at times to left ventricular hypertrophy [56], impairment of ventricular relaxation [57], and subendocardial ischemia in the presence or absence of coronary artery stenosis [58]. It is well appreciated that the aorta does not only provide a conduit function but plays important roles in regulating left ventricular performance, coronary blood flow, and normal arterial function throughout the entire cardiovascular system. Therefore, loss of vascular distensibility reduces the buffering function of the aorta manifested as elevated pulse pressure, which adds to load on the heart and likely damages the large and small vessels as well. Several studies have shown that disease states, aging, and pharmacological agents may alter the elastic properties of the aorta and that stiffening of the aorta may be associated with an increased incidence of cardiovascular events [59]. These effects may increase the susceptibility of the aging heart to ischemia and ventricular dysfunction. An increase in the stiffness of large conduit vessel may represent either a cause or a consequence of endothelial dysfunction and may explain why elevated pulse pressure is a new cardiovascular risk factor [60].

Regular physical activity is associated with reduced risk of cardiovascular disease [61]. In the Baltimore Longitudinal Study of Aging, it was found that aortic arterial pulse wave velocity increased progressively and that older adult males who performed endurance exercise on a regular basis demonstrated lower levels of aortic arterial pulse wave velocity than their sedentary peers did. Previous studies have reported that in endurance athletes, arterial stiffness is decreased by prolonged endurance training [62], and aortic distensibility is increased, particularly in those with the ACE II genotype. In addition, even a moderately intense exercise may be as brief as 10 min in duration is needed in order to elicit a decrease in resting blood pressure and may have potential benefits as a nonpharmacological aid to hypertension [63]. These effects represent an extracardiac adaptation to chronic prolonged training in athletes [64].

Arterial compliance is an important therapeutic target in individuals in whom stiffening of the proximal aortic circulation is thought to underlie systolic hypertension and increased cardiac work. This indicates a positive association between systemic arterial compliance and *fitness level* in healthy older people and an inverse association between systemic arterial compliance and systolic blood pressure. These findings are consistent with either acquisition of a more compliant circulation and lower blood pressure due to enhanced *physical activity* or that a more compliant arterial circulation and lower blood pressure permit greater athletic performance [65]. For healthy subjects between the ages of 25 and 65 years, there is an interactive effect between age and gender and an independent effect of physical training on peripheral vascular function [66]. It was suggested that interventions to improve aerobic capacity alleviate the stiffening of the arterial tree that accompanies normative aging [67].

Physical Activity in Hypertension

The high prevalence of hypertension in the modern industrialized society imposes an important public health problem, and therefore, prevention of hypertension is a major public health concern. Essential hypertension is a multifactorial disease, and it is very unlikely that only one causal factor is involved. Data indicates an association between baseline physical fitness and risk of future hypertension. Its pathogenesis is based on the interaction between genetic and environmental and lifestyle factors. Genetic variance has been shown in family and twin studies, but the exact nature of the postulated genetic defect remains largely unknown [68]. Therefore, emerging data suggest genetic links to the blood pressure reductions associated with acute and chronic exercise. *Physical activity* has been recommended in the prevention and treatment of hypertension [69]. A large body of evidence-based recommendations demonstrates that changes toward a more physically active lifestyle positively affect blood pressure in hypertensive individuals and otherwise healthy adults [70]. Meta-analysis of a number of longitudinal aerobic training studies in mild essential hypertensive subjects demonstrated an average reduction in resting systolic and diastolic blood pressures of 10.8 and 8.2 mmHg, respectively [71]. Therefore, participating in an exercise training program can be viewed as nonpharmacological approach for preventing and treating mild hypertension. High physical fitness is associated with lower blood pressure in both men and women [40]. Multiple regression evaluation demonstrated that sedentary individuals had a 62% increased risk of developing hypertension compared to their more trained peers. The proposed mechanisms for the blood pressure lowering effects of exercise include neurohumoral, vascular, and structural adaptations. Decreases in catecholamine and total peripheral resistance, improved insulin sensitivity, and alterations in vasodilators and vasoconstrictors are some of the postulated explanations for the antihypertensive effects of exercise [72]. These reductions in blood pressure are mediated through the significant decreases in circulating catecholamine, since the changes observed in blood pressure were not accompanied with changes in dietary habits, alcohol and caffeine consumption, or body weight loss.

A large body of data demonstrates that changes toward a more physically active lifestyle positively affect *blood pressure* response in *normotensive* and *hypertensive individuals* [73]. Exercise programs that primarily involve endurance activities prevent the development of hypertension and lower blood pressure in adults with normal blood pressure and those with hypertension. Meta-analysis of longitudinal *aerobic training* studies [74] in mild *essential hypertensive* subjects demonstrates an average reduction in resting *systolic* and *diastolic blood pressures* of 10.8 and 8.2 mmHg, respectively [75]. Therefore, participation in an exercise-training program may be viewed as a nonpharmacological approach for preventing and treating mild hypertension.

Previous studies have shown that a supervised *exercise program* leads to a decrease in *blood pressure* in humans with essential arterial hypertension [74]. Men in the high fitness group with resting systolic blood pressure above or equal to 140 mmHg had a lower death rate than their low-fitness, below-140-mmHg-resting-systolic-pressure counterparts. Nevertheless, even though the reduction in blood pressure due to *exercise training* was detected in *normotensive* and *hypertensive patients*, the magnitude of reduction in systolic and diastolic blood pressure at rest and during submaximal exercise are greater in hypertensive subjects [61]. At least 44 randomized controlled trials including 2,674 participants have studied the effect of aerobic *exercise training* on resting *blood pressure* [76]. The average reduction in systolic and diastolic blood pressure was 3.4 and 2.4 mmHg, respectively. Baseline blood pressure was an important determinant of the exercise effect. Average systolic and diastolic blood pressures decreased 2.6 and 1.8 mmHg in normotensive subjects and 7.4 and 5.8 mmHg in hypertensive subjects, respectively, suggesting that exercise may serve as the only therapy required in some mildly hypertensive subjects [11].

The mechanisms responsible for the reduction in *arterial pressure* has not been fully investigated, though a reduction in *sympathetic nerve activity* resultant from *exercise training* was suggested to lower arterial pressure [52]. However, the lack of change in muscle sympathetic nerve activity after training indicates that the lower arterial pressure is unrelated to a reduction in central sympathetic outflow. The failure of muscle sympathetic nerve activity to change at rest with *isometric training* is also typically observed with either forearm or leg dynamic exercise training [77].

Therefore, reductions in sympathetic outflow to skeletal muscle do not appear to be a prerequisite to lower arterial pressure in humans. However, it cannot be excluded that *sympathetic outflow* to other vascular beds (e.g., visceral regions) may be reduced and may contribute to the reduction in arterial pressure at rest [52].

Another possible mechanism for the reduction in *arterial pressure* is *peripheral vascular* adaptations because *aerobic* and *isometric exercises* elicit marked increases in muscle sympathetic nerve activity and *norepinephrine* release. Thus, vascular sensitivity to norepinephrine may be decreased with aerobic and isometric training [78, 79].

Finally, it is important to note that the indirect measurement of blood pressure is acceptable for systolic blood pressure during *aerobic* and *isometric exercises* and not at all at peak *anaerobic exercise*. Several studies have simultaneously compared intra-arterial and cuff measures during aerobic exercise [80, 81]. On the average, during dynamic exercise, the mean brachial intra-arterial systolic and diastolic blood pressures exceeded those means measured by the indirect conventional sphygmomanometer [81]. The direct intra-arterial method with the indirect conventional sphygmomanometer was compared at rest and during isometric exercise. It revealed that when utilizing large muscle mass during *isometric exercise*, the indirect method is not valid for the assessment of diastolic blood pressure [82]. The American Heart Association and the American College of Sports Medicine [83] have each endorsed moderate-intensity resistive training as a complement to aerobic exercise programs in the prevention, treatment, and control of hypertension. The rationale for resistive training as an adjunct to aerobic exercise for controlling blood pressure stems from multiple studies. Two meta-analyses by Cornelissen and Fagard and Kelley and Kelley of resistive training and hypertension are noteworthy [47, 84].

Exercise has been associated with antihypertensive benefits, but despite extensive research, the optimal exercise dose – training frequency, intensity, and time required to lower blood pressure and maintain normotensive status – remains unclear. Therefore, the correct exercise dose for the treatment of hypertension should be prescribed on an individual basis [85].

Aerobic training is not the only form of exercise found to decrease resting blood pressure. Strength training, in a form of circuit weight training, seems to produce the same effect on blood pressure as endurance training [86]. Recent studies have evaluated the safety and efficacy of circuit weight training in hypertensive patients [87]. Evidence for a blood pressure-lowering effect is much less compelling for this type of training than for aerobic endurance training. Recently, the American College of Sports Medicine [73] recommended resistance training to be an adjunct to an aerobic-based exercise program in the prevention, treatment, and control of hypertension [84].

How does physical activity produce the decrease in blood pressure in borderline hypertensive patients? Borderline hypertension is characterized by increased cardiac output and heart rate as a result of increased activity of the sympathetic nervous system [72]. One of the beneficial physical training outcomes seen in mild hypertensive patients is a reduction in sympathetic nervous system activity. This reduction in sympathetic nervous system activity causes a decrease in cardiac output and heart rate which then results in lower blood pressure.

References

1. Barlow CE, LaMonte MJ, Fitzgerald SJ, Kampert JB, Perrin JL, Blair SN. Cardiorespiratory fitness is an independent predictor of hypertension incidence among initially normotensive healthy women. Am J Epidemiol. 2006;163:142–50.
2. Wooten JS, Phillips MD, Mitchell JB, et al. Resistance exercise and lipoproteins in postmenopausal women. Int J Sports Med. 2011;32:7–13.
3. Sudano I, Roas S, Noll G. Vascular abnormalities in essential hypertension. Curr Pharm Des. 2011;17(28):3039–44.
4. Mikirova NA, Casciari JJ, Hunninghake RE, Beezley MM. Effect of weight reduction on cardiovascular risk factors and CD34-positive cells in circulation. Int J Med Sci. 2011;8:445–52.
5. Clarkson P, Montgomery HE, Mullen MJ. Exercise training enhances endothelial function in young men. J Am Coll Cardiol. 1999;33:1379–85.
6. Tjonna AE, Rognmo O, Bye A, Stolen TO, Wisloff U. Time course of endothelial adaptation after acute and chronic exercise in patients with metabolic syndrome-“a pilot study”. J Strength Cond Res. 2011;25(9):2552–8.
7. Luk TH, Dai YL, Siu CW, et al. Effect of exercise training on vascular endothelial function in patients with stable coronary artery disease: a randomized controlled trial. Eur J Cardiovasc Prev Rehabil. 2011. [Epub ahead of print].
8. Vona M, Codeluppi GM, Iannino T, Ferrari E, Bogousslavsky J, von Segesser LK. Effects of different types of exercise training followed by detraining on endothelium-dependent dilation in patients with recent myocardial infarction. Circulation. 2009;119:1601–8.
9. Glass CK, Witztum JL. Atherosclerosis: the road ahead. Cell. 2001;104:503–16.
10. Lowe DA, Alway SE. Animal models for inducing muscle hypertrophy: are they relevant for clinical applications in humans? J Orthop Sports Phys Ther. 2002;32:36–43.
11. Thompson PD, David Buchner D, Piña IL, et al. Exercise and physical activity in the prevention and treatment of atherosclerotic cardiovascular disease. A statement from the council on clinical cardiology (Subcommittee on Exercise, Rehabilitation, and Prevention) and the council on nutrition, physical activity, and metabolism (Subcommittee on Physical Activity). Circulation. 2003;107:3109–16.

12. Lee M, Sesso HD, Oguma Y, Paffenbarger Jr RF. Relative intensity of physical activity and risk of coronary heart disease. Circulation. 2003;107:1110–6.
13. Gibbons R, Balady G, Timothybricker J, et al. ACC/AHA 2002 guideline update for exercise testing: summary article a report of the American College of Cardiology/American Heart Association Task Force on practice guidelines. J Am Coll Cardiol. 2002;40: 1531–40.
14. Amir O, Yamin C, Sagiv M, et al. Acute incremental exercise to maximal performance does not cause alterations in serum oxidant levels of healthy young individuals. J Sports Med Phys Fitness. 2009;49: 105–11.
15. Sen CK. Oxidants and antioxidants in exercise. J Appl Physiol. 1995;79:675–86.
16. Wilund KR. Is the anti-inflammatory effect of regular exercise responsible for reduced cardiovascular disease? Clin Sci. 2007;112:543–55.
17. Sagiv M, Ben-Sira D, Goldhammer E. Beta-blockers, exercise, and the immune system in men with coronary artery disease. Med Sci Sports Exerc. 2002;34: 587–91.
18. Rauramaa R, Halonen P, Väisänen SB, et al. Effects of aerobic physical exercise on inflammation and atherosclerosis in men: the DNASCO study a six-year randomized, controlled trial. Ann Intern Med. 2004;140: 1007–14.
19. Napoli C, Williams-Ignarro S, de Nigris F, et al. Long-term combined beneficial effects of physical training and metabolic treatment on atherosclerosis in hypercholesterolemic mice. Proc Natl Acad Sci USA. 2004;101:8797–802.
20. Brown MD. Exercise and coronary vascular remodelling in the healthy heart. Exp Physiol. 2003;88:645–58.
21. Stefanick ML, Mackey S, Sheehan M, et al. Effects of diet and exercise in men and postmenopausal women with low levels of HDL cholesterol and high levels of LDL cholesterol. N Engl J Med. 1998;339:12–20.
22. Sagiv M, Sagiv M, Meckel Y, Ben-Sira D, Amir R. Effects of different sprint cycling bouts on left ventricular function in top cyclists. J Sports Med Phys Fitness. 2008;48:360–5.
23. Pesola GR, Pesola HR, Nelson MJ, Westfal RE. The normal difference in bilateral indirect blood pressure recordings in normotensive individuals. Am J Emerg Med. 2001;19:43–5.
24. Palatini P. Exercise haemodynamics in the normotensive and the hypertensive subject. Clin Sci (Lond). 1994;87:275–87.
25. MacDonald JR, MacDougall JD, Interisano SA, et al. Hypotension following mild bouts of resistance exercise and submaximal dynamic exercise. Eur J Appl Physiol Occup Physiol. 1999;79:148–54.
26. MacDonald JR. Potential causes, mechanisms, and implications exercise hypotension. J Hum Hypertens. 2002;16:225–36.
27. Halliwill JR, Taylor JA, Eckberg DL. Impaired sympathetic vascular regulation in humans after acute dynamic exercise. J Physiol. 1996;495:279–88.
28. Halliwill JR, Minson CT, Joyner MJ. Effect of systemic nitric oxide synthase inhibition on postexercise hypotension in humans. J Appl Physiol. 2000;89: 1830–6.
29. Halliwill JR. Mechanisms and clinical implications of post-exercise hypotension in humans. Exerc Sport Sci Rev. 2001;29:65–70.
30. Franklin PJ, Green DJ, Cable NT. The influence of thermoregulation mechanisms on post exercise hypotension in humans. J Physiol. 1993;470:231–41.
31. Senitko AN, Charkoudian N, Halliwill JR. Influence of endurance exercise training status and gender on postexercise hypotension. J Appl Physiol. 2002;92: 2368–74.
32. MacDougall JD, Tuxen D, Sale DG, Moroz JR, Sutton JR. Arterial blood pressure response to heavy resistance exercise. J Appl Physiol. 1985;58:785–90.
33. Narloch JA, Brandstater ME. Influence of breathing technique on arterial blood pressure during heavy weight lifting. Arch Phys Med Rehabil. 1995;76: 457–62.
34. Lentini AC, McKelvie RS, McCartney N, Tomlinson CW, MacDougall JD. Left ventricular response in healthy young men during heavy-intensity weight-lifting exercise. J Appl Physiol. 1993;75:2703–10.
35. Sagiv M, Ben-Sira D, Goldhammer E. Direct vs. indirect blood pressure measurement at peak anaerobic exercise. Int J Sports Med. 1999;20:275–8.
36. Brandão Rondon MU, Alves MJ, Braga AM, et al. Postexercise blood pressure reduction in elderly hypertensive patients. J Am Coll Cardiol. 2002;39: 676–82.
37. Tsuda M, Hatano K, Hayashi H, Yokota M, Hirai M, Saito H. Diagnostic value of postexercise systolic blood pressure response for detecting coronary artery disease in patients with or without hypertension. Am Heart J. 1993;125:718–25.
38. Nieman DC. The exercise-health connection. Champaign: Human Kinetics; 1998.
39. The sixth report of the Joint Committee on prevention, detection, evaluation, and treatment of high blood pressure (JNCVI). Public Health Service, National Institutes of Health, National Heart, Lung and Blood Institute, NIH Publication No. 98–4080, Nov 1997.
40. Joyner MJ. Baroreceptor function during exercise: resetting the record. Exp Physiol. 2006;91:27–36.
41. Raven PB, Fadel PJ, Ogoh S. Arterial baroreflex resetting during exercise: a current perspective. Exp Physiol. 2006;91:37–49.
42. Fadel PJ. Arterial baroreflex control of the peripheral vasculature in humans: rest and exercise. Med Sci Sports Exerc. 2008;40(12):2055–62.
43. Kamiya A, Michikami D, Fu Q, Niimi Y, Iwase S, Mano T, Suzumura A. Static handgrip exercise modifies arterial baroreflex control of vascular sympathetic outflow in humans. Am J Physiol Regul Integr Comp Physiol. 2001;281:R1134–9.
44. Sagiv M, Hanson P, Besozzi M, Nagle F. Left ventricular responses to upright isometric handgrip and

dead-lift in men with coronary artery disease. Am J Cardiol. 1985;55:1298–302.

45. Harris KA, Holly RG. Physiological response to circuit weight training in borderline hypertensive subjects. Med Sci Sports Exerc. 1987;19:246–52.
46. Blumenthal JA, Siegel WC, Appelbaum M. Failure of exercise to reduce blood pressure in patients with mild hypertension. Results of a randomized controlled trial. JAMA. 1991;266(15):2098–104.
47. Kelley GA, Kelley KS. Progressive resistance exercise and resting blood pressure: a meta-analysis of randomized controlled trials. Hypertension. 2000; 35:838–43.
48. Sagiv M, Ben-Sira D, Goldhammer E. Direct vs. indirect blood pressure measurement at peak anaerobic exercise. Int J Sports Med Sci Sports Exerc. 2000; 32:1197–201.
49. Sagiv M, Ben-Sira D, Sagiv M, Goldhammer E. Left ventricular function at peak all-out anaerobic exercise in older men. Gerontology. 2005;51:122–5.
50. Sagiv M, Sagiv M, Ben-Sira D. Weight lifting training and left ventricular function in adolescents subjects. J Sports Med Phys Fitness. 2007;47:329–34.
51. Sagiv M, Sagiv A, Ben-Sira D, Rudoy J, Soudry M. The effect of hypertension and aging on left ventricular function during isometric exercise. J Aging Phys Activ. 1996;4:69–79.
52. Ray CA, Carrasco DI. Isometric handgrip training reduces arterial pressure at rest without changes in sympathetic nerve activity. Am J Physiol Heart Circ Physiol. 2000;279:H245–9.
53. Boutouyrie P, Tropeano AI, Asmar R, et al. Aortic stiffness is an independent predictor of primary coronary events in hypertensive patients: a longitudinal study. Hypertension. 2002;39:10–5.
54. McEniery CM, Wilkinson IB, Avolio AP. Age, hypertension and arterial function. Clin Exp Pharmacol Physiol. 2007;34:665–71.
55. Benetos A, Waeber B, Izzo J, et al. Influence of age, risk factors, and cardiovascular and renal disease on arterial stiffness: clinical applications. Am J Hypertens. 2002;15:1101–8.
56. Stefanadis C, Dernellis J, Tsiamis E, et al. Aortic stiffness as a risk factor for recurrent acute coronary events in patients with ischaemic heart disease. Eur Heart J. 2000;21:390–6.
57. Kohno F, Kumada T, Kamabayashi M, et al. Change in aortic end-systolic pressure by alterations in loading sequence and its relation to left ventricular isovolumic relaxation. Circulation. 1996;93:2080–7.
58. Laurent S, Katsahian S, Fassot C, Tropeano AI, Gautier I, Laloux B, Boutouyrie P. Aortic stiffness is an independent predictor of fatal stroke in essential hypertension. Stroke. 2003;34:1203–6.
59. Kontopoulos AG, Athyros VG, Pehlivanidis AN, Demitriadis DS, Papageorgiou AA, Boudoulas H. Long-term treatment effect of atorvastatin on aortic stiffness in hypercholesterolaemic patients. Curr Med Res Opin. 2003;19:22–7.
60. Nigam A, Mitchell GF, Lambert J, Tardif JC. Relation between conduit vessel stiffness (assessed by tonometry) and endothelial function (assessed by flow-mediated dilatation) in patients with and without coronary heart disease. Am J Cardiol. 2003;92: 395–9.
61. Blair SN, Kohl 3rd HW, Barlow CE, Paffenbarger Jr RS, Gibbons LW, Macera CA. Changes in physical fitness and all-cause mortality. JAMA. 1995;273:1093–8.
62. Kakiyama T, Sugawara J, Murakami H, Maeda S, Kuno S, Matsuda M. Effects of short-term endurance training on aortic distensibility in young males. Med Sci Sports Exerc. 2005;37:267–71.
63. MacDonald JR, MacDougall JD, Hogben CD. The effects of exercise duration on post-exercise hypotension. J Hum Hypertens. 2004;14:125–9.
64. Tanriverdi H, Evrengul H, Kaftan A, et al. Effects of angiotensin-converting enzyme polymorphism on aortic elastic parameters in athletes. Cardiology. 2005; 104:113–9.
65. Cameron JD, Rajkumar C, Kingwell BA, Jennings GL, Dart AM. Higher systemic arterial compliance is associated with greater exercise time and lower blood pressure in a young older population. J Am Geriatr Soc. 1999;47:653–6.
66. Martin 3rd WH, Ogawa T, Kohrt WM, Malley MT, Korte E, Kieffer PS, Schechtman KB. Effects of aging, gender, and physical training on peripheral vascular function. Circulation. 1991;84:654–64.
67. Vaitkevicius PV, Fleg JL, Engel JH, et al. Effects of age and aerobic capacity on arterial stiffness in healthy adults. Circulation. 1993;88:1456–62.
68. Pescatello LS. Exercise and hypertension: recent advances in exercise prescription. Curr Hypertens Rep. 2005;7:281–6.
69. Fletcher GF, Balady G, Blair SN, et al. Statement on exercise: benefits and recommendations for physical activity programs for all Americans. A statement for health professionals by the Committee on Exercise and Cardiac Rehabilitation of the Council on Clinical Cardiology. Circulation. 1996;94:857–62.
70. Cléroux J, Feldman RD, Petrella RJ. Lifestyle modifications to prevent and control hypertension. 4. Recommendations on physical exercise training. Canadian Hypertension Society, Canadian Coalition for High Blood Pressure Prevention and Control, Laboratory Centre for Disease Control at Health Canada, Heart and Stroke Foundation of Canada. CMAJ. 1999;160(9 Suppl):S21–8.
71. Gordon NF, Scott CB, Wilkinson WJ, Duncan JJ, Blair SN. Exercise and mild essential hypertension. Recommendations for adults. Sports Med. 1990; 10:390–404.
72. Esler M, Kaye D. Increased sympathetic nervous system activity and its therapeutic reduction in arterial hypertension, portal hypertension and heart failure. J Auton Nerv Syst. 1998;72:210–9.
73. Pescatello LS, Franklin BA, Fagard R, Farquhar WB, Kelley GA, Ray CA. American College of Sports

Medicine position stand. Exercise and hypertension. Med Sci Sports Exerc. 2004;36:533–53.

74. Hagberg JM, Park JJ, Brown MD. The role of exercise training in the treatment of hypertension: an update. Sports Med. 2000;30:193–206.
75. Gordon NF, Scott CB, Wilkinson WJ, et al. Exercise and mild essential hypertension. Recommendations for adults. Sports Med. 1990;10:390–404.
76. Fagard RH. Exercise characteristics and the blood pressure response to dynamic physical training. Med Sci Sports Exerc. 2001;33(6 suppl):S484–92.
77. Ray CA. Sympathetic adaptations to one-legged training. J Appl Physiol. 1999;86:1583–7.
78. Ng AV, Callister R, Johnson DG, et al. Endurance exercise training is associated with elevated basal sympathetic nerve activity in healthy older humans. J Appl Physiol. 1994;77:1366–74.
79. Kingwell BA, Tran B, Cameron JD, et al. Enhanced vasodilation to ACh in athletes is associated with lower plasma cholesterol. Am J Physiol Heart Circ Physiol. 1996;270:H2008–13.
80. Gould BA, Hornung RS, Altman C, Cashman PMM, Rafferty EB. Indirect measurement of blood pressure during exercise testing can be misleading. Br Heart J. 1985;53:611–5.
81. Robinson TE, Sue DY, Huszczuk A, Weiler-Ravell D, Hansen JE. Intra-arterial and cuff blood pressure responses during incremental cycle ergometry. Med Sci Sports Exerc. 1988;20:142–9.
82. Sagiv M, Hanson PG, Ben-Sira D, Nagle FJ. Direct vs. indirect blood pressure at rest and during isometric exercise in normal subjects. Int J Sports Med. 1995; 16:514–8.
83. Pollock ML, Franklin BA, Balady GJ, et al. AHA Science Advisory: resistance exercise in individuals with and without cardiovascular disease: benefits, rationale, safety, and prescription: an advisory from the Committee on Exercise, Rehabilitation, and Prevention, Council on Clinical Cardiology, American Heart Association; Position paper endorsed by the American College of Sports Medicine. Circulation. 2000;101:828–33.
84. Cornelissen VA, Fagard RH. Effect of resistance training on resting blood pressure: a meta-analysis of randomized controlled trials. J Hypertens. 2005;23(2): 251–9.
85. Hamer M. The anti-hypertensive effects of exercise: integrating acute and chronic mechanisms. Sports Med. 2006;36:109–16.
86. Figueroa A, Park SY, Seo DY, Sanchez-Gonzalez MA, Baek YH. Combined resistance and endurance exercise training improves arterial stiffness, blood pressure, and muscle strength in postmenopausal women. Menopause. 2011;18:980–4.
87. Mota MR, Pardono E, Lima LC, Arsa G, Bottaro M, Campbell CS, Simões HG. Effects of treadmill running and resistance exercises on lowering blood pressure during the daily work of hypertensive subjects. J Strength Cond Res. 2009;23:2331–8.

Metabolic Cardiovascular Risk Factors

7

Lipoproteins

Endurance exercise is widely recommended in the treatment paradigm of various hyperlipoproteinemias for its putative anti-atherogenic action on circulating lipids and apolipoproteins (Fig. 7.1) and to improve cardiorespiratory fitness, which may lower atherosclerotic risk independent of lipids and other risk factors [1]. Support for this notion, however, is largely based on research in normocholesterolemic subjects. Training studies in hypercholesterolemic subjects are rare, and lipid results are inconclusive [2].

Aerobic fitness and exercise programs such as walking, jogging, and aerobics have been encouraged as a means to reduce *total cholesterol*, *low-density lipoprotein cholesterol* (*LDL-C*), and triglycerides while elevating high-density lipoprotein cholesterol (*HDL-C*). The association between serum cholesterol levels and the incidence of *ischemic heart disease* (IHD) has been demonstrated in experimental and epidemiological studies [3]. The relationship between *cholesterol* and ischemic heart disease is continuous, gradual, and highly intense. The predictive value of the cholesterol level decreases with age, and actually is low from the sixth decade of life on. The risk attributed to hypercholesterolemia is due to low-density lipoprotein cholesterol. When it involves large and medium-sized arteries, it is referred to as atherosclerosis.

Aerobic Exercise Effect on Lipoprotein

The hypothesis that *physical training* programs are beneficial to the heart is based on evidence that chronic repeated exercise may reduce the risk of developing *coronary artery disease* [4]. Studies have established that the blood level of high-density lipoprotein cholesterol is inversely associated with the incidence of coronary artery disease. On the other hand, reductions in low-density lipoprotein cholesterol produce definite further reductions in the incidence of heart attack, of revascularization, and of ischemic stroke; with each 1.0 mmol · L^{-1} reduction, the annual rate of these major vascular events drops by just over a fifth. Reduction of high-density lipoprotein cholesterol by 2–3 mmol · L^{-1} would reduce risk by about 40–50% [5]. A number of intervention studies have demonstrated that the lowering of high-density lipoprotein cholesterol by means of hypolipidemic agents is accompanied by significant reductions in *cardiovascular morbidity* and *mortality*, both in primary and secondary care [6]. Major interest in these epidemiologic findings among investigators in the field of sports medicine stems from the important role that physical activity plays in affecting the lipid and lipoprotein profile of circulating blood.

The first indication of the *high-density lipoprotein cholesterol* raising effect of *exercise*

M.S. Sagiv, *Exercise Cardiopulmonary Function in Cardiac Patients*,
DOI 10.1007/978-1-4471-2888-5_7, © Springer-Verlag London 2012

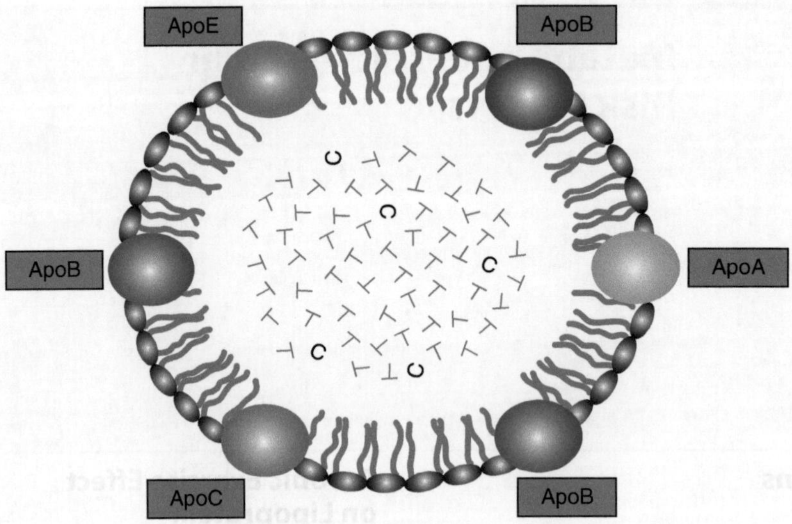

Fig. 7.1 Lipoprotein structure (chylomicron) ApoA, ApoB, ApoC, and ApoE (apolipoproteins); T (triacylglycerol); C (cholesterol); and green (phospholipids). A lipoprotein is a biochemical assembly that contains both proteins and lipids water-bound to the proteins. Many enzymes, transporters, structural proteins, antigens, adhesins, and toxins are lipoproteins. Examples include the high-density (HDL) and low-density (LDL) lipoproteins, which enable fats to be carried in the blood stream, the transmembrane proteins of the mitochondrion and the chloroplast, and bacterial lipoproteins

arose from an observation that highly trained athletes have lower levels of *low-density lipoprotein cholesterol* and higher level of high-density lipoprotein cholesterol than do sedentary persons matched to age and sex. This is also true following aerobic exercise training programs [7]. Disabled individuals, whose movement is further restricted, exhibit even lower levels of high-density lipoprotein cholesterol [8]. The levels of *lipoprotein* in individuals with different degrees of *physical training* vary with the type and mode of exercise. Previous studies found that the distance run per week is the best predictor of high-density lipoprotein cholesterol levels among runners [9]. Rotkis et al. compared 90 runners reporting mean weekly distance run of 13, 27, and 58 miles with 19 nonrunners. It has been found that in runners, mean high-density lipoprotein cholesterol was 47 mg · dL^{-1} in 28 runners, 53 mg · dL^{-1} in 30 runners, and 60 mg · dL^{-1} in 32 runners. Nineteen nonrunners had a mean high-density lipoprotein cholesterol level of 34 mg · dL^{-1} [10]. *Athletes* mainly engaged in *anaerobic training* have lower high-density lipoprotein cholesterol and *high-density lipoprotein cholesterol/total cholesterol ratios* when compared to endurance-trained subjects such as long-distance runners [11]. Nikkila have shown that in *anaerobic* sprinters, whose training program consisted mainly of short duration efforts, the serum *lipid* and *lipoprotein* levels were not elevated and there were no significant differences in *total cholesterol* or *triglycerides* between speed-skaters, *weight-lifters*, and inactive men [12]. Cross-sectional studies confirm that active women have higher high-density lipoprotein cholesterol levels than their sedentary counterparts. Apparently, the duration and frequency of aerobic exercise may be more important in altering high-density lipoprotein cholesterol than the intensity of the exercise. However, because of the confounding effects of diet, body composition, exogenous hormone use, contraceptive use, alcohol consumption, and age, the specific exercise recommendations for increasing high-density lipoprotein cholesterol have yet to be determined [13].

Strength Training Effect on Lipoprotein

There is a lack of well-controlled studies investigating the effect of *resistive training* intervention on lipid metabolism in individuals with normal lipoprotein-lipid profiles and those who are hypercholesterolemic. Some investigators reported *high-density lipoprotein cholesterol* values in male *strength-trained* athletes similar to those of endurance-trained athletes [14]; nevertheless, others suggested that caution may be warranted in recommending strength training for improving high-density lipoprotein cholesterol and triglycerides in adults. Cross-sectional evidence regarding the relation between muscle strength, resistive training, and plasma lipoprotein-lipid profiles is contradictory. When these factors are controlled, most studies show no improvement in lipid profiles after resistive training in either middle-aged or older adults. Future research should continue to examine the effects of strength training on lipids and lipoproteins in adults so as to determine optimal programs and populations in which strength training may have a positive effect [15]. Tucker and Silvester [16] studied 8,499 male employees of more than 50 companies and observed a reduced risk of hypercholesterolemia among individuals participating above 4 h in resistive training programs. In contrast, Kohl et al. [17] studied 1,193 women and 5,460 men and reported no significant association between muscle strength and total or low-density lipoprotein cholesterol for either gender. However, there was a direct association between both upper and lower body strength and triglyceride levels in men.

Although total cholesterol levels are lower in persons with high aerobic fitness compared to low aerobic fitness, it has not been conclusively demonstrated that exercise training lowers total cholesterol. Shoup and Durstine [18] suggested that it is possible that the resistive training does not generate conversion of high-density lipoprotein cholesterol subfraction high-density lipoprotein-2 cholesterol to high-density lipoprotein-3 cholesterol. The same applies for low-density lipoprotein cholesterol. Even though it appears that endurance training may decrease low-density lipoprotein cholesterol, there is little information about the biochemical mechanism producing this change. Nevertheless, one published and well-designed study indicated that 5 months of sustained resistance training significantly decreased total cholesterol and low-density lipoprotein cholesterol in women [19].

High-Density Lipoprotein

The evidence that blood levels of lipoprotein not only differ between persons of different activity levels, but are also affected by physical activity, is substantial [20]. Physical training is thus thought to be a stimulus for incrementing the level of high-density lipoprotein cholesterol and reducing triglycerides in the blood. The response of different lipoproteins to aerobic training is well-established, at least in males [21]. Aerobic training is associated with two of the major lipoproteins that transport cholesterol in plasma: high-density lipoprotein cholesterol, *very low-density lipoprotein (LVDL)* cholesterol, and possible low-density lipoprotein cholesterol. Moreover, the cholesterol composition of *high-density lipoprotein* cholesterol can vary in response to different modes of exercise [20]. Thompson et al. [22] have suggested that any level of continued running exercise may have a favorable effect on high-density lipoprotein cholesterol in adults. Thorland and Gilliam's [23] findings in 59 white *preadolescent* males indicated that higher *physical activity* is associated with lower triglycerides and higher *high-density lipoprotein cholesterol* and high-density lipoprotein cholesterol/total cholesterol ratio. However, initial levels of VO_{2max} are associated with the magnitude changes of serum lipids and lipoproteins. Subjects with greater $\mathrm{VO_{2max}}$ values are less likely to show a change in serum lipids and lipoproteins with training than individuals with lower initial $\mathrm{VO_{2max}}$. However, the fact that world class *marathon runners* are known to have exceptional high-plasma high-density lipoprotein cholesterol and relatively low *total cholesterol*, *low-density*

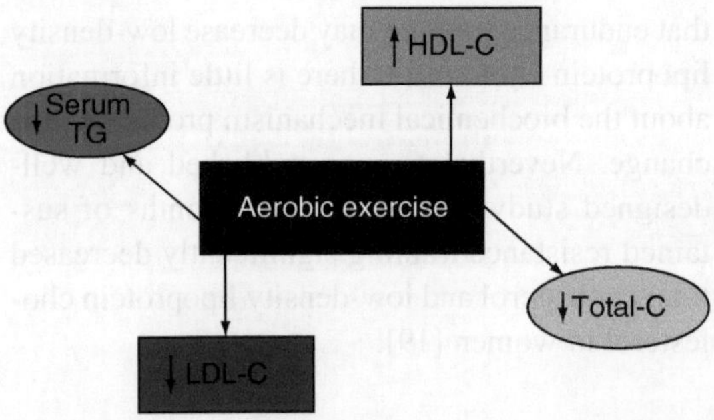

Fig. 7.2 Effect of aerobic exercise training on serum triglycerides (*TG*), total cholesterol (*TOTAL-C*), low-density lipoprotein cholesterol (*LDL-C*), and high-density lipoprotein cholesterol (*HDL-C*)

lipoprotein cholesterol and *triglycerides* concentration suggests that an individual who trains in regular *strenuous aerobic exercise* may alter serum lipids and lipoproteins, which in turn may reduce cardiovascular risk [2].

Angelopoulos et al. [24] have reported that previously sedentary men (Fig. 7.2) can expect an increase in high-density lipoprotein cholesterol and a reduction in low-density lipoprotein cholesterol and triglycerides as a result of an exercise program [25].

With respect to the dependency of lipoprotein cholesterol fraction changes on the intensity of training, Stein et al. [26] evaluated four intensity groups following 12 weeks of cycle ergometer training. Significant increases of high-density lipoprotein cholesterol were observed among the groups training at 75% and 85% of maximal heart rate, in comparison to controls, but not among those training at 65%. This leads to hypothesis that a minimum intensity equal to 75% maximal heart rate is required to increase high-density lipoprotein cholesterol levels. Halverstadt et al. [20] have confirmed earlier findings that changes in lipoproteins, particularly an increase in high-density lipoprotein cholesterol, can be achieved with moderate exercise. This is important since it has implications in the management of patients with proven coronary heart disease, who cannot perform strenuous exercise. Kodama et al. [27] conclude from their meta-analysis review that the minimum threshold needed to raise high-density lipoprotein cholesterol is 120 min · week^{-1} or approximately 900 kcal · week^{-1} of energy expenditure from aerobic exercise. Greater durations of cardiovascular exercise elicit impressive improvements in high-density lipoprotein cholesterol levels although at this time an optimal training dose in minutes or kcal · week^{-1} has not been identified.

According to Eapen et al. [28], low high-density lipoprotein cholesterol levels are actually the best predictor of coronary *heart disease risk* in women, regardless of whether *low-density lipoprotein* cholesterol levels and *triglycerides* are elevated or not. Estrogen, which reaches its peak during the childbearing years, usually raises high-density lipoprotein cholesterol. In women, moderate exercise may not have an identical effect on high-density lipoprotein cholesterol to that seen in men [29]. In postmenopausal women, a 2-year randomized trial of exercise showed no effect [30]. Recently, however, Stranska et al. [31] reported that 37 sedentary, nondiabetic women with physical activity protocol that included 60-min supervised trainings, intensity at 65% of VO_{2max}, were modified by the clamp heart rate test. Median of total training hours was 34 during 115 days (median), which is sufficient to elevate significantly mean high-density lipoprotein cholesterol. In a meta-analysis by Lokey and Tran of 27 longitudinal studies of exercise studies in women, a moderate reduction in total cholesterol and triglycerides was apparent. However, a significant increase in *high-density lipoprotein cholesterol* was not observed [32].

Exercise and High-Density Lipoprotein Cholesterol Synthesis

The primary hypothesis to explain the increase in high-density lipoprotein cholesterol levels by exercise focuses on the exercise-related increase in *lipoprotein lipase*, the key enzyme in triglyceride hydrolysis. Lipoprotein lipase is synthesized in adipocytes and muscle cells. It is released and transported to the capillary endothelium where it binds to the luminal surface. The accelerated catabolism of triglyceride-rich lipoproteins results in an increased transfer of surface components to high-density lipoprotein cholesterol, thus increasing high-density lipoprotein cholesterol mass. Other enzyme changes that might contribute to an increase in high-density lipoprotein cholesterol following exercise include the decrease in hepatic lipase and the increase in lecithin cholesterol acyl transferase. The hepatic lipase activity correlates inversely with physical fitness and with high-density lipoprotein-2 cholesterol [33]. Lecithin cholesterol acyl transferase activity is increased after a period of training in relation to changes in high-density lipoprotein cholesterol. The changes described in hepatic lipase and lecithin cholesterol acyl transferase activities result in increase high-density lipoprotein-2 cholesterol. The finding that the high-density lipoprotein-2 cholesterol level rather than high-density lipoprotein-3 cholesterol is affected by training supports this contention [21].

Increased synthesis of nascent high-density lipoprotein cholesterol might occur of the triglyceride-rich lipoprotein, implicated in forming nascent high-density lipoprotein cholesterol [34]. Alternatively, secretion of nascent high-density lipoprotein cholesterol by the intestine could be elevated. Ben Ounis et al. [35] reported an increase in *apoprotein AI* (Apo AI) synthesis following training period of 8 weeks in obese children. Morris et al. [36] reported on 142 cardiac rehabilitation patients a progressive increase in serum levels of apoprotein AI, over a training period of 6 months. Kiens and Lithell investigated seven young men exercising a single leg on modified bicycle ergometer for up to 2 h over 8 weeks, 3 days a week. A biopsy-associated comparison between the exercising and rested legs demonstrated an exercise-induced increase in the number of capillaries surrounding each muscle fiber, a 70% increase in lipoprotein lipase activity, and a decrease in arteriovenous very low-density lipoprotein cholesterol triglyceride concentration difference, with corresponding arteriovenous high-density lipoprotein cholesterol difference across the legs [37]. These observations demonstrate the key role of lipoprotein lipase in high-density lipoprotein cholesterol and very low-density lipoprotein cholesterol regulation and how exercise affects this regulation.

Obesity

Obesity, defined as excess of body fat, is a major and common health problem in the Western society and is primarily associated with sedentary lifestyle and aging with significant adverse health outcomes. Obesity is strongly associated with coronary artery disease and may be an independent risk factor; however, limited data are available on obesity intervention in coronary artery disease patients. Lavie et al. [38] demonstrated the benefits of cardiac rehabilitation and *exercise training* programs in obesity indices, exercise capacity, plasma lipids, behavioral characteristics, and quality of life in obese patients with coronary artery disease, which were particularly noted in a subgroup of obese patients who were more successful with weight reduction, suggesting that greater emphasis on more successful *weight reduction* programs is needed in preventive cardiology. In addition, obesity has significant adverse effects on various *coronary heart disease* risk factors, including increasing arterial pressure, promoting development of left ventricular hypertrophy, worsening *insulin resistance*, adversely affecting plasma lipids particularly increasing levels of *triglycerides*, reducing levels of *high-density lipoprotein cholesterol*, and leading to a more sedentary lifestyle [39]. Of interest, even if weight loss is minimal, obese individuals showing a good level of cardiopulmonary fitness are at reduced risk for cardiovascular mortality than lean but poorly fit subjects.

Overweight and *obesity* are highly prevalent in cardiac rehabilitation. Overweight and obese patients had a greater adverse *cardiovascular risk profile*, including a lower *exercise capacity* in the latter. Thus, targeted interventions toward weight management in contemporary *cardiac rehabilitation programs* are important. Although short-term outcomes appear promising, greater efforts to improve these outcomes and to support long-term management are needed [40]. However, pharmacotherapy agents are available for long-term use to enhance weight loss efforts for some patients [41]. Weight reduction in obese persons will reduce all of the coronary vascular disease risk factors associated with type 2 *diabetes mellitus* and will improve *hyperglycemia*. Despite adversely affecting all of these *risk factors*, *physical inactivity* seems to have an independent effect on cardiovascular disease risk, whereas obesity increases the risk partly through the modification of other risk factors [42]. Although data are available to indicate that *weight reduction* with dietary therapy or exercise improves lipid profiles and leads to increases in *high-density lipoprotein cholesterol*, along with reduction in *insulin resistance*, and that weight reduction in severe obesity reduces both *arterial pressure* and *left ventricular hypertrophy*, limited data are available on the effects of vigorous risk factor intervention in obese patients with known coronary artery disease. Evidence-based guidelines support intensive nutrition and behavioral counseling and *moderate aerobic exercise* [41]. A growing body of literature demonstrates that aerobic exercise, accompanied with or without weight loss, can lead to favorable changes in body composition including a reduction in abdominal adiposity [43].

Exercise in Obesity

When exercise is included in a *weight loss* therapy, greater improvements in body composition and metabolic outcomes may be evident. At the onset of *aerobic exercise*, there is a large increase in uptake and oxidation of fatty acids in skeletal muscle. It is also well recognized that *prolonged exercise* for several hours at a low intensity induces a gradual decrease in the respiratory quotient and hence enhanced *lipid utilization* at the expense of *carbohydrates* as energy fuel [44]. During an aerobic bout, when the exercise intensity reaches the *anaerobic threshold*, which is very low in untrained obese individual, a shift in fuel selection appears toward an increase in carbohydrate and decrease in fat utilization. Aerobic exercise training improves aerobic fitness, that is, VO_2, which has other important cardiovascular and metabolic implications [45]. Following endurance training with increased VO_{2max}, the anaerobic threshold is also increased and, therefore, a shift towards enhanced *lipid utilization* is evident at least when exercise is performed at the same absolute workload in the untrained and trained state [46]. Even though a change in lipid utilization under different conditions is well described, the regulatory mechanisms controlling fatty acid uptake and oxidation may depend on the availability of oxygen. Exercise intervention can improve *glucose uptake* in skeletal muscle and affect the metabolic pathways supplying ATP to the exercising muscles through exercise-mediated *lipolysis* in adipose tissue and mitochondrial biogenesis.

Insulin and catecholamine have pronounced metabolic effects on human adipose tissue metabolism. *Insulin* stimulates lipoprotein lipase and inhibits hormone-sensitive lipase; the opposite is true for *catecholamine* – its level is increased during exercise. Catecholamine-induced lipolysis is enhanced in visceral fat but decreased in subcutaneous fat. Numerous adaptive responses take place with physical training. These adaptations result in a more efficient system for oxygen transfer to muscle, which is now able to better utilize the unlimited lipid stores instead of the limited carbohydrate reserves available. To generate beneficial metabolic effects, the recommendation for *physical activity* of *moderate intensity* is 30–45 min, performed 3–5 times per week. Walking is likely to be the most successful because it is safe and accessible. It appears that as long as the increase in energy expenditure is sufficient, low- to moderate-intensity endurance exercise is likely to reach the aim [47].

At rest and during exercise, skeletal muscles are the main site of oxidation of free fatty acid (FFA). In resting conditions, free fatty acids are the predominant fuel used by skeletal muscle. During *low-intensity exercise*, *metabolism* is elevated several fold compared to resting conditions, and *fat oxidation* is increased. Endurance exercise training elicits many skeletal muscle adaptations, including an increased capacity for *oxidative metabolism* of *fatty acids* and *carbohydrates*. When the *exercise intensity* increases, fat oxidation increases further, until exercise intensities of about 65% VO_{2max}, after which a decline in the rate of fat oxidation is observed. A cycle protocol with 3-min stages and 35-W increments in work

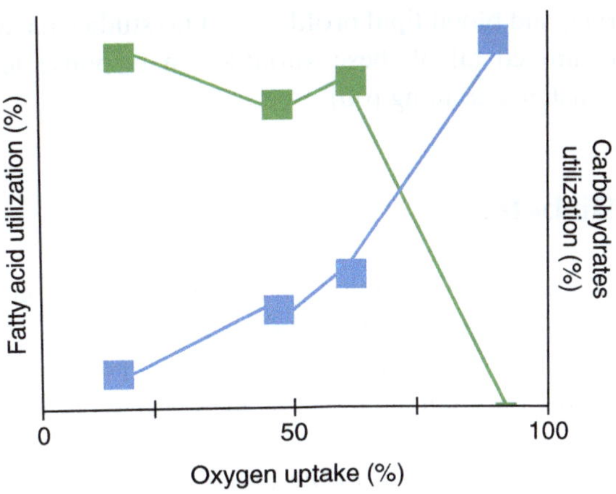

Fig. 7.3 Fat oxidation (*green*) and carbohydrate utilization (*blue*) as a function of exercise intensity in trained subjects. At low to moderate intensities, fat oxidation is the main source for energy production, peaked at 65% maximal oxygen uptake, and totally decreases around 85% maximal oxygen uptake

rate can be used to determine maximal fat oxidation. Fat oxidation rates are high over a large range of intensities. However, at exercise intensities above maximal fat oxidation around 65% VO_{2max}, *fat oxidation* rates drop markedly [48]. This is in contrast to *carbohydrate metabolism*, which increases as a function of the aerobic work rate. *Fat oxidation* is reduced at the high exercise intensities. At around 85% VO_{2max}, energy needed comes from carbohydrate metabolism only without breakdown of fatty acid (Fig. 7.3).

An increase in fatty acid oxidation is facilitated by increased capacities for fatty acid uptake into the myocyte [49], their subsequent mitochondrial transport, and -oxidation [50].

Subjects who regularly exercise aerobically 176 min · 3–4 week^{-1} lose significantly more weight than subject who did not exercise regularly. Subject who exercised more than 195 min · 3–4 week^{-1} may lose nearly 7% of its abdominal fat. *Aerobic exercise* lasting at 60–75% maximal work capacity at least 30 min · 3–4 week^{-1} may be adequate to maintain *cardiovascular health*, but it may not be enough to prevent unhealthful weight gain. Recommendations published in 2003 and 2004 suggest that 45–60 min · day^{-1} is necessary to prevent weight gain, and children may need more activity. Studies suggest that people who have trained for a long time develop more efficient mechanisms for burning fat and are able to stay leaner. Sometimes, exercise may even act as a mild *appetite suppressant*. With exercise training, these increments have been associated with the upregulation of membrane-associated fatty acid transport proteins, fatty acid-binding protein [51], fatty acid translocase [52], the mitochondrial transporter carnitine palmitoyltransferase I [53], and a key enzyme of β-oxidation, β-hydroxyacyl-CoA dehydrogenase [54].

The *molecular mechanisms* initiated by increased *physical activity* that enables the increased protein abundance of components of the fatty acids uptake and ß-oxidative pathways are undoubtedly complex. There are multiple steps important in the regulation of cellular protein, including gene transcription, mRNA stability, *protein translation rate*, translation efficiency, posttranslational modifications, and protein degradation. As a significant and sustained physiological stressor, it is not surprising that *endurance exercise* may regulate protein level by modifications at multiple sites. Many studies have now demonstrated that a bout of sustained muscular activity exerts the capacity to transiently activate the expression of many genes [55]. For example, *GLUT4*, hexokinase, and uncoupling protein (UCP)-3 *gene expression* are observed to peak from within 30 min to 3 h after exercise [56]. It seems that enhanced *fat oxidation* after *exercise training* is most closely associated with the *genes* involved in regulating fatty acid uptake across the plasma membrane and across the mitochondrial membrane.

In the literature, a debate exists over the independent and combined effects of *dieting* and increased *physical activity* on improving *metabolic risk factors*. Recently, it has been suggested by Redman et al. that exercise plays an equivalent role to caloric restriction in terms of energy balance [45]. Therefore, it has been suggested that physical activity is an important adjunct to caloric restriction for achieving and maintaining weight loss. The National Weight Control Registry enrolled 3,000 individuals who lost >10% of their body weight and maintained this weight loss for at least 1 year [57].

Resistive Exercise Training Effect on Obesity

Resistance training programs can increase *fat-free mass* and decrease the percentage of body fat. One of the outstanding benefits of resistance exercise, as it relates to weight loss, is the positive impact of increasing energy expenditure during the exercise session and somewhat during recovery, and on maintaining or increasing fat-free body mass while encouraging the loss of fat body weight. It is more likely that body composition is affected and controlled by resistance training programs using the larger muscle groups and greater total volume [58]. Although many training variables contribute to the performance and cellular and molecular adaptations to resistance exercise, relative intensity (% 1 repetition maximum (%1RM)) appears to be an important factor. In general, relative intensity appears to account for 18–35% of the variance for the hypertrophy response to *resistance exercise* [59]. Volume in resistance training is equal to the total workload, which is directly proportional to the energy expenditure of the work bout. Total volume is determined by the total number of repetitions (repetitions × sets) performed times the weight of the load (total repetitions × weight). Often total volume is calculated by multiplying the number of sets · repetitions · load. For example, three sets of 12 repetitions with 20–25 kg would be expressed, 3 · 12 · 25 = 900 kg of volume. An impressive finding to highlight with resistance training is that the energy expenditure following the higher total volume workouts appears to be elevated, compared to other forms of exercise, and, thus, further contributes to weight loss objectives. Furthermore, studies evaluating the impact of high-intensity resistance exercise on body composition and other physiological adaptations during weight loss have reported inconsistent findings [60]. However, one has to keep in mind that there are limitations with research examining the physiological effects of *resistive training* associated with various forms of *weight loss*. Only few studies have simultaneously reported data on body composition, exercise performance (muscular strength, endurance, power), metabolic rate, and blood lipid profiles, and no studies have examined all of these variables in response to resistance training [60].

Diabetes

Diabetes is a condition characterized by raised levels of sugar in the blood stream. It comes in two main forms: type 1 and type 2. Type 2 is by far the most common, and is generally related to insulin resistance which is a failure of the body to respond adequately to the blood sugar-lowering effects of insulin. An important risk factor for cardiovascular disease and diabetes is glucose tolerance. High blood glucose and high insulin levels can also have a deleterious effect on hypertension and blood lipids. Circulatory disorders associated with diabetes include coronary heart disease, stroke, peripheral arterial disease, cardiomyopathy, and congestive heart failure. Diabetes generally results in early death from cardiovascular diseases [61]. The prevalence of type 2 diabetes increases with age [62], and aging is associated with a reduction in muscle strength and metabolic control, both of which are influenced by the progressive age-related decline in muscle mass [63]. Human muscle strength declines at the rate of 12–14% per decade after the age of 50 years [64]. This loss of strength with age is due to many factors but is primarily attributed to a loss of muscle mass bringing to sarcopenia [65].

The elevated blood glucose levels and increased levels of glycosylated hemoglobin (HbA1c) observed with these disorders are known to increase the risk of microvascular and macrovascular complications that can cause a variety of other health issues, from hypertension and blindness to kidney failure and heart disease [66]. Diabetes, particularly type 2, is reaching epidemic proportions throughout the world, as more and more cultures adopt Western dietary habits. Diabetes type 2, glucose intolerance, and insulin resistance are central features of coronary artery disease risk, being strongly related to hypertension and dyslipidemia, proinflammatory markers, thrombogenic factors, and endothelial dysfunction. These abnormalities increase with age and represent the early stages of cardiovascular disease that precede the clinical manifestations of cardiovascular disease [67]. Both genetic and environmental factors have been implicated in the etiology of type 1 and 2 diabetes. A serious complication of diabetes is the increase in fracture risk observed in both type 1 and type 2 diabetic patients. The long-term complications associated with type 2 diabetes are both microvascular and macrovascular in nature. Hyperglycemia is present in both type 1 and 2 diabetes, and it alters bone matrix proteins such as collagen I through nonenzymatic glycation, which can decrease bone toughness and increase fracture risk even in the absence of bone loss, resulting from a lack of insulin or reduced insulin sensitivity [68]. Hyperglycemia alone may further inhibit insulin secretion. There is a strong genetic predisposition for those types of diabetes although the exact genetic defects are not currently well defined [69]. Diabetes is one of the leading causes of death and disability in the United States with type 2 diabetes accounting for 90–95% of all diabetic cases. In type 1 diabetes, the final common pathway is beta-cell destruction by autoimmune processes, which leads to insulin deficiency. Type 2 diabetes is characterized by varying degrees of insulin resistance and relative insulin deficiency.

Abnormalities in glucose metabolism such as insulin resistance, glucose intolerance, and diabetes mellitus are central features of the metabolic syndrome and generally arise when there is limited availability of insulin or impaired response to available insulin. The importance of maintaining low blood glucose levels is further evidenced by the findings of Khaw et al. [70], which estimated that 1% increase in glycated hemoglobin (HbA_{1C}) among study's subjects with glycated hemoglobin values of 5–6.9% were associated with a 28% increase in the risk of death independent of age, blood pressure, serum cholesterol, and body mass index. Unfortunately, the diagnosis of type 2 diabetes is often delayed for years after the onset of the disease. Abnormalities in central and peripheral parameters of cardiovascular structure and function result in type 2 diabetes and hypertension. Evidence for an exercise training benefit is strongest for improvements in endothelial vasodilator function and left ventricular diastolic function [71]. The goal of treatment in type 2 diabetes is to achieve and maintain near-normal blood glucose levels and optimal lipid levels, in order to prevent or delay the microvascular, macrovascular, and neural complications. This protective effect can be seen in exercise, the most in individuals at highest risk for developing type 2 diabetes. The risk of developing diabetes was reduced by 24% following an energy expenditure of 2,000 calories per week through exercise. However, this assertion is based more on a lack of randomized controlled trials rather than data to the contrary. Insulin secretion is reduced during exercise and does not play a major role in euglycemia during exercise. The current evidence, even though not fully confirmed in randomized trials, suggests major benefit of exercise is its effect on the heart and the associated reduction in death from heart disease. In addition to lowering the risk of heart disease in type 2 diabetes, exercise helps to decrease the chances of developing diabetes [71].

Exercise's Effects on Diabetes

During exercise, the liver is able of transform stored glycogen, via glycogenolysis as well as synthesizing new glucose from glycerol, pyruvate, and lactic acid in a process called gluconeogenesis. Training may elicit favorable changes in lipid metabolism and can bring about improvements in the regulation of hepatic glucose output, which is especially relevant to diabetes mellitus [72]. *Aerobic exercise* is proving to have significant benefits for people with both type 1 (diabetes juvenile) and type 2 (non-insulin-dependent diabetes mellitus). Aerobic exercise has significant and particular benefits for people with type 1 diabetes. It increases sensitivity to insulin, lowers blood pressure, improves cholesterol levels, and decreases body fat. In type 2 diabetes, moderate aerobic exercise can lower blood sugar levels and improve insulin sensitivity. Strength training, which increases muscle and reduces fat, may be particularly helpful for people with diabetes.

A distinction should be made between the acute effects of exercise and chronic training effects. Physical activity abnormal insulin secretion and peripheral insulin resistance are primary factors that influence the acute effects of physical activity on metabolic responses in those with type 2 diabetes. Single bout of exercise can increase insulin sensitivity for at least 16 h post-exercise in healthy as well as diabetes mellitus subjects [72]. Up to 2 h after exercise, glucose uptake is in part elevated due to insulin-independent mechanisms, probably involving a contraction-induced increase in the amount of GLUT4 associated with the plasma membrane and T tubules. The effect of an acute bout of exercise on insulin action is lost within a few days, and the benefit of a single bout of physical activity is short-lived for persons with type 2 diabetes. Acute exercise also enhances insulin-stimulated GLUT4 translocation and increases in muscle GLUT4 protein content.

Chronic aerobic activity using large muscle groups, such as walking, running, or swimming, produces cardiovascular adaptations that increase exercise capacity, endurance, and skeletal muscle strength. Habitual physical activity also prevents the development of coronary artery disease and reduces symptoms in patients with established cardiovascular disease and diabetes [73]. In addition, aerobic exercise training reduces total and abdominal fat. These changes in body composition mediate improvements in insulin sensitivity and blood pressure and may improve endothelial vasodilator function [71]. These changes can be especially important for those with borderline diabetes. Potential mechanisms through which exercise could improve cardiovascular health include decreased systemic inflammation, improved early diastolic filling (reduced diastolic dysfunction), improved endothelial vasodilator function, increase arteriovenous oxygen content differences, and decreased abdominal visceral fat accumulation [71].

Aerobic exercise training results in preferential loss of fat from the central regions of the body and should, therefore, contribute significantly in preventing or alleviating insulin resistance [74]. The mechanism for these benefits is that exercising muscles are more sensitive to circulating insulin. They thus take up blood sugar more easily and use sugar more effectively. Additionally, training may elicit favorable changes in lipid metabolism bringing about improvements in the regulation of hepatic glucose output, which is especially relevant to diabetes mellitus [72]. In addition, physical training potentiates the effect of exercise on insulin sensitivity through multiple adaptations in glucose transport and metabolism. Blood glucose reduction during physical activity is attributed to an attenuation of hepatic glucose production, whereas muscle glucose utilization increases normally.

Aerobic exercise also improves blood cholesterol levels and blood pressure control. This benefit occurs regardless of weight loss. Exercise program reduces triglyceride levels by 20%, increases high-density lipoprotein cholesterol significantly, and decreases blood pressure.

Aerobic exercise lasting 150 min · week^{-1} or 500 kcal · week^{-1} in energy expenditure of moderate intensity of physical activity or at least 90 min · week^{-1} of vigorous aerobic exercise was associated with a 6% decreased incidence of type 2 diabetes [75, 76]. Moderate-intensity aerobic exercise increases glucose uptake by 2–3 mg · kg^{-1} · min^{-1} above usual requirements (70-kg person, 8.4–12.6 g · h^{-1} of exercise). During high-intensity aerobic exercise, glucose uptake increases by 5–6 mg · kg^{-1} · min^{-1}; however, exercise of this intensity cannot usually be sustained for long intervals. Traditionally, diabetic patients have been encouraged to train aerobic exercises such as walking, running, cycling, and swimming.

Weight training is usually not promoted much for diabetics. However, prolonged aerobic exercise or sufficiently intense exercise can result in an imbalance leaning toward a higher rate of muscle utilization than hepatic output, at which point glucose levels fall along with the onset of fatigue. Due to the limited information on the role of *resistance training* for older patients with type 2 diabetes, it has been recommended that resistance training programs use moderate weights and high repetitions [77]. Muscle contraction increases glucose uptake in skeletal muscle [78], thereby forming the basis for recommending resistive training for individuals with abnormal glucose metabolism. In the absence of contraindications, the American Diabetes Association recommends resistive training for those with type 2 diabetes [79]. These recommendations are supported by evidence that resistive training is an integral component in the therapeutic management of glycemic control in both young and older type 2 diabetics [80]. The American Diabetes Association recommends performing resistance exercise three times a week, using three sets of 8–10 repetitions without developing fatigue. The American College of Sports Medicine has also recommended the use of progressive resistive training as part of a well-rounded exercise program for individuals with type 2 diabetes [81]. Studies demonstrated that improvement in insulin sensitivity correlates with increasing muscle mass following resistive training, due to the utilization of insulin-independent mechanisms to increase glucose uptake by the contracting muscles [82]. Aerobic exercise uses large muscle groups for extended periods of time, but whole-body resistive training programs may provide equally high or higher recruitment of muscle mass over a comparable period of time. However, the effect of resistive training is controversial. Several months of weight-lifting training has been found to significantly lower the insulin response to a glucose challenge without affecting glucose tolerance, and to increase the rate of glucose clearance during a euglycemic clamp [74]. Both aerobic and resistance training have been shown to be of benefit for the control of diabetes; however, resistance training may have greater benefits for glycemic control than aerobic training may have. Skeletal muscle is the primary metabolic recipient for glucose and triglyceride metabolism and is an important determinant of resting metabolic rate. Accordingly, it has been hypothesized that resistance exercise training and subsequent increases in muscle mass may reduce multiple cardiovascular disease risk factors.

Improved glycemic control and decreased HbA1c levels are important for reducing the microvascular and macrovascular complications of diabetes; each percentage point reduction in HbA1c was associated with a 35% reduction in microvascular complications [83]. In a recent study though, the effects of a mix of aerobic and resistance training were tested in a group of type 2 diabetics. The results were very encouraging indeed [84]. Combined physical activity and modest weight loss have been shown to lower type 2 diabetes risks by up to 58% in high-risk populations. Most benefits of physical activity on diabetes management are realized through acute and chronic improvements in insulin action, accomplished with both aerobic and resistance training [85]. Although both aerobic and resistance types of exercise have been shown to be associated with a decreased risk of type 2 diabetes [86], either aerobic or resistance training alone improves glycemic control in type 2 diabetes, but the improvements are greatest with combined aerobic and resistance training.

Several studies suggest that glucose transport is rate limiting for glucose uptake into muscle during exercise. Mechanism suggested for improving glycemic control during exercise is the muscle increases GLUT4 translocation and therefore glucose uptake. Skeletal muscle expresses multiple isoforms of glucose transporters [86]. During exercise, the most important of these is GLUT4, because systemic [87] and muscle-specific GLUT4 knockout abolishes contraction-stimulated glucose uptake [88]. Signaling of molecular mechanisms responsible for the increase in glucose transport and GLUT4 translocation during muscle contraction is still known. It is generally accepted that it arise from local factors within the contracting skeletal muscle [89]. This mechanism involves activation of AMP-activated protein kinase (AMPK). It has previously been reported that exercise causes an increase in glucose uptake in skeletal muscle and also an increase in 5′ AMP-activated protein kinase activity, due to an increase in the translocation of GLUT4 to surface membranes [90]. Other possible mechanisms involve in metabolic homeostasis is the signaling via nitric oxide, reactive oxygen species, as well as a physical mechanism caused by the contraction itself. The major glucose transporter protein expressed in skeletal muscle is GLUT4. Total GLUT4 content in skeletal muscle from individuals with diabetes mellitus is normal; however, it was suggested that translocation of GLUT4 to the plasma membrane is decreased in response to insulin stimulation. Kennedy et al. [91] suggested that the translocation of GLUT4 is an important cellular mechanism through which exercise enhances skeletal muscle glucose uptake in individuals with diabetes mellitus. Thus, physical exercise can be important in the treatment of both *diabetes mellitus* and *juvenile diabetes*. In skeletal muscle and adipocytes, insulin-stimulated glucose transport has been known to occur through the translocation of glucose transporter (GLUT 4) from the intracellular pool to the plasma membrane [92]. The intracellular pathways that lead to contraction and insulin-stimulated GLUT4 translocation seem to be different, allowing the attainment of a maximal effect when acting together. Insulin utilizes a phosphatidylinositol 3-kinase-dependent mechanism, whereas the exercise signal may be initiated by calcium release from the sarcoplasmic reticulum or from autocrine- or paracrine-mediated activation of glucose transport [92].

Before beginning a program of physical activity that is more vigorous than brisk walking, people with diabetes should be assessed for conditions that might contraindicate certain types of exercise or predispose to injury: severe autonomic neuropathy, severe peripheral neuropathy, preproliferative or proliferative retinopathy [61]. Physical activity is one of the principal therapies to acutely lower blood glucose in type 2 diabetes due to its synergistic action with insulin in insulin-sensitive tissues.

It is well established that patients with a diagnosis of type 2 diabetes have low maximal oxygen uptake values when compared with healthy age-matched controls. In studies with athletes and in patients with type 2 diabetes and their first-degree relatives, a close relationship has been demonstrated between maximal oxygen uptake and whole-body, insulin-stimulated glucose uptake [93]. Oxygen delivery to peripheral tissues in type 2 diabetic individuals may be impaired during acute bouts of graded exercise, as the rate of oxygen uptake during submaximal and maximal workloads is significantly lower than age- and activity-matched persons without diabetes [94]. Hence, functional capacity of those with type 2 diabetes is frequently lower than age-matched nondiabetic counterparts. Acute bouts of physical activity can favorably change abnormal blood glucose and insulin resistance. A cluster randomized trial found that diet alone, exercise alone, and combined diet and exercise were equally effective in reducing the progression from impaired glucose tolerance to diabetes [95]. Thus, exercise is a logical treatment modality because it improves insulin sensitivity by diminishing resistance and increases maximal oxygen uptake; this can be especially important for those with borderline diabetes.

For improving glycemic control, with weight maintenance, and reduce the risk of cardiovascular disease, the American Diabetes Association recommends at least 150 min per week of moderate-intensity physical activity (50–70% of maximum heart rate) or at least 90 min per week of vigorous aerobic exercise (more than 70% of reserved heart rate). Exercise at least 3 days a week, and without more than two consecutive days without exercising [96]. Therefore, patients with diabetes should be encouraged to perform 30–60 min of moderate-intensity aerobic activity such as brisk walking on most (preferably all) days of the week [96]. Resistive training induced improvements in glycemic control; however, it appears to be intensity dependent, with beneficial effects occurring when subjects train at 70–90% of the 1 repetition maximum strength (1-RM). Heavy-resistance strength training may be associated with a decrease in glycosylated hemoglobin and cholesterol in type I diabetic men and women regardless of age, following training, in addition to increasing overall strength [97]. Either aerobic or resistance training alone improves glycemic control in diabetes mellitus, but the improvements are greatest with combined aerobic and resistive training [98]. Strength training targeting all of the major muscle groups, which increases muscle and reduces fat, is also helpful for people with diabetes, who are able to do this type of exercise.

References

1. Crouse SF, O'Brien BC, Grandjean PW, Lowe RC, Rohack JJ, Green JS. Effects of training and a single session of exercise on lipids and apolipoproteins in hypercholesterolemic men. J Appl Physiol. 1997;83: 2019–28.
2. Durstine JL, Grandjean PW, Davis PG, Ferguson MA, Alderson NL, DuBose KD. Blood lipid and lipoprotein adaptations to exercise: a quantitative analysis. Sports Med. 2001;31:1033–62.
3. Lahoz C, Mostaza JM. Atherosclerosis as a systemic disease. Rev Esp Cardiol. 2007;60:184–95.
4. King AC, Haskell WL, Young DR, Oka RK, Stefanick ML. Long-term effects of varying intensities and formats of physical activity on participation rates, fitness, and lipoproteins in men and women aged 50 to 65 years. Circulation. 1995;91:2596–604.
5. Baigent C, Blackwell L, Emberson J, et al. Cholesterol Treatment Trialists' (CTT) Collaboration, Efficacy and safety of more intensive lowering of LDL cholesterol: a meta-analysis of data from 170,000 participants in 26 randomised trials. Lancet. 2010;376:1670–81.
6. Baigent C, Keech A, Kearney PM, Blackwell L, Buck G, Pollicino C, et al. Efficacy and safety of cholesterol-lowering treatment: prospective meta-analysis of data from 90,056 participants in 14 randomised trials of statins. Lancet. 2005;366:1267–78.
7. Marrugat J, Elosua R, Covas MI, Molina L, Rubies-Prat J. Amount and intensity of physical activity, physical fitness, and serum lipids in men. The MARATHOM Investigators. Am J Epidemiol. 1996;143:562–9.
8. Phillips WT, Kiratli BJ, Sarkarati M, et al. Effect of spinal cord injury on the heart and cardiovascular fitness. Curr Probl Cardiol. 1998;23:641–716.
9. Stefanick ML, Mackey S, Sheehan M, et al. Effects of diet and exercise in men and postmenopausal women with low levels of HDL cholesterol and high levels of *LDL cholesterol*. N Engl J Med. 1998;339:12–20.
10. Rotkis HB, Cote R, Coly E, Wilmore JH. Relationship between high density lipoprotein cholesterol and weekly running mileage. J Cardiac Rehabil. 1982;2: 109–12.
11. Petridou A, Lazaridou D, Mougios V. Lipidemic profile of athletes and non-athletes with similar body fat. Int J Sport Nutr Exerc Metab. 2005;15:425–32.
12. Nikkilä EA, Taskinen MR, Rehunen S, Harkonen M. Lipoprotein lipase activity in adipose tissue and skeletal muscle of runners: relation to serum lipoproteins. Metabolism. 1978;27:1661–7.
13. Taylor PA, Ward A. Women, high-density lipoprotein cholesterol, and exercise. Arch Intern Med. 1993;153:1178–84.
14. Hernan Jimenez O, Ramírez-Velez R. Strength training improves insulin sensitivity and plasma lipid levels without altering body composition in overweight and obese subjects. Endocrinol Nutr. 2011;58: 169–74.
15. Kelley GA, Kelley KS. Impact of progressive resistance training on lipids and lipoproteins in adults: another look at a meta-analysis using prediction intervals. Prev Med. 2009;49:473–5.
16. Tucker LA, Silvester LJ. Strength training and hypercholesterolemia: an epidemiologic study of 8499 employed men. Am J Health Promot. 1996;11:35–41.
17. Kohl III HW, Gordon NF, Scott CB, Vaandrager H, Blair SN. Musculoskeletal strength and serum lipid levels in men and women. Med Sci Sports Exerc. 1992;24:1080–7.
18. Shoup EE, Durstine JL. Acute circuit weight lifting and its effects on postheparin lipoprotein lipase activity. Med Sci Sports Exerc. 1991;23:4–9.
19. Boyden TW, Pamenter RW, Going SB, et al. Resistance exercise training is associated with decreases in serum low-density lipoprotein cholesterol levels in premenopausal women. Arch Intern Med. 1993;153:97–100.
20. Halverstadt A, Phares DA, Wilund KR, Goldberg AP, Hagberg JM. Endurance exercise training raises high-density lipoprotein cholesterol and lowers small low-density lipoprotein and very low-density lipoprotein independent of body fat phenotypes in older men and women. Metabolism. 2007;56:444–50.
21. Sagiv M, Goldbourt U. Influence of physical work on high density lipoprotein cholesterol: implications for the risk of coronary heart disease. Int J Sports Med. 1994;15:261–6.
22. Thompson PD, Tsongalis GJ, Seip RL, et al. Apolipoprotein E genotype and changes in serum lipids and maximal oxygen uptake with exercise training. Metabolism. 2004;53:193–202.
23. Thorland WG, Gilliam TB. Comparison of serum lipids between habitually high and low active preadolescent males. Med Sci Sports Exerc. 1981;13:316–21.
24. Angelopoulos TJ, Sivo SA, Kyriazis GA. Do age and baseline LDL cholesterol levels determine the effect of regular exercise on plasma lipoprotein cholesterol and apolipoprotein B levels? Eur J Appl Physiol. 2007;101:621–8.
25. Kelley GA, Kelley KS, Franklin B. Aerobic exercise and lipids and lipoproteins in patients with cardiovascular disease: a meta-analysis of randomized controlled trials. J Cardiopulm Rehabil. 2006;26:131–44.
26. Stein RA, Michielli DW, Glanz MD, Sardy H, Cohen A, Goldberg N, Brown CD. Effects of different exercise training intensities on lipoprotein cholesterol fractions in healthy middle-aged men. Am Heart J. 1990;119:277–83.
27. Kodama S, Tanaka S, Saito K, et al. Effect of aerobic exercise training on serum levels of high-density lipoprotein cholesterol: a meta-analysis. Arch Intern Med. 2007;167:999–1008.
28. Eapen DJ, Kalra GL, Rifai L, Eapen CA, Merchant N, Khan BV. Raising HDL cholesterol in women. Int J Womens Health. 2010;1:181–91.
29. Joseph LJ, Davey SL, Evans WJ, Campbell WW. Differential effect of resistance training on the body

composition and lipoprotein-lipid profile in older men and women. Metabolism. 1999;48:1474–80.
30. Cauley JA, Kriska AM, LaPorte RE, Sandler RB, Pambianco GA. Two year randomized exercise trail in older women: effects on HDL-cholesterol. Atherosclerosis. 1987;66:247–58.
31. Stranska Z, Matoulek M, Vilikus Z, Svacina S, Stransky P. Aerobic exercise has beneficial impact on atherogenic index of plasma in sedentary overweigh and obese women. Neuro Endocrinol Lett. 2011; 32:102–8.
32. Lokey EA, Tran ZV. Effects of exercise training on serum lipid and lipoprotein concentrations in women: a meta-analysis. Int J Sports Med. 1989;10:419–29.
33. Goldberg AP, Busby-Whitehead MJ, Katzel LI, Krauss RM, Lumpkin M, Hagberg JM. Cardiovascular fitness, body composition, and lipoprotein lipid metabolism in older men. J Gerontol A Biol Sci Med Sci. 2000;55:M342–9.
34. Corvilain B. Lipoprotein metabolism. Rev Med Brux. 1997;18:3–9.
35. BenOunis O, Elloumi M, Makni E, Zouhal H, Amri M, Tabka Z, Lac G. Exercise improves the ApoB/ApoA-I ratio, a marker of the metabolic syndrome in obese children. Acta Paediatr. 2010;99:1679–85.
36. Morris R, Digenio A, Padayachee GN, Kinnear B. The effect of a 6-month cardiac rehabilitation programme on serum lipoproteins and apoproteins A1 and B and lipoprotein a. S Afr Med J. 1993;83: 315–8.
37. Kiens B, Lithell H. Lipoprotein metabolism influenced by training-induced changes in human skeletal muscle. J Clin Invest. 1983;83:558–64.
38. Lavie CJ, Milani RV. Effects of cardiac rehabilitation, exercise training, and weight reduction on exercise capacity, coronary risk factors, behavioral characteristics, and quality of life in obese coronary patients. Am J Cardiol. 1997;79:397–401.
39. Lavie CJ, Ventura HO, Messerli FH. Left ventricular hypertrophy its relationship to obesity and hypertension. Postgrad Med. 1992;91:131–43.
40. Bader DS, Maguire TE, Spahn CM, O'Malley CJ, Balady GJ. Clinical profile and outcomes of obese patients in cardiac rehabilitation stratified according to National Heart, Lung, and Blood Institute criteria. J Cardiopulm Rehabil. 2001;21:210–7.
41. Meires J, Christie C. Contemporary approaches to adult obesity treatment. Nurse Pract. 2011;36:37–46.
42. Hu G, Tuomilehto J, Silventoinen K, Barengo N, Jousilahti P. Joint effects of physical activity, body mass index, waist circumference and waist-to-hip ratio with the risk of cardiovascular disease among middle-aged Finnish men and women. Eur Heart J. 2004;25:2212–9.
43. Giannopoulou I, Ploutz-Snyder LL, Carhart R, Weinstock RS, Fernhall B, Goulopoulou S, Kanaley JA. Exercise is required for visceral fat loss in postmenopausal women with type 2 diabetes. J Clin Endocrinol Metab. 2005;90:1511–8.
44. Windecker S, Allemann Y, Billinger M, et al. Effect of endurance training on coronary artery size and function in healthy men: an invasive follow up study. AJP Heart. 2002;282:H2216–23.
45. Redman LM, Heilbronn LK, Martin CK, Alfonso A, Smith SR, Ravussin E. Effect of calorie restriction with or without exercise on body composition and fat distribution. J Clin Endocrinol Metab. 2007;92: 865–72.
46. Helge JW, Wulff B, Kiens B. Impact of a fat-rich diet on endurance in man: role of the dietary period. Med Sci Sports Exerc. 1998;30:456–61.
47. Poirier P, Després JP. Exercise in weight management of obesity. Cardiol Clin. 2001;19:459–70.
48. Achten J, Gleeson M, Jeukendrup AE. Determination of the exercise intensity that elicits maximal fat oxidation. Med Sci Sports Exerc. 2002;34:92–7.
49. Ibrahimi A, Bonen A, Blinn WE, et al. Muscle-specific overexpression of FAT/CD36 enhances fatty acid oxidation by contracting muscle, reduces plasma triglycerides and fatty acids, and increases plasma glucose and insulin. J Biol Chem. 1999;274:26761–6.
50. Tunstall RJ, Mehan KA, Wadley GD, Collier GR, Bonen A, Hargreaves M, Cameron-Smith D. Exercise training increases lipid metabolism gene expression in human skeletal muscle. Am J Physiol Endocrinol Metab. 2002;283:E66–72.
51. Kiens B, Kristiansen S, Jensen P, Richter EA, Turcotte LP. Membrane associated fatty acid binding protein (FABPpm) in human skeletal muscle is increased by endurance training. Biochem Biophys Res Commun. 1997;231:463–5.
52. Bonen A, Dyck DJ, Ibrahimi A, Abumrad NA. Muscle contractile activity increases fatty acid metabolism and transport and FAT/CD36. Am J Physiol Endocrinol Metab. 1999;276:E642–9.
53. Berthon PM, Howlett RA, Heigenhauser GJF, Spriet LL. Human skeletal muscle carnitine palmitoyltransferase I activity determined in isolated intact mitochondria. J Appl Physiol. 1998;85:148–53.
54. Spina RJ, Chi MM-Y, Hopkins MG, Nemeth PM, Lowry OH, Holloszy JO. Mitochondrial enzymes increase in muscle in response to 7–10 days of cycle exercise. J Appl Physiol. 1996;80:2250–4.
55. Baar K, Blough E, Dineen B, Esser K. Transcriptional regulation in response to exercise. Exerc Sport Sci Rev. 1999;27:333–79.
56. Kraniou Y, Cameron-Smith D, Misso M, Collier G, Hargreaves M. Effects of exercise on GLUT-4 and glycogenin gene expression in human skeletal muscle. J Appl Physiol. 2000;88:794–6.
57. Vuori IM. Dose–response of physical activity and low back pain, osteoarthritis, and osteoporosis. Med Sci Sports Exerc. 2001;33(6 suppl):S551–86.
58. Stone MH, Fleck SJ, Triplett NT, Kraemer WJ. Health- and performance-related potential of resistance training. Sports Med. 1991;11:210–31.
59. Fry AC. The role of resistance exercise intensity on muscle fibre adaptations. Sports Med. 2004;34:663–79.

60. Kraemer WJ, Volek SJ, Clark KL, et al. Physiological adaptations to a weight-loss dietary regimen and exercise programs in women. J Appl Physiol. 1997; 83:270–9.
61. Buse JB, Ginsberg HN, Bakris GL, et al. Primary prevention of cardiovascular diseases in people with diabetes mellitus. A scientific statement from the American Heart Association and the American Diabetes Association. Circulation. 2007;115:114–26.
62. Dunstan DW, Zimmet PZ, Welborn TA, De Courten MP, et al. The rising prevalence of diabetes and impaired glucose tolerance: the Australian diabetes, obesity and lifestyle study. Diabetes Care. 2002;25:829–34.
63. Evans WJ. Effects of exercise on body composition and functional capacity of the elderly. J Gerontol A Biol Sci Med Sci. 1995;50A:147–50.
64. Lindle R, Metter E, Lynch N, et al. Age and gender comparisons of muscle strength in 654 women and me aged 20–93. J Appl Physiol. 1997;83:1581–7.
65. Frontera WR, Hughes VA, Lutz KJ, Evans WJ. A cross-sectional study of muscle strength and mass in 45- to 78-yr-old men and women. J Appl Physiol. 1991;71:644–50.
66. Ingelsson E, Sullivan LM, Murabito JM, et al. Prevalence and prognostic impact of subclinical cardiovascular disease in individual with the metabolic syndrome and diabetes. Diabetes. 2007;56:1718–26.
67. Harris MI, Flegal KM, Cowie CC, et al. Prevalence of diabetes, impaired fasting glucose, and impaired glucose tolerance in US adults: the Third National Health and Nutrition Examination Survey, 1988–1994. Diabetes Care. 1998;21:518–24.
68. McCabe L, Zhang J, Raehtz S. Understanding the skeletal pathology of type 1 and 2 diabetes mellitus. Crit Rev Eukaryot Gene Expr. 2011;21:187–206.
69. Villeneuve LM, Natarajan R. The role of epigenetics in the pathology of diabetic complications. Am J Physiol Renal Physiol. 2010;299:F14–25.
70. Khaw KT, Wareham N, Luben R, et al. Glycated haemoglobin, diabetes, and mortality in men in Norfolk cohort of European prospective investigation of cancer and nutrition (EPICNorfolk). BMJ. 2001;322:1–6.
71. Stewart KJ. Exercise training and the cardiovascular consequences of type q diabetes and hypertension: possible mechanisms for improving cardiovascular health. JAMA. 2002;288:1622–31.
72. Borghouts LB, Keizer HA. Exercise and insulin sensitivity: a review. Int J Sports Med. 2000;21:1–12.
73. Thompson PD, David Buchner D, Piña IL, et al. Exercise and physical activity in the prevention and treatment of atherosclerotic cardiovascular disease. A statement from the Council on Clinical Cardiology (Subcommittee on Exercise, Rehabilitation, and Prevention) and the Council on Nutrition, Physical Activity, and Metabolism (Subcommittee on Physical Activity). Circulation. 2003;107:3109–16.
74. Ivy JL. Role of exercise training in the prevention and treatment of insulin resistance and non-insulin-dependent diabetes mellitus. Sports Med. 1997;24:321–36.
75. Knowler WC, Barrett-Connor E, Fowler SE, Hamman RF, Lachin JM, Walker EA, Nathan DM. Reduction in the incidence of type 2 diabetes with lifestyle intervention or metformin. N Engl J Med. 2002; 346:393–403.
76. Warburton DER, Nicol CW, Bredin SSD. Health benefits of physical activity: the evidence. CMAJ. 2006;174:801–9.
77. American Diabetes Association. Diabetes mellitus and exercise (Position Statement). Diabetes Care. 2000;23 Suppl 1:S50–4.
78. Holloszy JO, Hansen PA. Regulation of glucose transport into skeletal muscle. Rev Physiol Biochem Pharmacol. 1996;128:99–193.
79. Braith RW, Stewart KJ. Resistance exercise training its role in the prevention of cardiovascular disease. Circulation. 2006;113:2642–50.
80. Ibanez J, Izquierdo M, Arguelles I, et al. Twice-weekly progressive resistance training decreases abdominal fat and improves insulin sensitivity in older men with type 2 diabetes. Diabetes Care. 2005;28:662–7.
81. Albright A, Franz M, Hornsby G, Kriska A, Marrero D, Ullrich I, Verity LS. American College of Sports Medicine position stand: exercise and type 2 diabetes. Med Sci Sports Exerc. 2000;32:1345–60.
82. Pereira LO, Lancha Jr AH. Effect of insulin and contraction up on glucose transport in skeletal muscle. Prog Biophys Mol Biol. 2004;84:1–27.
83. Manley S. Haemoglobin A1c: a marker for complications of type 2 diabetes: the experience from the UK Prospective Diabetes Study (UKPDS). Clin Chem Lab Med. 2003;41:1182–90.
84. Balducci S, Zanuso S, Nicolucci A, et al. Effect of an intensive exercise intervention strategy on modifiable cardiovascular risk factors in subjects with type 2 diabetes mellitus: a randomized controlled trial: the Italian Diabetes and Exercise Study (IDES). Arch Intern Med. 2010;170:1794–803.
85. Colberg SR, Albright AL, Blissmer BJ, et al. Exercise and type 2 diabetes: American College of Sports Medicine and the American Diabetes Association: joint position statement. Exercise and type 2 diabetes. Med Sci Sports Exerc. 2010;42:2282–303.
86. Ploug T, Ralston E. Anatomy of glucose transporters in skeletal muscle. Effects of insulin and contractions. Adv Exp Med Biol. 1998;441:17–26.
87. Ryder JW, Kawano Y, Galuska D, et al. Postexercise glucose uptake and glycogen synthesis in skeletal muscle from GLUT4-deficient mice. FASEB J. 1999;13:2246–56.
88. Rose AJ, Richter EA. Skeletal muscle glucose uptake during exercise: how is it regulated? Physiology. 2005;20:260–70.
89. Richter EA. Glucose utilization. In: Handbook of physiology. Exercise: regulation and integration of multiple systems. Bethesda: American Physiological Society; 1996. p. 913–51.
90. Kraczek EJK, Hirshman MF, Goodyear LJ, Winder WW. 5′ AMP-activated protein kinase activation

causes GLUT4 translocation in skeletal muscle. Diabetes. 1999;48:1667–71.
91. Kennedy JW, Hirshman MF, Gervino EV, et al. Acute exercise induces GLUT4 translocation in skeletal muscle of normal human subjects and subjects with type 2 diabetes. Diabetes. 1999;48:1192–7.
92. Miura T, Suzuki W, Ishihara E, Arai I, Ishida H, Seino Y, Tanigawa K. Impairment of insulin-stimulated GLUT4 translocation in skeletal muscle and adipose tissue in the Tsumura Suzuki obese diabetic mouse: a new genetic animal model of type 2 diabetes. Eur J Endocrinol. 2001;145:785–90.
93. Seibek M, Vestergaard H, Burchardt H, et al. Insulin resistance and maximal oxygen uptake. Clin Cardiol. 2003;26:515–20.
94. Regensteiner JG, Bauer TA, Reusch JEB, et al. Abnormal oxygen uptake kinetic responses in women with type II diabetes mellitus. Physiology. 1998; 85:310–7.
95. Pan XR, Li GW, Hu YH, et al. Effects of diet and exercise in preventing NIDDM in people with impaired glucose tolerance: the Da Qing IGT and Diabetes Study. Diabetes Care. 1997;20:537–44.
96. Kamalesh M, Feigenbaum H, Sawada S. Challenge of identifying patients with diabetes mellitus who are at low risk for coronary events by use of cardiac stress imaging. Am Heart J. 2004;147:561–3.
97. Durak EP, Jovanovic-Peterson L, Peterson CM. Randomized crossover study of effect of resistance training on glycemic control, muscular strength, and cholesterol in type I diabetic men. Diabetes Care. 1990;13:1039–43.
98. Sigal RJ, Kenny GP, Boulé NG, et al. Effects of aerobic training, resistance training, or both on glycemic control in type 2 diabetes: a randomized trial. Ann Intern Med. 2007;147:357–69.

Cardiopulmonary Function in Elderly

8

Aging Considerations

Overall cardiovascular function at rest in most healthy elderly individuals is adequate to meet the body's need for pressure and flow. The resting heart rate and heart size are essentially not different in younger vs. older adults, but heart wall thickness increases modestly, due largely to an increase in myocyte size [1]. Atherosclerosis and arteriosclerosis progressively decrease the tissue oxygen supply and cell constituents change with aging, as a consequence, most biological functions show a progressive, age-related deterioration [2]. *Aging* is a complex process involving many variables: genetics, lifestyle factors, and chronic diseases that interact with one another, greatly influencing the manner in which the individual ages. Participation in regular *physical activity* both aerobic and resistive exercises elicits a number of favorable responses that contribute to healthy aging. Much has been learned recently regarding the adaptability of various biological systems as well as the ways that regular exercise can influence them. The functional capacity of the cardiopulmonary system, as assessed by VO_{2max}, declines with advancing age in *trained* and *untrained individuals* (Figs. 8.1 and 8.2). This reduction results in a decrease in physiological functional capacity that would contribute to a loss of independence, increased incidence of disability, and reduced quality of life with age. The primary aging process, itself genetically associated, occurs both independently of lifestyle and in the absence of disease [3].

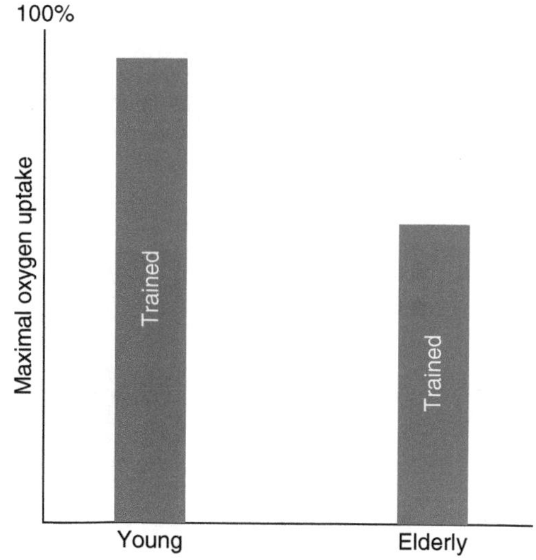

Fig. 8.1 The decrease in maximal oxygen uptake with age is due to the reduced cardiopulmonary function and peripheral factors in the elderly

Accordingly, one may expect *maximal cardiac output* to decrease with aging irrespective of lifestyle because of *genetic factors* (Fig. 8.3). Reduced $(a\text{-}v)O_2$ at maximal effort is the second factor associated with decrease with aging of VO_{2max} [4].

The evidence, that VO_{2max} is limited by *cardiac output*, the oxygen-carrying capacity, and in some cases the *pulmonary system*, is nowadays undeniable. This statement pertains to healthy subjects performing whole-body, dynamic exercise [5]. However, in diverse populations and elderly, incremental exercise exposes the subjects

M.S. Sagiv, *Exercise Cardiopulmonary Function in Cardiac Patients*,
DOI 10.1007/978-1-4471-2888-5_8, © Springer-Verlag London 2012

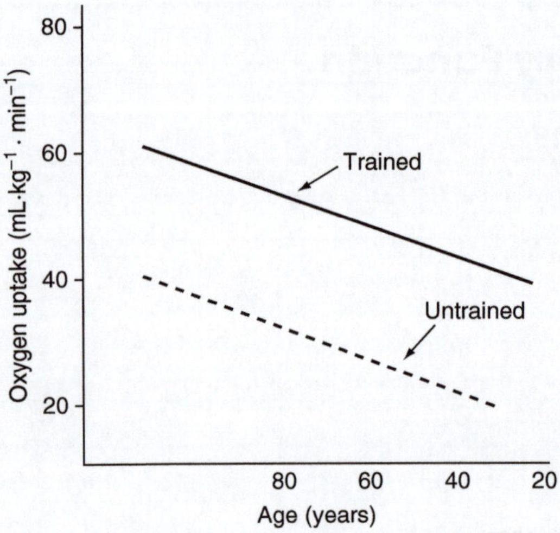

Fig. 8.2 The decrease in maximal oxygen uptake with age due to inactivity. An elderly that exercises regularly also has a decreased maximal oxygen uptake; however, the slope of the decrement is less steeped compared to the untrained individual

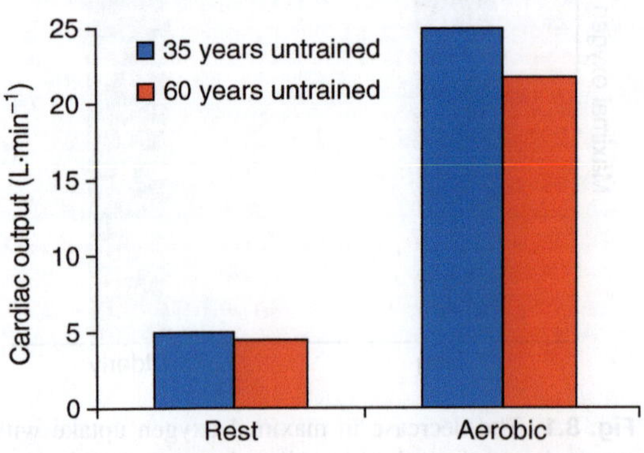

Fig. 8.3 Comparison between young untrained individual with aged individual in cardiac output. The decrease in maximal oxygen uptake with age and inactivity may be explained by the reduced cardiac output

to a relatively high degree of load, which may alter *left ventricular contractility* and *function* [6]. This has the effect of placing a large load on the left ventricle, which might have significant effects on oxygen delivery to the working muscles.

Since metabolic demands during incremental exercise are increased over time, elderly may have different rate of reaction for energy supply between *oxygen delivery and extraction* [6].

The changes in structure and function of the *cardiovascular system* result in VO_{2max} decline, which is the best single indicator of physical working capacity. Whether maximal cardiac output actually decreases with primary aging depends on many interactive factors. During short bursts of graded *maximal aerobic exercise*, reductions in peak work rate, *heart rate*, and *left ventricular emptying* but higher *blood pressure* and *total peripheral resistance* occur in healthy older vs. younger humans [7].

Changes in cardiac structure occur with increasing age. Cardiac function is also altered, partially by the increase in *blood pressure* that accompanies aging. The cardiovascular alterations that occur with *aging* in some ways parallel the changes that occur with deconditioning, including a lower VO_{2max}, maximal cardiac output, *end-diastolic volume* index, lower stroke volume index, and lower cardiac index. Resting *heart rate*, *ejection fraction*, and peak ejection rate remain unchanged with aging [8]. The loss of elasticity of the great arteries, and in particular the aorta which becomes tortuous and wider, results in an increase of impedance at ejection. At systole time, pressure rises in the whole cardiovascular system, so that the *left ventricle* is subjected to an increase of parietal tension to which it adapts itself by hypertrophy which normalizes this tension. Ejection fraction and end-systolic volume are thus preserved, and the systolic function at rest globally remains unmodified by age [9].

It is estimated that mean fall in *cardiac output* is 0.23–0.35 L · min^{-1} per decade. Normalization of the cardiac output for differences in body surface area does not eliminate the effects of aging.

However, several of the changes noted with aging are related to disuse and normalize with increased activity [8]. Peak endurance performance is maintained until approximately 35 years of age, followed by modest decreases until 50–60 years of age, with progressively steeper declines thereafter.

Aging influence on *work capacity* and physical performance and during exercise suggests that there are aging changes in the *heart*, *lung*, and *skeletal muscles* that reduce physical performance with advancing age. *Heart rate* dynamics, which depend on sympathetic nervous activity, are sensitive to physical activity than to age, but VO_{2peak}, as estimated by the age-associated decline in maximum heart rate, is unrelated to *physical training* status [10]. A reduction in lactate threshold contributes to the reduction in endurance performance with aging, although this may be secondary to decreases in VO_{2peak}.

In response to *exercise stress*, the age-related reduction in physiological reserves causes a loss of regulatory or homeostatic balance. This, combined with another consequence of age-related changes, namely an increased perception of effort associated with *submaximal exercise*, sets, especially to a patient unbeknown to the above, a vicious cycle leading to decreased *exercise capacity*, resulting in an elevated perception of effort, subsequently causing avoidance of activity, and finally feeding back to increase the severity of the age-related declines secondary to disuse.

The primary aging process, which has first a *genetic component*, occurs in the absence of disease and independent of lifestyle [11]. Since in the elderly the VO_{2max} during exercise can be 9–10 times that at rest, there must be other factors involved than cardiac since the *cardiac output* can only increase by a factor of four- to fivefold. At least in part, this increased oxygen delivery to tissues is accomplished by increased oxygen extraction by exercising muscles and an increase in (a-v) O_2 by a factor of twofold, resulting in a 15-fold increase in oxygen delivery to exercising muscles. If oxygen transport is indeed limited by *maximal cardiac output*, this may be calculated as the product of *maximal heart rate* and *(a-v)O_2*, and *maximal stroke volume*. The second possible cause that may reduce VO_{2max} with aging is the reduced (a-v) O_2 at maximal effort. The elderly are not generally *anemic* and the *red blood cell* content is usually well maintained, although it may decrease in subjects with a large VO_{2max} [12].

However, the longitudinal rate of decline in peak VO_2 in healthy adults is not constant across the age span in healthy persons, as assumed by cross-sectional studies, but accelerates markedly with each successive age decade, especially in men, regardless of *physical activity* habits. The accelerated rate of decline of *peak aerobic capacity* has substantial implications with regard to functional independence and quality of life, not only in healthy older persons, but particularly when disease-related deficits are superimposed [13].

Age Effect on Oxygen Uptake

Improvements in cardiovascular and respiratory function that accompany growth suggested that VO_{2max} similarly increases. Studies in *males* have shown that the VO_{2max} peaks between the ages of 17–25 years and then decreases. Studies on *females* have found the same trend, although in females the decrease begins at a much younger age, generally aged between 12 and 15 years which is thought to come about due to an assumption of a sedentary lifestyle. VO_{2max} when expressed in $L \cdot min^{-1}$ is lower in *adolescents* than in adults at similar levels of training. This is attributable primarily to an adolescent's lower maximal cardiac capacity. When VO_{2max} values are expressed to reflect the difference in body size between children and adults, there is no difference in aerobic capacity. One study followed a group of 12-year-old boys through to the age of 20 – half of which were trained, the other half untrained but active. Relative to body weight, no differences in VO_{2max} were found between the groups, suggesting that training had no influence on VO_{2max}. However, when VO_{2max} was expressed relative to body surface area, there was a significant difference between groups, and VO_{2max} did indeed increase in proportion to training [14].

VO_2 declines with *aging*, and it was estimated that the rate of this decline is on average 1% per year or approximately 10% per decade after the age of 25 in sedentary subjects [13]. One large cross-sectional study found the average decrease was $0.46\ mLO_2 \cdot kg^{-1} \cdot min^{-1}$ per year in men and $0.54\ mLO_2 \cdot kg^{-1} \cdot min^{-1}$ in *women* [15]. However, this deterioration might not be necessarily due to the aging process, since the trend to increase body weight constitutes by itself an explanation to the decrease in the relative VO_{2max} despite the

maintenance of its absolute values. Usually, the decline in age-related VO_2 can be accounted for by a reduction in *maximum heart rate*, *maximal stoke volume*, that is, cardiac output, and $(a\text{-}v)O_2$ [16].

Regarding the age influence on former *elite athletes*, it has been shown that VO_2 declines by 43% from ages 23 to 50 (from 70 to 40 $mLO_2 \cdot kg^{-1} \cdot min^{-1}$) when they stop training after their careers are over [17]. In some cases, the relative decline is greater than for the average population – as much as 15% per decade or 1.5% per year [18]. However in comparison, master athletes who continue to keep fit only show a decrease of 5–6% per decade or 0.5–0.6% per year [18]. When they maintain the same relative intensity of training, a decrease of only 3.6% over 25 years has been reported and most of that was attributable to a small increase in bodyweight. It seems that training per se can slow down the age-induced decline rate of VO_2, becoming however less effective after the age of about 50 [19].

Aging Effect on Pulmonary Function

Healthy *aging* causes reductions in *lung elastic recoil*, *vital capacity*, *diffusion surface* area, and *chest wall compliance*. Accordingly, in highly fit elderly individuals, significant *expiratory flow* limitation with an accompanying increase *ventilatory work* begins during *submaximal exercise* at V_E values of the 70–80 $L \cdot min^{-1}$ range [20]. At *rest* and *during exercise*, *coronary artery disease patients* do not exhibit difficulties regarding the pulmonary capacity [21]. Aging is associated with a progressive deterioration in the structure and function of the pulmonary circulation. The older adult demonstrates several alterations in the *ventilatory response* to exercise relative to the young adult. These differences are primarily caused by the aging-induced loss of *elastic recoil* of the lung, which reduces *expiratory airflow* rates along the effort-independent portion of the maximal volitional flow-volume envelope. Following a 6-year period of *aerobic training* in active, and highly *trained older adults* (mean age 67–73 years), suggests that habitual *physical activity* and high aerobic capacity modify neither the normal deterioration in resting lung function nor the increased levels of ventilatory work during exercise that occur with *healthy aging* over the sixth and seventh decades of life [22]. Despite these distinctions in the response to exercise in the aged adult, *alveolar ventilation* is adequate for CO_2 elimination even during maximal exercise, and arterial oxygen homeostasis is generally maintained [23]. Thus, elderly appears able to maintain alveolar ventilation at a level that allows maintenance of arterial blood gases within normal limits, even during *heavy exercise*. This ability to maintain adequate gas exchange likely occurs because age-related reductions in the maximal metabolic demand of exercise occur at a rate equal to or greater than the rate of deterioration in ventilatory reserve [24].

Muscle Mass and Cardiopulmonary Function

Muscle mass influences myocardium function since both organs and lungs are connected by a closed circuit vessels. Therefore, any reduction in *muscle mass* (sarcopenia) that reduces its function, such as decline in oxygen extraction ability during dynamic endurance exercise due to *sarcopenia*, will in turn increase *heart rate* in order to have the *cardiac output* needed to deliver more oxygen to the working muscles. The increase in heart rate is reflected by the Fick equation. Thus, physical work capacity declines with advancing age, but the extent to which this can be attributed to a decrement in *cardiac reserve* is not certain. Part of the age-related decline in VO_{2max} appears to be due to peripheral oxygen extraction ability rather than central circulatory factors, for example, to a decrease in muscle mass with age during exercise, the ability to direct blood flow to muscles, and the ability of muscle to utilize oxygen [1]. Previously, a positive correlation between VO_2 and *muscle mass* has been shown [25]. *Mitochondrial density* was found to be lower in *skeletal muscle* of older individuals, which could further diminish capacity for endurance work. Thus, it may be that the aging-related *atrophy* of skeletal muscle (Fig. 8.4) plays some role in the

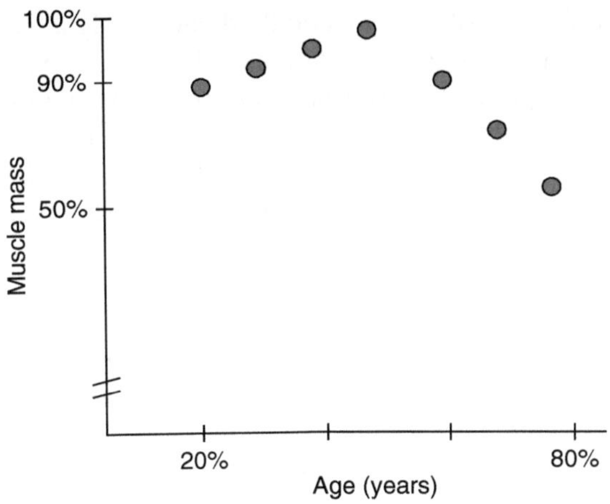

Fig. 8.4 For endurance performance, the key problem associated to aging is the gradual decline in muscle mass. The missing muscle makes it more difficult to perform a powerful physical activity. Muscles reach their maximum size during their 25th year of life, grow smaller by about 10% between the ages of 25 and 50, and then decline by 45% over the next three decades

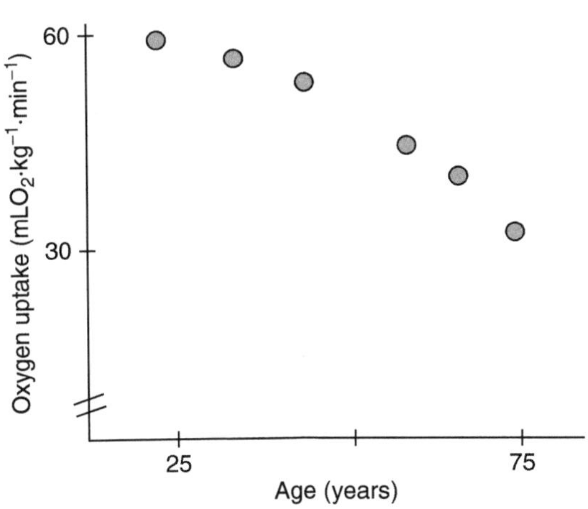

Fig. 8.5 The gradual decline in maximal oxygen uptake makes it more difficult to perform at high levels of physical activity. Maximal oxygen uptake reaches its maximum at the age of 21–25 years; it decreases between the ages of 25 and 75 by 38%

aging-related decline in *aerobic capacity*. The alterations in skeletal muscle structure and function after prolonged periods of *physical inactivity* are initiated by the chronic lack of mechanical stimulus of sufficient intensity, which is the result of a series of biochemical and metabolic interactions spanning from cellular to tissue/organ level. Reduced activation of skeletal muscle alters the *gene expression* of *myosin heavy chain isoforms* to meet the functional demands of reduced mechanical load, which results in *muscle atrophy* and reduced capacity to process *fatty acids*.

In contrast, chronic loading results in the opposite pattern of adaptations [25]. However, others [26] do not support a causal role for muscular atrophy in the decline in VO_{2max} during aging (Fig. 8.5). It seems that the related changes in VO_{2max} are dependent on number of factors including the onset of disease and level of *physical activity*.

Muscle mass may decline by 25% between the ages of 50 and 75 years [27], which translates into an atrophy or decrement in type II fibers and a tendency toward an increase or the maintenance of type I fibers [28]. In accordance, previous findings confirmed that metabolically healthy persons have a greater mass of lean tissue from diverse compartments [29] as well as more visceral fat [30]. Thus, muscle atrophy will reduce the ability of the muscle to generate force which will compel the recruitment of more motor units. This will increase the load on the *myocardium* by increasing *heart rate* and as a consequence increase in *myocardial oxygen demand*. George et al. [31] have indicated that the best scaling variable for *cardiac function* would be one that represents the most metabolically active tissues in the body, that is, muscle or lean body mass. It has been suggested that lean body mass [32] and the allometric model [31] represent the most appropriate normalization for cardiac structures and functions.

Influence of Physical Activity on Exercise Performance

During *isometric maneuver*, an increase in heart rate is produced by isometric contraction, when both the percentage of *maximal force* is increased and the muscle mass involved is greater. Thus, during sustained isometric contractions, the greater the number of *motor units* activated, the greater the activation of muscle's afferent nerve fibers. This suggests that the increase in *heart rate* is related to the muscle mass and the percentage of maximal force exerted. With sarcopenia, the muscle recruits more motor units in order to generate the needed force, and for that reason, heart rate increases without proportion to the effort applied.

The lowest rates of decline in VO_{2max} with age are found in those who remain disease free and continue to maintain high levels of *physical activity*. No significant decline in the VO_{2max} over a 10-year period was found in a group of competitive master athletes who maintained their training intensity and continued to compete. The annual rate of decay in VO_{2max} in the general population is estimated to be 0.4–0.5 $mLO_2 \cdot kg^{-1} \cdot min^{-1}$ per year. The highest rates of decline in VO_{2max} are in those individuals that have reduced their levels of physical activity as they age. *Aerobic capacity* is associated with peripheral vascular reserve in *men*, but not *women*, and *aging* is accompanied by a more pronounced sex difference in this relationship [33]. Through endurance training, a high level of physical capacity can be maintained late in life. The superior *cardiovascular function* of the veteran athletes, compared with the *untrained* controls, was due to both better systolic and diastolic *left ventricular function*. *Myocardial perfusion* defects in athletes should be judged with caution, as this finding is common in veteran athletes as well as healthy young ones. On the whole, it appears that the *physical activity* level plays a dominant role in maintaining cardiovascular fitness, but it does not protect from cardiovascular disease at the individual level. Regular exercise not only reduces the risk for coronary heart disease but also makes the individual better prepared to manage a potential myocardial infarction [34].

Aerobic Exercise Capacity

Aerobic exercise capacity declines approximately 10% per decade in cross-sectional studies; in longitudinal studies, however, this decline is accelerated in the elderly. Reductions in *peak heart rate* and peripheral oxygen utilization but not *stroke volume* appear to mediate the age-associated decline in *aerobic capacity*. Deficits in both cardiac *β-adrenergic receptor* density and in the efficiency of postsynaptic β-adrenergic signaling contribute significantly to the reduced cardiovascular performance *during exercise* in older adults. Although these cardiovascular aging changes are considered natural, they lower the threshold for the development of *cardiovascular disease*, which affects the majority of older adults.

The ability of older persons to function independently is dependent largely on the maintenance of sufficient *cardiopulmonary* and, thus, aerobic capacity and strength to perform daily activities. *Blood plasma volume* decreases with the *onset of exercise* due the increase in blood pressure and changes in intramuscular osmotic pressures forcing water from the vascular compartment to the interstitial space. This reduced plasma volume in turn increases the concentration of *hemoglobin*. Although no extra red blood cells have been produced, the greater concentration of hemoglobin per unit of blood significantly increases the blood's oxygen-carrying capacity. Even though oxygen delivery to the working muscle may be reduced, and since metabolic demand during incremental exercise is increased over time to maximum, elderly may maintain the energy supply due to the balance between oxygen delivery and extraction. Although peak aerobic capacity is widely recognized to decline with age, its rate of decline has been estimated primarily from cross-sectional studies that may provide misleading, overly optimistic estimates of aging changes. The longitudinal rate of decline in VO_{2peak} in healthy adults is not constant across the age span in healthy persons, as assumed by cross-sectional studies, but accelerates markedly with each successive age decade, especially in men, regardless of physical activity habits. The accelerated rate of decline of peak aerobic capacity and cardiovascular function has substantial implications with regard to functional independence, not only in healthy older persons, but particularly when disease-related deficits are superimposed [35].

Cardiac Changes and Cardiac Output

The *cardiopulmonary* system structure appears to be influenced by age, disease, and the level of physical activity. Some changes are independent of gender, disease, and level of *physical activity*. Other structural changes such as an increase in the *left ventricular mass* appear to be dependent on both *gender* and the level of physical activity. In the left ventricle, modest concentric wall thickening occurs due to cellular hypertrophy, but cavity size does not change. In the *cardiovascular system*, morphological and physiological changes have been identified in the elderly. The morphological changes typically do not produce clinical signs of cardiac dysfunction during life. In the elderly, there is a modest increase in *left ventricular thickness*, probably resulting from the observed increase in *systolic blood pressure*. Except for increased tortuosity, cross-sectional area, and degree of atherosclerosis, there are no clear age-associated changes in coronary arteries. However, studies in this area are limited. In normal subjects during exercise, the cardiac function is modified by age. Maximum *heart rate* is reduced in the elderly, whereas the *stroke volume* increases more than in younger subjects, which maintains the appropriate *cardiac output*. Only the maximum exercise level (VO_{2max}) decreases with age, mainly because of the decrease of skeletal muscle mass.

In normal subjects at rest, neither heart rate nor ejection fraction is influenced by age. *Left ventricular compliance* appears to decrease with *aging*, which may contribute to the high incidence of *heart failure* in the *elderly*. However, whether this change is an inevitable consequence of senescence or rather secondary to reduced physical activity is unknown. Prolonged, sustained endurance training preserves ventricular compliance with aging and may help to prevent heart failure in the elderly [36].

Aging is associated with a shift in mechanism by which *cardiac output* is maintained during submaximal exercise. In spite of the elderly having lower *early diastolic filling rate* during submaximal exercise, *end-diastolic volume* is maintained and even increased as a function of age. However, while the early diastolic filling rate is reduced, an enhanced *atrial* contribution to *left ventricular filling* in elderly individuals maintains filling volume at a normal level. Filling of the left ventricle seems to continue to rely, at rest as at exercise, on atrial compensation. However, the delay and slowing down of *left ventricular relaxation time*, due to *left ventricular hypertrophy*, to the reflection waves and to other changes in cardiac muscle physical properties during senescence reduce the importance of the initial phase of left ventricular filling [9]. As a result, older subjects appear to have a greater reliance on the *Frank-Starling mechanism* for the maintenance of *cardiac output* during *submaximal exercise*. The mechanism for the change in maximal *limb conduction* with age is not well understood. Therefore, at peak exercise, older individuals tend to increase end-diastolic volume and end-systolic volume compared with younger subjects [9].

With advancing *age*, changes occur in both the central and peripheral circulation that can affect compliance in arteries and arterioles and blood pressure and ultimately alter the vascular response to exercise [37]. *Cardiac output* at peak exercise is reduced in the older persons due to reduced *maximal heart rate* without change in *stroke volume*. The decrease of maximal heart rate associated with advanced age is similar for the sedentary person, the average active person, and the top athlete. The mechanism underlying the decreased maximal heart rate may be associated with diminished response to *adrenergic regulation* of the heart and circulation [38].

Although older subjects rely on changes in *stroke volume* by dilatation of the left ventricle during intermediate and maximal exercise to partially maintain cardiac output, and to *compensate* for the reduction in *heart rate* [39], maximal stroke volume is decreased due to reduced *preload* (circulating blood volume associated with physical inactivity) and increase in *afterload*. Thus, perfusion of the working muscles via many regulatory mechanisms is reduced. *Older* individuals tend to increase *end-diastolic volume and end-systolic volume* compared with younger subjects [9]. Cardiac output therefore is globally maintained with age during a dynamic effort. Though, some elderly individuals exhibit cardiac dilatation which produces an increased stroke volume sufficient to counter the well-known age-related decrease in exercise heart rate, such that high levels of cardiac output can be maintained during exercise. Still, in these individuals, the exercise-induced reduction in end-systolic volume and increase in ejection fraction is less than in younger individuals [1].

During *isometric exercise*, which in the elderly results in a higher rise in blood pressure, the ejection fraction decreases, the *end-systolic volume* increases, and the initial filling decreases but is compensated by a greater contribution of the atrium: *atrial filling fraction*. Thus, cardiac work at rest and during exercise is well preserved in the aging man due to secondary homeostatic adaptations which counterbalance the primary age-related changes. The principal primary changes are loss of elasticity of the great vessels and reduction of efficacy in response to adrenergic stimulation. The principal secondary adaptations are left ventricular hypertrophy, increased atrial contribution, and, during exercise, intervention of Starling's mechanism [9].

Heart Rate Response

The decrease of *maximal heart rate* associated with advanced age is similar for the sedentary person, the average active person, and the top athlete. In humans, maximal heart rate peaks at around 10 years of age and decreases by approximately beat · min^{-1} · year^{-1} (Fig. 8.6). This suggests that maximal heart rate does not adapt to *chronic exercise* [40]. The mechanisms underlying the decreased maximal heart rate are unknown. The changes may be attributed to the heart itself rather than to neural input. An example for the input ability of the nervous system in the elderly is the manifestation of *ventricular arrhythmias*. Cardiac responses to ß-adrenergic *sympathetic stimulation* decline with aging as does the heart rate response to *parasympathetic* withdrawal, but the extent to which other responses to parasympathetic withdrawal decrease is less clear.

The responses to parasympathetic withdrawal as well as sympathetic stimulation decline with aging, and both contribute to the reduced cardiovascular responses to stress with advancing age [41]. Moreover, changes in the number of pacemaker cells and volume of the sinoatrial node result from aging [1]. Other investigations suggested that there is an age-related decline in maximal heart rate which could be associated with decreased sympathetic drive [42] due to diminished response to adrenergic regulation of the heart and circulation.

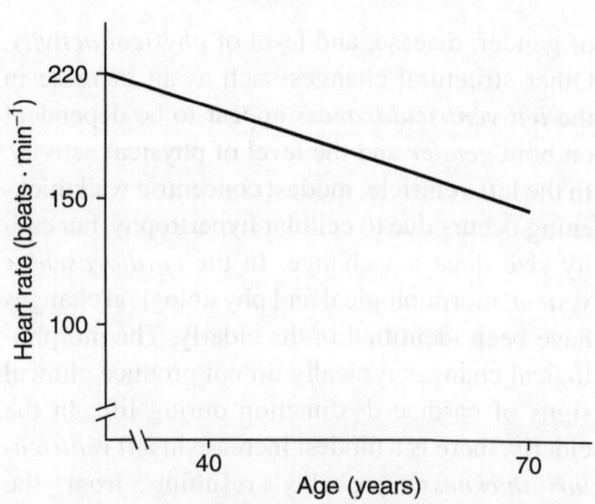

Fig. 8.6 Maximal heart rate predicted is age-related. Maximal heart rate generally declines with age from about 220 beats · min^{-1} in childhood to about 160 beats · min^{-1} at age 60. This fall in heart rate is fairly linear, decreasing by approximately 1 beat · min^{-1} · year^{-1}. There is no strong evidence to suggest that training influences the decline in maximal heart rate

The classical equation for the calculation of maximal heart rate based on age is as follows (8.1):

$$\text{Peak rate} = (220\ \text{beats} \cdot \text{min}^{-1} - \text{age in years} \quad (8.1)$$

This implies a maximum of about 155 beats · min^{-1} at age 65 years [43]. However, research suggests that a well-motivated 65-year-old can attain a rate of 170 beats · min^{-1} or more during uphill treadmill running [44].

Stroke Volume Response

Stroke volume during exercise is regulated by a highly integrated mechanism involving alterations in *inotropic state* and concomitant changes in cardiac loading conditions. Although during submaximal exercise the stroke volume responses of young subjects and old are similar, the old tend to augment stroke volume during exercise more through cardiac dilatation, with an increase in *left ventricular end-diastolic volume* but without much change in *ejection fraction*, whereas the young rely more on an increase in the ejection fraction with no cardiac dilatation, but an elderly person has difficulty in sustaining stroke volume as maximal effort is approached [45], due to reduced sensitivity to catecholamine which blunts the inotropic increase of myocardial contractility during vigorous exercise.

Although older subjects rely on changes in *stroke volume* by increasing of the *left ventricular end-diastolic volume* during intermediate and *maximal exercise* to partially maintain *cardiac output*, and to compensate for the reduction in heart rate [9], maximal stroke volume is decreased due to reduced preload and circulating blood volume associated with *physical inactivity* and increase in *afterload*, and hence, reducing the perfusion of the working muscles via many regulatory mechanisms. Age appears to be associated with an increase in the *total peripheral resistance* independent of change in maximal limb *blood flow*. However, studies suggested that age is associated with a decrease in the maximal conductance of the vascular bed of the calf.

Stroke Volume Response to Training

The larger peak exercise stroke volume in the elderly in response to training appears to be mediated by at least two mechanisms. One is the combination of chronic adaptations, that is, left ventricular hypertrophy due to volume overload and the Frank-Starling mechanism as evidenced by a strong correlation between left ventricular end-diastolic volume and stroke volume at peak exercise. Despite the significant cardiovascular changes that occur in the response to a single bout of exercise with aging, adaptations to *chronic exercise training* are not different with aging and include improvements of left ventricular contractility with or without concomitant reduction of afterload, left ventricular systolic performance, maximal workload and increases in ejection fraction, stroke volume index, and cardiac index at peak exercise. This adaptation takes place owing to an increase of cardiac volume and through Starling's mechanism which ensures a greater ejection volume [9]. The enhanced response to training is reflected by a larger increase in *stroke volume* and significantly higher peak exercise *left ventricular ejection fraction indices*. This may be due to the reduced left ventricular wall stress at peak exercise because systolic blood pressure and left ventricular geometry are likely to change during exercise along with increased sensitivity to *catecholamine* in the trained state [46]. The change in left ventricular wall stress is due to the increased ventricular filling that causes marked decreases in wall stress. The stress–strain characteristics of left ventricular myocardium are dependent on the previous contraction and could be related to the pattern of filling throughout diastole. Major modification of diastolic dynamics at rest is compensated, at the end of diastole, by a more vigorous contraction of the left atrium, which increases its contribution to left ventricular filling. The global filling volume is thus preserved and the end-diastolic volume remains appropriate, these two conditions being necessary to start off a normal ejection [9].

Left Ventricular Function During Aerobic Exercise

At rest, *aging*, independent of cardiovascular diseases, may slightly affect left ventricular cavity dimension, *fractional shortening* of the *minor semiaxis*, and *velocity of circumferential* fiber shortening. Others suggested that age-related deterioration in cardiovascular function is usually attributed to structural and functional changes in the myocardium and associated blood vessels, leading to impairment of *left ventricular systolic function*, increased *afterload*, and blunted *inotropic* and chronotropic responses to catecholamine [47]. Although systolic pressure at rest increases with age, the resting end-systolic volume and ejection fraction are not altered, due partly to the increase in left ventricular thickness. However, aging in the normal male is associated with altered left ventricular *diastolic filling*, increased aortic root diameter, and *left ventricle hypertrophy* but little change in *left ventricular contractility*

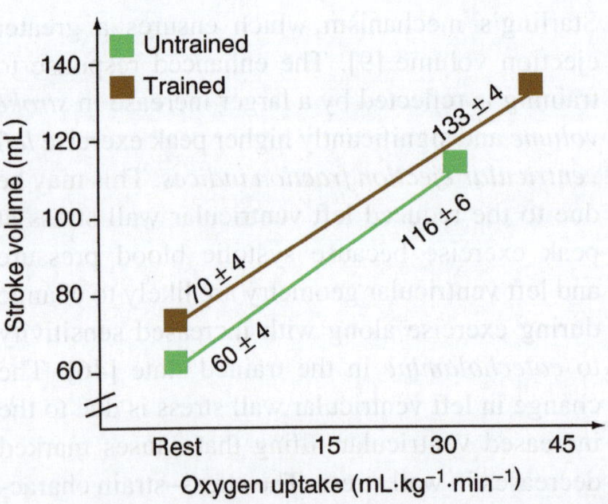

Fig. 8.7 At rest and during exercise, stroke volume values at various workloads (mean ± SD) were significantly greater in the trained elderly compared to that of the untrained elderly

ability in the resting state. The observed change in left ventricular pump performance is related to smaller left ventricular chamber size and higher *total peripheral resistance* in older subjects [48]. In contrast to systolic function, which is relatively well preserved with advancing age, *left ventricular diastolic function* declines steadily after age 30 years [49]. Pulsed Doppler analysis of *mitral inflow* showed a significant age-related decline in the *peak early filling velocity* and in the *ratio of early and late diastolic filling velocity*, while *peak late diastolic flow velocity* and duration of *isovolumic relaxation* increased significantly [50]. The age-associated decline in diastolic function occurs even in the absence of cardiovascular disease and is thought to be a major reason why the incidence of diastolic *heart failure* increases exponentially with age.

By endurance training, a high level of physical capacity can be maintained late in life. The superior cardiovascular function in the veteran athletes, compared with the untrained controls, is due to both better systolic and diastolic left ventricular function (Fig. 8.9). *Myocardial perfusion* defects in athletes should be judged with caution, as this finding is common both in veteran athletes and, as previously shown, in young athletes [34]. As ejection fraction is partially afterload dependent, a lower peripheral resistance in the trained compared with the untrained

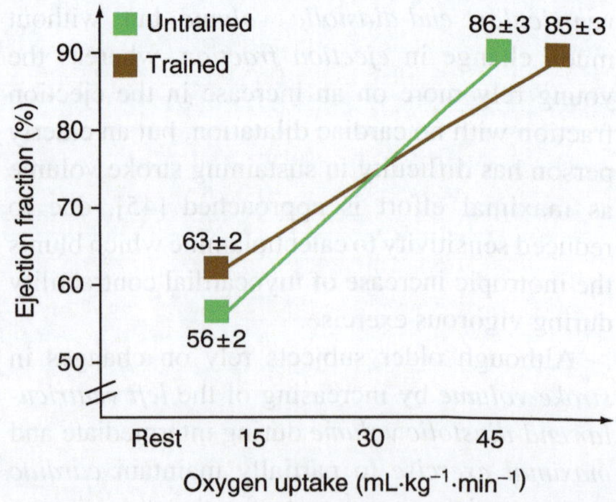

Fig. 8.8 At rest and during exercise, ejection fraction values at various workloads (mean ± SD) were significantly greater in the trained elderly compared to the untrained elderly

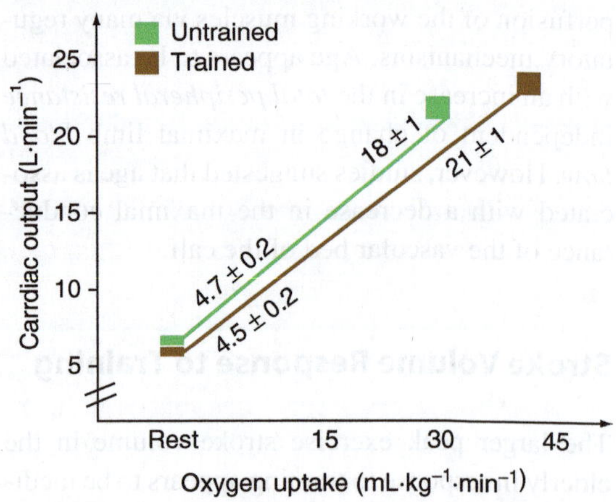

Fig. 8.9 At rest and during exercise, cardiac output values at various workloads (mean ± SD) were significantly higher in the trained elderly compared to the untrained elderly

(Fig. 8.7) during exercise could also contribute to the higher ejection fraction values seen in the athletes.

In healthy trained and untrained elderly, the normal responses through aerobic dynamic exercise are increased left ventricular contractility ejection fraction (Fig. 8.8) indices, stroke volume, end-diastolic volume and cardiac output, and a slight decrease in left ventricular end-systolic volume without any *wall motion abnormalities* [51].

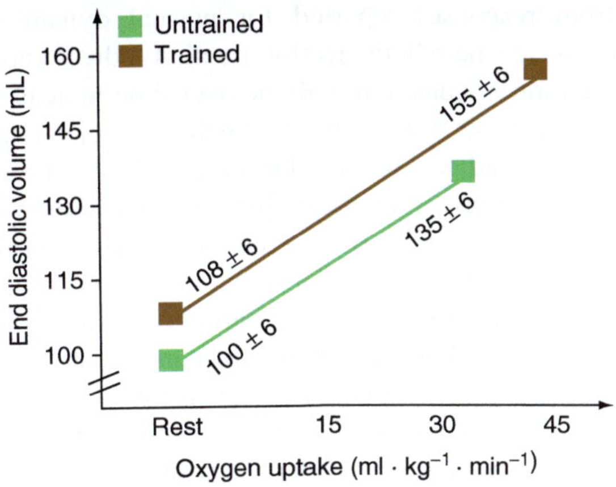

Fig. 8.10 At rest and during exercise, end-diastolic volume values at various workloads (mean ± SD) were significantly greater in the trained elderly compared to the untrained elderly

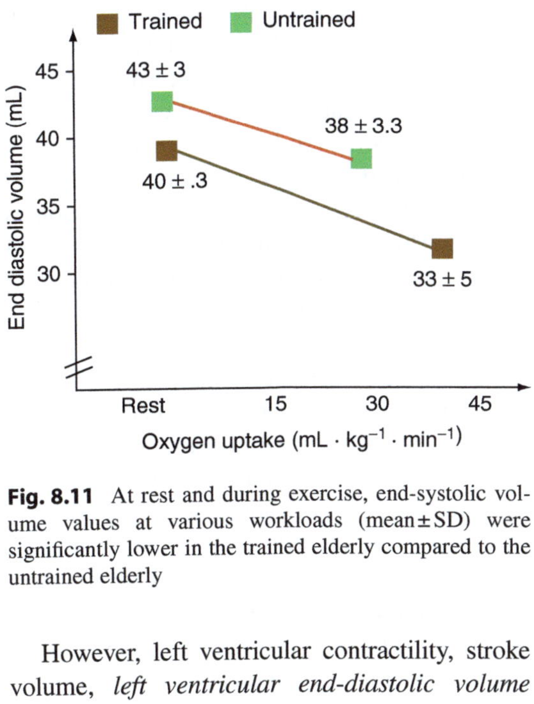

Fig. 8.11 At rest and during exercise, end-systolic volume values at various workloads (mean ± SD) were significantly lower in the trained elderly compared to the untrained elderly

However, left ventricular contractility, stroke volume, *left ventricular end-diastolic volume* (Fig. 8.10), and cardiac output are all significantly higher in the trained elderly compared to untrained ones; while *left ventricular end-systolic volume* (Fig. 8.11) is lower, left ventricular contractility state and function differ at peak all-out anaerobic effort compared with maximal aerobic effort [52].

During the aerobic effort, left ventricular contractility and function increase likely due to the relatively lower afterload opposing the ejection of the left ventricle [53, 54]. This low *afterload* is known to be mediated through the peripheral *autoregulation mechanism* occurring in the active muscles. Thus, left ventricular ejects against *volume overload*. Such lower afterload allows *cardiac output* to increase as a result of increases in *ejection fraction*, *stroke volume* [55], and heart rate [56].

Left Ventricular Function During Anaerobic Exercise

It has been assumed that *anaerobic* type of activity is potentially dangerous for the older population, due to *hypoxia* and a seemingly inappropriate blood pressure response [57]. This has the effect of placing a large load on the left ventricle which affects on *systolic function*. There are many constraints upon peak ventricular function in the *elderly*. *Venous filling* is impaired by poor peripheral venous tone, varicosities, and a slow relaxation of the ventricular wall. At peak anaerobic bout, *left ventricular function* remains stable in *young subjects* and decreases significantly in older men. The magnitude of left ventricular function was related to age and not to absolute work load. *Left ventricular contractility* and left ventricular function are decreased most likely due to the relatively higher afterload opposing the ejection of the left ventricle [58]. Such afterload does not allow cardiac output to increase as a result of decrease in stroke volume and mimics the increase in myocardium *inotropic state* [6]. The decrease in *stroke volume* during anaerobic exercise in the older subjects is due to reduced end-diastolic volume.

It seems that in the older men, compared with the young subjects, the observed lower left ventricular function at peak anaerobic challenge is due, at least partially, to the greater elevation in systolic, diastolic, and *mean blood pressures*, and to the demeaning reduction in *total peripheral resistance*, due to greater concentrations of vasoactive substances owing to tissue *hypoxia* and *acidosis*. This may force the left ventricle to eject blood against a relatively higher pressure. This, coupled with low, peak heart rate, could result in a low overall *cardiac output*.

All-out anaerobic effort in healthy subjects do not produce the expected increase in the left ventricular end-diastolic volume, ejection fraction, stroke volume, and cardiac output, while left ventricular end-systolic volume remains unchanged from resting values [6] seemingly because of the mild decrease in total peripheral resistance. Left ventricular contractility is increased significantly from resting values during all-out anaerobic effort; however, at peak aerobic exercise contractility of the left ventricle is further significantly increased compared to values obtained at peak all-out anaerobic effort [6]. This may suggest that the increase in left ventricular inotropic state is not adequate to increase *left ventricular end-diastolic volume* and reduce *left ventricular end-systolic volume*, and thus ejection fraction remains unchanged during all-out anaerobic exercise [59].

Left Ventricular Function During Isometric Exercise

During *dynamic exercise*, the normal response to an increase in afterload is an increase in the *systolic blood pressure over left ventricular end-systolic volume ratio*. In the *elderly* during *isometric exercise*, the systolic blood pressure over left ventricular end-systolic volume ratio increases significantly from resting values [47]. The ratio increase during isometric exercise maneuver is similar to that seen during dynamic exercise in the elderly. This suggests that healthy elderly respond to isometric exercise by increasing left ventricular contractility in response to an increase in afterload. During *dead lift bout*, in normal elderly subject *left ventricular end-diastolic volume* and *left ventricular end-systolic volume* does not change from resting values [60]. No significant change in mean values for *ejection fraction* indices and the ratio of *change in volume over time* from rest to isometric exercise. The unchanged ejection fraction indices and the ratio of change in volume over time response during the isometric maneuver are markedly different from responses reported for normal dynamic exercise where both ejection fraction indices and the ratio of change in volume over time increase significantly from rest. The unchanged ejection fraction indices may be due to the effects of an acute increase in *afterload* [61]. The physiological effects of resistive exercise training involve changes in left ventricular function and hemodynamic alterations at rest and during exercise [62]. It has been shown that hearts of normal subjects engaged in predominantly pressure overload activities such as weight lifting exercise develop a concentric left ventricular hypertrophy.

Cardiovascular and Physical Performance

Several cardiac changes accompany the normal *aging process*, including prolongation of excitation-contraction and relaxation, increased *afterload*, increased vascular and myocardial stiffness, and decreased catecholamine sensitivity [63]. *Left ventricular systolic performance* is well maintained with aging under resting conditions. However, during exercise, systolic function is reduced. This response may be mediated, at least in part by age-associated reductions in *ß-adrenergic receptor* sensitivity or density, reducing the *inotropic state* response of the myocytes to a standard dose of *catecholamine* [7]. In addition, the decreased responsiveness of cardiovascular tissues to β-adrenergic stimulation is the reduced ability of the atrium to dilate. The peripheral vasculature, however, does not show decreased vasodilatation by the vasodilatating stimuli of nitrates, indicating that the vascular changes are receptor-mediated rather than intrinsic, therefore increasing *blood pressure* and *mean arterial blood pressure* progressively with age, both at rest and *during exercise*. This rise in *total peripheral resistance* may affect left ventricular loading conditions which in turn may mask or mimic changes in left ventricular volumes and diastolic and systolic functions. Left ventricular compliance appears to decrease with aging, which may contribute to the high incidence of heart failure in the elderly. However, whether this change is an inevitable consequence of senescence or rather secondary to reduced physical activity is unknown [36]; therefore, left ventricular contractility appears to be diminished with age.

Compared to the young individuals, older subjects have a greater *end-systolic volume* and a lower *ejection fraction* during submaximal exercise. The mechanism(s) for the decrease in left ventricular contractility with age are unclear; however, increased *afterload*, and/or decreased responsiveness to *adrenergic stimulation*, has been suggested. In addition to that, maximal *isometric contractile properties* of left ventricular muscle are altered in old humans [36]. Left ventricular contraction duration is prolonged and may result from a decrease in the rate of calcium transport by cardiac sarcoplasmic reticulum [64]. Similarly, the *isotonic contractile properties* are altered with *aging*, leading to change in two variables of isotonic contraction: velocity of shortening and relaxation time. These changes in the isometric phase and isotonic phase contracting cardiac muscle lower *peak filling* of the heart in elderly humans. Endurance exercise training enhances *inotropic state* of the left ventricle in older men; after training, elderly increased *ejection fraction* during exercise due to a significant decreased end-systolic volume. In addition, training increased the ratio of the end-systolic pressure–volume [65].

Diastolic left ventricular filling has been shown to be affected not only by ventricular property, but also by aging [66]. Therefore, aging is associated with a shift of left ventricular filling from early to late, decreasing the passive/active phases of filling ratio during diastole. Thus the heart relies more on *atrial filling*, and an increase in isovolumic relaxation time indicating *left ventricular diastolic dysfunction*. In older patients with isolated systolic hypertension, concentric left ventricular hypertrophy is common. Diastolic dysfunction, including the presence of a Doppler filling pattern of impaired relaxation, has been observed in >80% of older hypertensives [67].

Most available studies have been cross-sectional rather than longitudinal, comparing older, highly trained athletes with their more sedentary peers. In addition, some prior studies have been confounded by the failure to rigorously exclude underlying occult disease or by relatively mild training protocols.

Training effect on cardiopulmonary function and muscle metabolism performance of the heart as a pump has been a major element in testing the idea that exercise ameliorates the aging process. Exercise training was associated with health benefits and specifically with decreased cardiovascular mortality in two large observational studies [68, 69]. Hull et al. [70] suggested that following training, the mechanism most likely to be involved is a change in the cardiac autonomic balance, producing an increase, or a relative dominance, of the *vagal component*. It has been long known that *exercise training* reduces resting and submaximal *heart rate* and thus increasing *left ventricular filling time* and hence *stroke volume*.

Alterations in left ventricular structure and *systolic function* are a well-described and accepted component of the response to physical conditioning. This is true if elderly or younger subjects are engaged in similar endurance training. Both age groups demonstrated cardiac changes previously documented to occur with exercise training, including lower heart rates, larger *ventricular cavities*, lower *left ventricular wall stresses*, and higher passive/active ratio. Despite the occurrence of structural and functional changes in response to exercise in the older individuals' hearts, the older hearts were significantly different in some respects from those of their younger counterparts, suggesting that some aspects of normal aging were unaltered by exercise training.

The training effect on cardiopulmonary function during submaximal exercise of a fixed absolute work rate is similar for younger and older individuals. Although many studies have shown a decrease in functional capacity and VO_{2max} among the elderly, it generally did not involve physically older men. Tanaka and Seals [4] reported on the slow decline of VO_{2max} in older ("Masters") athletes striving to maintain or even improve upon the performance they achieved at younger ages, but declines in athletic performance are inevitable with aging. Tanaka and Seals [4] have shown a progressive reduction in VO_{2max} that appears to be the primary mechanism associated with declines in endurance performance with age. The degree of the VO_{2max} improvement with training in the elderly, expressed in relative terms, appears to be comparable to that demonstrated by younger subjects. Given their impressive peak performance capability and physiological function capacity, Masters athletes remain an attractive model of successful aging. The increased maximal oxygen uptake in the active subjects may be due to an increase in mitochondrial respiratory capacity.

Aging of the Arteries

Important changes occur in the cardiovascular system with advancing age, even in apparently healthy individuals. Thickening and stiffening of the large arteries develop due to collagen and calcium deposition and loss of elastic fibers in the medial layer. These arterial changes cause *systolic blood pressure* to rise with age, while diastolic blood pressure generally declines after the sixth decade [37]. However, as large arteries dilate, wall tension and pulsatile stresses increase and exacerbate artery wall degeneration, thus initiating feedback, whereby increased *hypertension* leads to further degeneration [71]. Many cross-sectional studies have demonstrated a significant relationship between age and aortic stiffness, although the age-related changes observed in peripheral arteries appear to be less marked [72]. Age is the main clinical determinant of large artery stiffness, seen in elderly persons with isolated systolic hypertension characterized by fissuring and fracturing of the elastin protein, collagen proliferation, and calcium deposition, frequently associated with a widened and torturous aorta [71].

In response to a stress, the age-related reduction in physiological reserves causes a loss of regulatory or homeostatic balance. This, combined with another consequence of age-related changes, namely an increased perception of effort associated with submaximal work, sets, especially to a patient unbeknown to the above, a vicious cycle leading to decreased exercise capacity, resulting in an elevated perception of effort, subsequently causing avoidance of activity, and finally feeding back to an exacerbation of the age-related declines secondary to disuse.

Aging-related, environmental, and *genetic factors* are responsible for structural and functional changes of the arterial wall, leading to decreased elasticity and increased stiffness [73]. Aging is also associated with structural and functional changes of the vessel wall, which result in decreased vascular distensibility and elevated arterial stiffness [74]. There are several possible explanations for the influence of aging on the loss of elasticity of central arteries. The most likely explanation appears to be age-associated structural changes in the arterial wall. Aging is associated with a decrease in elastin and an increase in collagen and connective tissues in the arterial wall [4].

In patients with aortic stenosis, senescence profoundly influences the pattern of hypertrophic growth and diastolic function. Patients with pressure overload are characterized by more severe hypertrophy and interstitial fibrosis, as well as more severe impairment of relaxation, myocardial stiffness, and filling indices [65]. The aorta stiffens during senescence, as indicated by an increase in arterial pulse wave velocity [75]. Pulse pressure, measured as the difference between systolic blood pressure and diastolic blood pressure, rises markedly after the fifth decade due to arterial stiffening with age, which results in a progressive rise in systolic blood pressure and fall in diastolic blood pressure as the elastic capacity of the aorta diminishes [76]. Pulse pressure may be increased because of a larger forward pressure wave or an earlier or larger wave reflection [77].

The Baltimore Longitudinal Study of Aging [75] found that aortic arterial pulse wave velocity increased progressively with age in 50 healthy *females* (26–96 years) in whom only modest age-related increases in blood pressure were observed. This is noteworthy since elastic properties of arteries are not necessarily uniform [78], and aging has been reported to have different effects on the stiffness of peripheral arteries such as brachial and radial arteries and central arteries in men [79]. This may increase cardiovascular morbidity and mortality because of an elevation of systolic blood pressure, which raises left ventricular *afterload*, and because of a decrease in *diastolic blood pressure*, which alters coronary perfusion [80].

The loss of elasticity of the great arteries results in an increase of impedance at ejection. Thus, *aging* is associated with higher *mean arterial blood pressures*. Aging-related, environmental, and genetic factors are responsible for structural and functional changes of the arterial wall, leading to decreased elasticity and increased stiffness [81]. There are several possible explanations for the influence of aging on the loss of elasticity of central arteries. The most likely explanation appears to be age-associated structural changes in the arterial wall.

Many cross-sectional studies have demonstrated a significant relationship between age and *aortic stiffness*, although the age-related changes observed in peripheral arteries appear to be less marked [22]. Aging is also associated with structural and functional changes of the vessel wall, which result in decreased vascular distensibility and elevated arterial stiffness [74]. Age is the main clinical determinant of large artery changes, seen in elderly persons with isolated systolic hypertension characterized by fissuring and fracturing of the elastin protein, collagen proliferation, and calcium deposition, frequently associated with a widened and torturous aorta [82]. As large arteries dilate, wall tension and pulsatile stresses increase and exacerbate artery wall degeneration, thus initiating feedback, whereby increased hypertension leads to further degeneration [71].

Pulse pressure, measured as the difference between systolic blood pressure and diastolic blood pressure, rises markedly after the fifth decade of life due to arterial stiffening with age, which results in a progressive rise in *systolic blood pressure* and fall in *diastolic blood pressure* as the elastic capacity of the aorta diminishes [76]. Pulse pressure may be increased because of a larger forward pressure wave or an earlier or larger wave reflection [77]. In addition, arterial pulse wave velocity is increasing progressively with age in healthy females aged 26–96 years [75].

1. *At systole time*, *pressure* rises in the whole cardiovascular system so that the left ventricle is subjected to an increase of parietal tension to which it adapts itself by hypertrophy which normalizes this tension. The *aorta stiffens* during senescence, as indicated by an increase in arterial pulse wave velocity [75]. *Arterial compliance* is an important therapeutic target in *older individuals* in whom stiffening of the *proximal aortic* circulation is thought to underlie *systolic hypertension* and increased cardiac work. This indicates a positive association between systemic arterial compliance and *fitness level* in healthy older people and an inverse association between systemic arterial compliance and systolic blood pressure. These findings are consistent with either acquisition of a more compliant circulation and lower blood pressure due to enhanced *physical activity* or that a more compliant arterial circulation and lower blood pressure permit greater athletic performance [83]. For healthy subjects between the ages of 25 and 65 years, there is an interactive effect between age and gender and an independent effect of physical training on peripheral vascular function [80]. It was suggested that interventions to improve aerobic capacity alleviate the stiffening of the arterial tree that accompanies normative aging [75].

Training Effect on Cardiovascular Function

Following lifelong regular and intense training 70- to 80-year-old endurance-trained athletes have an aerobic capacity comparable to that of untrained young men and markedly higher than that of healthy age-matched controls. However, compared with young endurance athletes, the *veteran athletes* had a 40% lower pulmonary VO_2. Most available studies have been cross-sectional rather than longitudinal, comparing older, highly trained athletes with their more sedentary peers.

In addition, some prior studies have been confounded by the failure to rigorously exclude underlying occult disease or by relatively mild training protocols. For the most part, it is unclear whether cardiovascular adaptations to training differ with aging, because prior longitudinal studies of downloaded cardiovascular training adaptations in the elderly have not examined both young and old groups. Despite the alterations in *cardiac function* with aging, relatively marked adaptations to training occur in the old group, which did not differ qualitatively or quantitatively from those seen in younger men [41]. Thus, the age-dependent decline in physical capacity can largely be retarded by endurance training but not stopped.

Dynamic *aerobic exercise training* results in profound adaptations of the cardiovascular and neuromuscular system that enhance the *delivery of oxygen* to the *mitochondria* enable a tighter regulation of muscle metabolism. Performance of the *heart as a pump* has been a major element in testing the idea that exercise counteracts senescence. Exercise training was associated with change in the cardiac autonomic balance, producing an increase, or a relative dominance, of the *vagal component*. It has long been known that exercise training reduces resting and *submaximal heart rate*.

The *physiological effect* of exercise training involves changes in *left ventricular function* and hemodynamic alterations at rest and during exercise (Table 8.1). Physiological responses differ, depending upon whether they result from a *pressure overload* and increased *total peripheral resistance* or from a *volume overload*. Dynamic aerobic exercise training programs induce *enlargement of cardiac* dimensions, an increase in *left ventricular mass*, heart weight-to-body weight ratio, *left ventricular contractility*, and VO_2. The *eccentric left ventricular hypertrophy* that characterizes these changes is still physiological despite the fact that at times the degree of hypertrophy approaches that seen in *hypertrophic cardiomyopathy*. *Resistive muscle contraction training* involves large muscle mass that produces a characteristic increase in systolic and diastolic blood pressure (*pressor response*), increasing *mean arterial blood pressure* and thereby increasing *afterload*. In such cases, hypertrophy of the left ventricle may be associated with abnormalities of the left ventricular diastolic and systolic functions. The consequent effect is an increased large pressure load on the left ventricle. Specifically, minor *left ventricular systolic* dysfunction was observed in some healthy elderly subjects during exercise, with increased afterload. These minor changes, however, may be attributed to aging alone. This is not true in elderly subjects engaged in prolonged resistive training whose left *ventricular systolic function* is reduced even at rest. During *resistive maneuver* such as *dead lift*, the different patterns found at rest are indeed more prominent. Furthermore, in young weight lifters, although overload training causes left ventricular hypertrophy, the modification is physiological rather than *left ventricular pathological*.

Table 8.1 Cardiovascular changes induced following dynamic aerobic exercise training during submaximal and maximal efforts in elderly subjects

	Mode of exercise		
Variable	Rest	Submaximal	Maximal
Systolic blood pressure	↓	↓	↓
Diastolic blood pressure	↓	↓	↓
Stroke volume	↑	↑	→
Heart rate	↓	↓	↑
Cardiac output	→	→	↑
Total peripheral resistance	→	→	↓
Arteriovenous O_2 difference	→	→	↑
Contractility	→	→	→↑

Aged subjects engaged in *resistive training* both at rest and during exercise have shown changes in left *ventricular systolic function* changes such as acceleration times, ratios of acceleration time/flow, stroke volume, cardiac output, and total peripheral resistance as compared with normal older men and young ones. It is likely that these changes in the elderly are function related and are reduced compared to normal young subjects. It is clear that the arterial impedance may differ in older as compared with young populations and be primarily responsible for these changes.

Prolonged *dynamic aerobic* training causes similar alterations in left ventricular structure and function in the young and elderly as well. This is true where elderly or younger subjects are engaged in similar endurance training. Both age groups demonstrated cardiac changes previously documented to occur with exercise training, including lower *heart rates*, larger ventricular cavities, lower wall stresses, increased *contractility* state, and higher *E*/*A* ratio. The similarity in the structural and functional changes between the groups belies the major difference between them: the magnitude of the changes. The latter may suggest that some aspects of normal aging remain unaltered by exercise training.

Although the effects of *training* on cardiovascular function are relatively well described in young subjects, little is known regarding the changes that occur with training in older subjects; however, with time, it has become clear that older subjects can adapt to exercise training [84]. A longitudinal study suggested that the reduced maximal *ejection fraction* response seen in healthy older subjects may improve with training, but this has not been confirmed [84].

Endurance training results in an increase in the maximal conductance independent of age. In untrained elderly individuals, the changes in *left ventricular volumes* during exercise may be due to reduced left ventricular contractility, diastolic and systolic left ventricular functions, and loading conditions. The failure to augment left ventricular contractility in the sedentary older subjects may be the cause of reduced diastolic and systolic functions.

Table 8.1 summarizes some of the changes associated with training on cardiovascular and hemodynamic variables. Endurance exercise training in the elderly decreased resting and submaximal exercise heart rate and systolic and diastolic blood pressure, while stroke volume is increased. Marked changes are notable in the elderly subjects during maximal effort in which stroke volume, cardiac output, left ventricular contractility, and VO_2 are increased, while total peripheral resistance and systolic and diastolic blood pressure decreased, thus lowering afterload which in turn facilitate left ventricular systolic and diastolic function.

In addition, if the level of training stimulus in terms of duration, frequency, and intensity is adequate, older individuals can also exhibit improvement in aerobic work capacity [22]. The mechanisms underlying the training-induced augmentation of exercise capacity remain obscure. In young and middle-aged subjects, the increase in VO_2 capacity after training is generally attributed to both enhanced *left ventricular performance* resulting in augmented maximal *cardiac output* (central adaptations) and increased oxygen extraction by working skeletal muscle reflected in widening of the $(a\text{-}v)O_2$: peripheral adaptations [4, 36]. Studies in both human and animal hearts indicate that contractile function is unaffected by age while at rest; though the ability to increase *cardiac contractile* force during strenuous activities, such as exercise, declines with age [85]. It seems that there are age-related modifications in the expression, regulation, and function of a number of proteins essential to excitation-contraction coupling in the heart. This indicates that these changes in excitation-contraction coupling proteins disrupting Ca^{++} homeostasis contribute to decrease in peak contraction and prolongation of contraction duration observed in myocytes from aged hearts [85]. However, elderly subjects can adapt to *endurance exercise training* if the level of training stimulus is adequate as evidenced by significant improvement of maximal aerobic exercise capacity consistent with recent observations [84]. The increase in VO_{2max} in these men appears to be mediated primarily by central adaptations as reflected by enhancement of left ventricular systolic performance and larger *stroke volume* at peak exercise. Though, the smaller increase in heart rate during *the submaximal exercise* at a given exercise intensity observed in the trained state is also compatible with concomitant peripheral adaptations. The lack of increase in the peak exercise (a-v)O_2 after training is most likely due to the mode of exercise and possibly inadequate sample size [35].

Exercise Training for Elderly with CAD

Elderly patients are at high risk of disability following a coronary event or hospitalization for heart failure. Complications of *myocardial infarction* (MI) and myocardial revascularization procedures are more frequent at elderly age with prolongation of hospitalization predisposing to deconditioning. As a result, more than half of patients eligible for cardiac rehabilitation are older than age 65 [86]. Older patients constitute a high percentage of those with diagnosed *coronary artery disease* and are at high risk for disability after a coronary event. Older patients with coronary artery disease have higher rates of disability than younger *coronary artery disease patients*, partly based on lower levels of skeletal muscle strength. However, *older patients* with coronary artery disease have exercise trainability comparable to that of younger patients participating in similar *exercise rehabilitation*, with elderly male and female patients showing comparable improvement [87]. *Exercise training* has been shown to reverse the decline in muscle strength and aerobic power that occurs in older patients with coronary artery disease. Exercise training is an important intervention that can reverse the decline in peak aerobic power [88] and muscle strength that occurs in older individuals with coronary artery disease. However, referral to and participation in exercise rehabilitation is less frequent for older patients, especially for *older women* [2]. Few studies have examined the effect that exercise training has on altering VO_{2peak} in older women with coronary artery disease [88, 89]. Hung et al. [90] have found that 12–26 weeks of aerobic training resulted in a 5–30% increase in peak oxygen uptake in older women (age range, 53–82 years) with coronary artery disease. It was found that 8 weeks of aerobic training resulted in a 12% increase VO_{2peak}. This improvement is due to an increase in *stroke volume* and/or *(a-v)*O_2, as the oxygen pulse during peak exercise was significantly higher after training [91]. In addition, older coronary artery disease patients can effectively increase body strength with a combined *resistive-aerobic* exercise program in the early post-myocardial infarction period [92]. Individual that goes through combined aerobic and strength training has significant increases in peak aerobic power, distance walked in 6 min, and lower extremity strength. No significant complications or adverse outcomes of exercise training in older patients have been described in any study. Thus, not unlike that found in healthy older women, the increase in VO_{2peak} associated with exercise training in older women with coronary artery disease appears to be due to an increase in peak (a-v)O_2 [93]. Consequently, older coronary artery disease patients of both genders should be strongly encouraged to participate in exercise-based cardiac rehabilitation. Whether exercise training is associated with a reduction of morbidity or mortality in the elderly coronary artery disease patients is controversial [94], although in the British Regional Heart Study, men with coronary artery disease with a mean age of 63 years who engaged in light-to-moderate *physical activity* had a significantly lower all-cause mortality over the 5-year follow-up than did their sedentary counterparts [95].

Exercise Benefits for Hypertensive Elderly

There is increasing evidence that regular training initiated as early as young adulthood, but even during old age, can achieve a high level of activity, thereby influencing the aging process. Thus, it is appropriate to perceive physical activity as a medical prescription for the aging population [96]. Regular physical activity is associated with reduced risk of cardiovascular disease including hypertension [97]. In the Baltimore Longitudinal Study of Aging, it was found that *aortic arterial pulse wave velocity* increased progressively and that older adult males who performed *endurance exercise* on a regular basis demonstrated lower levels of aortic arterial pulse wave velocity than their sedentary peers did. Previous studies have reported that in endurance athletes, *arterial stiffness* is decreased by prolonged endurance training [98], and aortic distensibility is increased, particularly in those with the ACE II genotype. In addition, even a moderately intense exercise may be as brief as 10 min in duration that is needed in order to elicit a decrease in resting blood pressure and may have potential benefits as a nonpharmacological aid to hypertension [99]. These effects represent an extracardiac adaptation to chronic prolonged training in athletes [100].

Arterial compliance is an important therapeutic target in older individuals in whom stiffening of the proximal aortic circulation is thought to underlie systolic hypertension and increased cardiac work. This indicates a positive association between *systemic arterial compliance* and *fitness level* in healthy *older people* and an inverse association between systemic arterial compliance and *systolic blood pressure*. These findings are consistent with either acquisition of a more compliant circulation and lower blood pressure due to enhanced *physical activity* or that a more compliant arterial circulation and lower blood pressure permit greater athletic performance [83]. For healthy subjects between the ages of 25 and 65 years, there is an interactive effect between age and gender and an independent effect of physical training on peripheral vascular function [101]. It was suggested that interventions to improve aerobic capacity alleviate the stiffening of the arterial tree that accompanies normative aging [75].

Pulmonary Exercise's Benefits

The *aged lung* is more fragile in the face of respiratory and systemic diseases than the *pulmonary system* of young adults. Both *male* and *female* elderly subjects have lower lung function testing scores than the adult subjects, with this difference more marked in females. *Aging* is accompanied by numerous structural and functional changes in the lung, chest wall respiratory muscles, bronchopulmonary system, and vasculature. Functional modifications are concern mainly in respiratory changes, pulmonary circulation, adaptation to exercise, biochemical system, and pulmonary defenses [102]. Age in itself is not a risk factor of respiratory failure, but elderly individuals have an increased risk of mortality for both acute respiratory failure (the failing lung) and exacerbated chronic ventilatory failure (the failing pump). Four major changes appear to affect lung function, *pulmonary mechanics*, and *respiratory flow* rates as aging occurs: (a) a decrease in *elastic recoil* of the lung tissue, and to a lesser extent a stiffening of the chest wall, (b) a decrease in intervertebral space, (c) an apparent loss of respiratory muscle strength, and (d) a decrease in PaO_2 and an increase in the *alveolar to arterial gradient*. In addition, the respiratory centers are less sensitive. Residual volume, closing volume, and function residual capacity increase, whereas vital capacity and *forced expiratory volume* in 1 s (FEV_1) progressively decrease [103]. In addition, the flow-volume curve becomes more convex to the volume axis at low lung volume. Mechanical ventilatory constraints are progressive with aging, elderly subjects demonstrating marked mechanical ventilatory constraints *during exercise*.

The impact of these constraints on exercise tolerance could not be determined and remains unclear. These result in a reduction of *arterial oxygen partial pressure*, maximal voluntary ventilation, force expiratory volumes, *total lung capacity*, vital capacity and *pulmonary diffusing capacity*, and increases in functional residual capacity, residual volume *physiological dead space*, and time required for mixing inhaled air [103]. However, in theory, the aforementioned age-related changes in the pulmonary circulation may conspire to make elderly individuals more susceptible to gas exchange abnormalities during exercise. Yet, despite the erosion in *ventilatory reserve* with aging, the healthy older adult appears able to maintain *alveolar ventilation* at a level that allows maintenance of arterial blood gases within normal limits, even during *heavy exercise*. This ability to maintain adequate gas exchange likely occurs because age-related reductions in the maximal metabolic demand of exercise occur at a rate equal to or greater than the rate of deterioration in ventilatory reserve [63].

McClaran et al. [46] suggested that in contrast to implications from cross-sectional data, longitudinal findings demonstrate that habitual physical activity and high aerobic capacity modify neither the normal deterioration in resting lung function nor the increased levels of *ventilatory work* during exercise that occur with healthy aging over the sixth and seventh decades of life.

The older adult demonstrates several alterations in the ventilatory response to exercise relative to the young adult. These differences are primarily caused by the aging-induced loss of elastic recoil of the lung, which reduces *expiratory airflow rates* along the effort-independent portion of the maximal volitional expiratory boundary of the maximal flow-volume envelope [23]. This in turn increases the severity of expiratory airflow limitation and induces dynamic lung hyperinflation during exercise. The consequences of this age-associated decrease in elastic recoil on the pulmonary circulation are speculative, but an age-associated decline in elastic recoil may influence *pulmonary vascular resistance* and *cardiac output*, in addition to its impact on the work and oxygen cost of breathing [24]. Despite these distinctions in the response to exercise of the aged adult, alveolar ventilation is adequate for CO_2 elimination even during maximal exercise, and arterial oxygen homeostasis is generally maintained [23].

Table 8.2 reveals that *breathing efficiency* is improved in the elderly following an endurance training program, seen by the V_E decrement during submaximal and maximal efforts. Therefore, V_E/VO_2 ratio is decreased as well as the V_E/VCO_2, suggesting reduction in muscle respiratory work. These changes include increased maximal ventilation and reduction in *lactic acid* levels due to the VO_2 increase.

Table 8.2 Changes in pulmonary function induced following endurance training in healthy elderly subjects

	Mode of exercise		
Variable	Rest	Submaximal	Maximal
Maximal voluntary ventilation	→	—	—
Oxygen uptake	→	→	↑
Minute ventilation	→	↓	↓
Ventilation/oxygen uptake	→	↓	↓
Ventilation/carbon dioxide	→	→	↓
Lactic acid	→	↓	↓

Metabolic Improvements

The most important adaptive response of skeletal muscle to endurance exercise is an augmentation of *respiratory capacity* with increases in the ability to oxidize pyruvate, fatty acids, and ketones. As a result of increases in the levels of the enzymes of the malate-aspartate shuttle, there is also an enhancement of the capability for mitochondrial oxidation of the reducing equivalents generated in the cytoplasm during glycolysis. The rise in muscle respiratory capacity results from an increase in muscle *mitochondria* and an alteration in mitochondrial composition. This makes skeletal muscle mitochondria more like heart mitochondria in their enzyme pattern. When previously sedentary individuals are retested at the same absolute submaximal work rate after adapting to *endurance exercise*, their endurance is found to be markedly increased. However, metabolic factors do not appear to determine the magnitude of VO_{2max}.

The changes in muscle oxidative potential may play a major role in the *elderly capacity* to perform submaximal work. As an example, in physically conditioned young subjects, submaximal work performance increased by 300%, while VO_{2max} increased by 19% [85].

References

1. Lakatta EG. Changes in cardiovascular function with aging. Eur Heart J. 1990;11(Suppl C):22–9.
2. Shephard RJ. Physical activity and aging. 2nd ed. London: Croom Helm Publishing; 1987.
3. Hawkins S, Wiswell R. Rate and mechanism of maximal oxygen uptake decline with aging: implications for exercise training. Sports Med. 2003;33:877–88.
4. Tanaka H, Seals DR. Endurance exercise performance in Masters athletes: age-associated changes and underlying physiological mechanisms. J Physiol. 2008;586:55–63.
5. Basset Jr DR, Howley ET. Limiting factors for maximum oxygen uptake and determinants of endurance performance. Med Sci Sports Exerc. 2000;32:70–84.
6. Sagiv M, Ben-Sira D, Goldhammer E, Soudry M. Left ventricular contractility and function at peak aerobic and anaerobic exercises. Med Sci Sports Exerc. 2000; 32:1197–201.
7. Correia LC, Lakatta EG, O'Connor FC, et al. Attenuated cardiovascular reserve during prolonged submaximal cycle exercise in healthy older subjects. J Am Coll Cardiol. 2002;40:1290–7.
8. Bortz WM. Disuse and aging. JAMA. 1982;248:1203–8.
9. Swine C. Aging of heart function in man (French). Presse Med. 1992;21:1216–21.
10. Fukuoka Y, Nakagawa Y, Ogoh K, Shiojiri T, Fukuba Y. Dynamics of the heart rate response to sinusoidal work in humans: influence of physical activity and age. Clin Sci (Lond). 2002;102:31–8.
11. Lamin A, Reddy S, Comai L. Farnesylation and aging. Exp Cell Res. 2012;318:1–7.
12. Stathokostas L, Jacob-Johnson S, Petrella RJ, Paterson DH. Longitudinal changes in aerobic power in older men and women. J Appl Physiol. 2004;97:781–9.
13. Fleg JL, Morrell CH, Bos AG, Brant LJ, Talbot LA, Wright JG, Lakatta EG. Accelerated longitudinal decline of aerobic capacity in healthy older adults. Circulation. 2005;112:674–82.
14. Sjodin B, Svedenhag J. Oxygen uptake during running as related to body mass in circumpubertal boys: a longitudinal study. Eur J Appl Physiol Occup Physiol. 1992;65:150–7.
15. Ishida K, Katayama K, Akima H, Iwase S, Sato K, Hotta N, Miyamura M. Effects of deconditioning on the initial ventilatory and circulatory responses at the onset of exercise in man. Adv Exp Med Biol. 2010;669:319–22.
16. Rossiter HB, Kowalchuk JM, Whipp BJ. A test to establish maximum O_2 uptake despite no plateau in the O_2 uptake response to ramp incremental exercise. J Appl Physiol. 2006;100:764–70.
17. Huang YC, O'Brien SR, MacIntyre NR. Intrabreath diffusing capacity of the lung in healthy individuals at rest and during exercise. Chest. 2002;122:177–85.
18. Tolle J, Waxman A, Systrom D. Impaired systemic oxygen extraction at maximum exercise in pulmonary hypertension. Med Sci Sports Exerc. 2008;40:3–8.
19. Wilmore JH, Costill DL. Physiology of sport and exercise: rate of reaction. 3rd ed. Champaign: Human Kinetics; 2005.
20. Guenette JA, Witt JD, McKenzie DC, Road JD, Sheel AW. Respiratory mechanics during exercise in endurance-trained men and women. J Physiol. 2007;581: 1309–22.
21. Dufour Doiron M, Prud'homme D, Boulay P. Time-of-day variation in cardiovascular response to maximal exercise testing in coronary heart disease patients taking a beta-blocker. Appl Physiol Nutr Metab. 2007;32:664–9.
22. McClaran SR, Babcock MA, Pegelow DF, Reddan WG, Dempsey JA. Longitudinal effects of aging on lung function at rest and exercise in healthy active fit elderly adults. J Appl Physiol. 1995;78:1957–68.
23. Johnson BD, Badr MS, Dempsey JA. Impact of the aging pulmonary system on the response to exercise. Clin Chest Med. 1994;15:229–46.
24. Taylor BJ, Johnson BD. The pulmonary circulation and exercise responses in the elderly. Semin Respir Crit Care Med. 2010;31:528–38.
25. Dash RK, Dibella 2nd JA, Cabrera ME. A computational model of skeletal muscle metabolism linking cellular adaptations induced by altered loading states to metabolic responses during exercise. Biomed Eng Online. 2007;6:14–42.
26. Pollack ML, Foster C, Knapp D, Rod JL, Schmidt DH. Effect of age and training in aerobic capacity and body composition of master athletes. J Appl Physiol. 1987;62:725–31.
27. Balagopal P, Ljungqvist O, Nair KS. Skeletal muscle myosin heavy-chain synthesis rate in healthy humans. Am J Physiol. 1997;272:E45–50.
28. Doherty TJ. Invited review: aging and sarcopenia. J Appl Physiol. 2003;95:1717–27.
29. Karelis AD, Faraj M, Bastard JP, et al. The metabolically healthy but obese individual presents a favorable inflammation profile. J Clin Endocrinol Metab. 2005;90:4145–50.
30. Aubertin-Leheudre M, Audet M, Goulet ED, Dionne IJ. HRT provides no additional beneficial effect on sarcopenia in physically active postmenopausal women: a cross-sectional, observational study. Maturitas. 2005;51:140–5.
31. George KP, Gates PE, Birch KM, Campbell IG. Left ventricular morphology and function in endurance trained female athletes. J Sports Sci. 1999;17:633–42.
32. Roman MJ. How best to identify prognostically important left ventricular hypertrophy: a cut to the chase. J Am Coll Cardiol. 1997;29:648–50.
33. Ridout SJ, Parker BA, Smithmyer SL, Gonzales JU, Beck KC, Proctor DN. Age and sex influence the balance between maximal cardiac output and peripheral vascular reserve. J Appl Physiol. 2010;108:483–9.
34. Bouvier F, Saltin B, Nejat M, Jensen-Urstad M. Left ventricular function and perfusion in elderly endurance athletes. Med Sci Sports Exerc. 2001;33:735–40.
35. Bogaard HJ, Woltjer HH, Dekker BM, van Keimpema AR, Postmus PE, de Vries PM. Haemodynamic

response to exercise in healthy young and elderly subjects. Eur J Appl Physiol Occup Physiol. 1997;75:435–42.

36. Arbab-Zadeh A, Dijk E, Prasad A. Effect of aging and physical activity on left ventricular compliance. Circulation. 2004;110:1799–805.
37. Fleg JL, Strait J. Age-associated changes in cardiovascular structure and function: a fertile milieu for future disease. Heart Fail Rev. 2011 Aug 2. [Epub ahead of print].
38. Krzemiński K, Kruk B, Nazar K, Ziemba AW, Cybulski G, Niewiadomski W. Cardiovascular, metabolic and plasma catecholamine responses to passive and active exercises. J Physiol Pharmacol. 2000;51:267–78.
39. Borlaug BA, Melenovsky V, Russell SD, Kessler K, Pacak K, Becker LC, Kass DA. Impaired chronotropic and vasodilator reserves limit exercise capacity in patients with heart failure and a preserved ejection fraction. Circulation. 2006;114:2138–47.
40. Tate CA, Hyek MF, Taffet GE. Mechanisms for the responses of cardiac muscle to physical activity in old age. Med Sci Sports Exerc. 1994;26:561–7.
41. Stratton JR, Levy WC, Caldwell JH, Jacobson A, May J, Matsuoka D, Madden K. Effects of aging on cardiovascular responses to parasympathetic withdrawal. J Am Coll Cardiol. 2003;41:2077–83.
42. Karas M, Larochelle P, LeBlanc RA, Dubé B, Nadeau R, Champlain J. Attenuation of autonomic nervous system functions in hypertensive patients at rest and during orthostatic stimulation. J Clin Hypertens (Greenwich). 2008;10:97–104.
43. Camarda SR, Tebexreni AS, Páfaro CN, Sasai FB, Tambeiro VL, Juliano Y, Barros Neto TL. Comparison of maximal heart rate using the prediction equations proposed by Karvonen and Tanaka. Arq Bras Cardiol. 2008;91:311–4.
44. Shephard RJ. Health and aerobic fitness. Champaign: Human Kinetics; 1993.
45. Murias JM, Kowalchuk JM, Paterson DH. Mechanisms for increases in VO_{2max} with endurance training in older and young women. Med Sci Sports Exerc. 2010;42:1891–8.
46. McLaren PF, Nurhayati Y, Boutcher SH. Stroke volume response to cycle ergometry in trained and untrained older men. Eur J Appl Physiol. 1997;75:537–42.
47. Sagiv M, Goldhammer E, Abinader EG. Aging and the effect of increased after-load on left ventricular contractile state. Med Sci Sports Exerc. 1988;20:281–4.
48. Slotwiner DJ, Devereux RB, Schwartz JE, et al. Relation of age to left ventricular function in clinically normal adults. Am J Cardiol. 1998;82:621–6.
49. Benjamin EJ, Levy D, Anderson KM, et al. Determinants of Doppler indexes of left ventricular diastolic function in normal subjects (the Framingham Heart Study). Am J Cardiol. 1992;70:508–15.
50. Badano L, Carratino L, Giunta L, Calisi P, Lucatti A. Age-induced changes in the cardiovascular system in normal subjects (Italian). G Ital Cardiol. 1992;22:1023–34.
51. Rodheffer RJ, Gerstenblith G, Becker LC, Fleg JL, Weisfeldt ML, Lakatta EG. Exercise cardiac output is maintained with advancing age in healthy human subjects: cardiac dilatation and increased stroke volume compensate for a diminished heart rate. Circulation. 1984;69:203–13.
52. Sagiv M, Ben-Sira D, Sagiv M, Goldhammer E. Left ventricular function at peak all-out anaerobic exercise in older men. Gerontology. 2005;51:122–5.
53. Calabrò R, Pisacane C, Pacileo G, Russo MG. Hemodynamic effects of a single oral dose of enalapril among children with asymptomatic chronic mitral regurgitation. Am Heart J. 1999;138:955–61.
54. Dawson EA, Shave R, Whyte G, et al. Preload maintenance and the left ventricular response to prolonged exercise in men. Exp Physiol. 2007;92:383–90.
55. Sullivan MJ, Cobb FR, Higginbotham MB. Stroke volume increases by similar mechanisms during upright exercise in normal men and women. Am J Cardiol. 1991;67(16):1405–12.
56. Foster C, Gal RA, Port SC, Schmidt DH. Left ventricular ejection fraction during incremental and steady state exercise. Med Sci Sports Exerc. 1995;27:1602–6.
57. Sagiv M, Ben-Sira D, Goldhammer E. Direct vs. indirect blood pressure measurement at peak anaerobic exercise. Int J Sports Med. 1999;20:275–8.
58. Andersen K, Vik-Mo H. Increased left ventricular emptying at maximal exercise after reduction in afterload. Circulation. 1984;69:492–6.
59. Poole DC, Gaesser GA, Hogan MC, Knight DR, Wanger PD. Pulmonary and leg VO_2 during submaximal exercise: implications for muscular efficiency. J Appl Physiol. 1992;72:805–10.
60. Sagiv M, Ben-Sira D, Rudoy J. Cardiovascular response during upright isometric dead lift in young, older, and elderly healthy men. Int J Sports Med. 1988;9:134–6.
61. Sagiv M, Hanson P, Besozzi M, Nagle F. Left ventricular responses to upright isometric handgrip and deadlift in men with coronary artery disease. Am J Cardiol. 1985;55:1298–302.
62. Sagiv M, Fisher N, Yaniv A, Rudoy J. Effect of running versus isometric training programs on healthy elderly at rest. Gerontology. 1989;35:72–7.
63. Donal E, Rozoy T, Kervio G, Schnell F, Mabo P, Carré F. Comparison of the heart function adaptation in trained and sedentary men after 50 and before 35 years of age. Am J Cardiol. 2011;108(7):1029–37.
64. Janowski E, Berríos M, Cleemann L, Morad M. Developmental aspects of cardiac Ca(2+) signaling: interplay between RyR- and IP(3)R-gated Ca(2+) stores. Am J Physiol Heart Circ Physiol. 2010;298:H1939–50.
65. Lorell BH, Carabello BA. Left ventricular hypertrophy pathogenesis, detection, and prognosis. Circulation. 2000;102:470–9.
66. Schulman SP, Lakatta EG, Fleg JL, Lakatta L, Becker LC, Gerstenblith G. Age-related decline in left ventricular filling at rest and exercise. Am J Physiol. 1992;263:H1932–8.

67. Zabalgoitia M, Rahman SN, Haley WE, et al. Comparison in systemic hypertension of left ventricular mass and geometry with systolic and diastolic function in patients <65 to ≥65 years of age. Am J Cardiol. 1998;82:604–8.
68. Sandvik L, Erikssen J, Thaulow E, Erikssen O, Mundal R, Rodahl K. Physical fitness as a predictor of mortality among healthy, middle-aged Norwegian men. N Engl J Med. 1993;328:574–5.
69. Paffenbarger RS, Hyde RT, Wing AL, Lee J, Jung DL, Kampert JB. The association of changes in physical activity level and other lifestyle characteristics with mortality among men. N Engl J Med. 1993;328:538–45.
70. Hull SS, Vanoli E, Adamson PB, Verrier RL, Foreman RD, Schwartz PJ. Exercise training confers anticipatory protection from sudden death during acute myocardial ischemia. Circulation. 1994;89:548–52.
71. Nichols WW, O'Rourke MF. MacDonald's blood flow in arteries. 4th ed. London: Arnold, Hodder Headline Group; 1998.
72. McEniery CM, Wilkinson IB, Avolio AP. Age, hypertension and arterial function. Clin Exp Pharmacol Physiol. 2007;34:665–71.
73. Laurent S, Katsahian S, Fassot C, et al. Aortic stiffness is an independent predictor of fatal stroke in essential hypertension. Stroke. 2003;34:1203–6.
74. Avolio AP, Chen SG, Wang RP, et al. Effects of aging on changing arterial compliance and left ventricular load in a northern Chinese urban community. Circulation. 1983;68:50–8.
75. Vaitkevicius PV, Fleg JL, Engel JH, et al. Effects of age and aerobic capacity on arterial stiffness in healthy adults. Circulation. 1993;88:1456–62.
76. Franklin SS, Gustin IV W, Wong ND, et al. Hemodynamic patterns of age-related changes in blood pressure. Circulation. 1997;96:308–15.
77. Mitchell GF, Lacourcière Y, Ouellet JP, et al. Determinants of elevated pulse pressure in middle-aged and older subjects with uncomplicated systolic hypertension: the role of proximal aortic diameter and the aortic pressure-flow relationship. Circulation. 2003;108:1592–8.
78. Kelly R, Hayward C, Avolio A, et al. Noninvasive determination of age-related changes in the human arterial pulse. Circulation. 1989;80:1652–9.
79. O'Rourke M. Arterial haemodynamics and ventricular-vascular interaction in hypertension. Blood Press. 1994;3:33–7.
80. Mattace-Raso FU, van der Cammen TJ, Hofman A, et al. Arterial stiffness and risk of coronary heart disease and stroke: the Rotterdam Study. Circulation. 2006;113:657–63.
81. Laurent S, Kingwell B, Bank A, et al. Clinical applications of arterial stiffness: therapeutics and pharmacology. Am J Hypertens. 2002;5:453–8.
82. Seals DR, Desouza CA, Donato AJ, Tanaka HJ. Habitual exercise and arterial aging. J Appl Physiol. 2008;105:1323–32.
83. Cameron JD, Rajkumar C, Kingwell BA, et al. Higher systemic arterial compliance is associated with greater exercise time and lower blood pressure in a young older population. J Am Geriatr Soc. 1999;47:653–6.
84. Ehsani AA, Ogawa T, Miller TR, Spina RJ, Jilka SM. Exercise training improves left ventricular systolic function in older men. Circulation. 1991;83:96–103.
85. Fares E, Howlett SE. Effect of age on cardiac excitation-contraction coupling. Clin Exp Pharmacol Physiol. 2010;37:1–7.
86. Pasquali SK, Alexander KP, Peterson ED. Cardiac rehabilitation in the elderly. Am Heart J. 2001;142:748–55.
87. Ades PA, Waldmann ML, Gillespie C. A controlled trial of exercise training in older coronary patients. J Gerontol A Biol Sci Med Sci. 1995;50A:M7–11.
88. Kirwan LD, Mertens DJ, Kavanagh T, et al. Exercise training in women with heart disease: influence of hormone replacement therapy. Med Sci Sports Exerc. 2003;35:185–92.
89. Ades PA, Waldmann ML, Polk DM, et al. Referral patterns and exercise response in the rehabilitation of female coronary patients aged greater than or equal to 62 years. Am J Cardiol. 1992;69:1422–5.
90. Hung C, Daub B, Black B, Quinney A, Haykowsky M. Exercise training improves overall physical fitness and quality of life in older women with coronary artery disease. Chest. 2004;126:1026–31.
91. Ades PA, Waldmann ML, Meyer WL, et al. Skeletal muscle and cardiovascular adaptations to exercise conditioning in older coronary patients. Circulation. 1996;94:323–30.
92. Fragnoli-Munn K, Savage PD, Ades PA. Combined resistive-aerobic training in older patients with coronary artery disease early after myocardial infarction. J Cardiopulm Rehabil. 1998;18:416–20.
93. Spina RJ, Ogawa T, Kohrt WM, et al. Differences in cardiovascular adaptations to endurance exercise training between older men and women. J Appl Physiol. 1993;75:849–55.
94. Thompson PD, Buchner D, Piña IL, et al. Exercise and physical activity in the prevention and treatment of atherosclerotic cardiovascular disease. Circulation. 2003;107:3109–16.
95. Wannamethee SG, Shaper AG, Walker M. Physical activity and mortality in older men with diagnosed coronary heart disease. Circulation. 2000;102:1358–63.
96. Leach RE. Aging and physical activity. Orthopade. 2000;29:936–40.
97. Blair SN, Kohl HW, Barlow CE, et al. Changes in physical fitness and all-cause mortality. JAMA. 1995; 273:1093–8.
98. Kakiyama T, Sugawara J, Murakami H, et al. Effects of short-term endurance training on aortic distensibility in young males. Med Sci Sports Exerc. 2005; 37:267–71.
99. MacDonald JR, MacDougall JD, Hogben CD. The effects of exercise duration on post-exercise hypotension. J Hum Hypertens. 2004;14:125–9.

100. Tanriverdi H, Evrengul H, Kaftan A, et al. Effects of angiotensin- converting enzyme polymorphism on aortic elastic parameters in athletes. Cardiology. 2005;104:113–9.
101. Martin 3rd WH, Ogawa T, Kohrt WM, Malley MT, Korte E, Kieffer PS, Schechtman KB. Effects of aging, gender, and physical training on peripheral vascular function. Circulation. 1991;84:654–64.
102. Kammoun S, Rekik WK, Ayoub A. The aging lung: structural and functional modifications related to aging. Tunis Med. 2001;79:10–4.
103. Rossi A, Ganassini A, Tantucci C, Grassi V. Aging and the respiratory system. Aging (Milano). 1996; 8:143–61.

9 Exercise and Sudden Death

Physical Inactivity and Cardiovascular Disease

Physical inactivity is increasingly recognized as modifiable behavioral risk factor for cardiovascular diseases. Available data do not provide clear evidence that withdrawal of physical activity increases *coronary artery disease* risk, although results from the Harvard Alumni Study suggest that college athletic activity is not protective in later years without lifelong physical activity [1]. Lack of physical activity is among the risk factors that are considered to have adverse effects on the progression of coronary *atherosclerosis*. Risk of first myocardial infarction was found to be related inversely to energy expenditure reported by 16,936 Harvard male alumni, aged 35–74 years, of whom 572 experienced myocardial infarction in 117,680 person-years of follow-up. Stairs climbed, blocks walked, strenuous sports played all opposed risk. Men with energy expenditure below 2,000 $Kcal \cdot wk^{-1}$ were at 64% higher risk than classmates with higher index. Numerous observational studies in both men and women have demonstrated that both regular exercise and *physical fitness* are associated with reduced *risk factors* of coronary events and coronary death. Recent epidemiological studies indicate that individuals who maintain a physically active lifestyle are much less likely to develop impaired glucose tolerance and non–insulin-dependent diabetes mellitus. Moreover, it was found that the protective effect of *physical activity* was strongest for individuals at highest risk of developing non–insulin-dependent diabetes mellitus [2]. Physical inactivity is a major underlying cause of death, disease, and disability. Preliminary data from a World Health Organization study on risk factors suggest that inactivity, or sedentary lifestyle, is one of the ten leading global causes of death and disability [3]. The risk of heart problems due to physical inactivity is related to fitness level and the intensity of the activity performed. For example, someone who is not physically fit is at higher risk for a myocardial infarction during vigorous activity than a person who is physically fit. In the vast majority of the *sudden cardiac death* cases, the underlying cause is advanced *coronary heart disease*, which in large proportion of the cases has been asymptomatic and has allowed regular strenuous training. Attempts to prevent the complications by special large-scale screening programs would be ineffective and individual counseling limited by lack of resources [4]. These measures should, however, be used in selected groups and individuals. Even if all available measures at present were used, the cardiovascular complications of physical activity could not be totally prevented. Fortunately, preliminary evidence suggests that at population level, the cardiovascular hazards of physical activity are outweighed by its cardiovascular benefits. Subgroup of patients who are particularly at higher risk of exercise-related sudden death may be identified in different ways, such as pre-participation history taking, physical examination, and/or supplementary cardiac evaluation. Limitations exist because current diagnostic tools are not

M.S. Sagiv, *Exercise Cardiopulmonary Function in Cardiac Patients*,
DOI 10.1007/978-1-4471-2888-5_9, © Springer-Verlag London 2012

sufficient to predict a coronary artery plaque with potential risk of disruption and/or an acute thrombotic occlusion. Proper and cost-effective methods for identification of younger subjects with cardiac structural problems or genetic ion channel diseases are still controversial [5]. Physical inactivity is a term used to denote a type of sedentary lifestyle that includes less than 150 min of moderate physical activity or less than 60 min of *vigorous physical activity* per week [6]. Sedentary lifestyle includes little or no vigorous physical exercise which contributes to many preventable causes of death. Cardiovascular diseases remain the biggest cause of deaths worldwide. Premature deaths from cardiovascular disease range from 4% in high-income countries to 42% in low-income countries. In recent years, cardiovascular risk in women has been increasing and has killed more women than breast cancer. Rainwater et al. [7] demonstrated that vascular injury accumulates from adolescence, making primary prevention efforts necessary from childhood. By the time that heart problems are detected, the underlying cause, that is, atherosclerosis, is usually significantly advanced, having progressed for decades. There is therefore increased emphasis on preventing atherosclerosis by modifying risk factors, such as healthy eating and exercise.

Population-based studies show that the precursors of *heart disease* start in adolescence. The process of *atherosclerosis* evolves over decades, and begins as early as childhood. The pathobiological determinants of atherosclerosis in youth study demonstrated that intimal lesions appear in all the aortas and more than half of the right coronary arteries of youths aged 7–9 years. However, most adolescents are more concerned about other risks such as HIV, accidents, and cancer than cardiovascular disease [8]. This is extremely important considering that one in three people will die from complications attributable to atherosclerosis. In order to stem the tide, education and awareness that cardiovascular disease poses the greatest threat and measures to prevent or reverse this disease must be taken.

Obesity and diabetes mellitus are often linked to cardiovascular disease [9], as are a history of chronic kidney disease and hypercholesterolemia. In fact, cardiovascular disease is the most life threatening of the diabetic complications, and diabetics are two- to fourfold more likely to die of cardiovascular-related causes than nondiabetics [10]. Overweight and obesity is clearly multifactorial, but ultimately it is determined by the long-term balance between energy intake and expenditure.

Are Exercise and Sudden Death Causally Related?

For middle-aged and older adults, the risk of heart problems due to *physical activity* is related to *coronary heart disease*. Individuals who have coronary heart disease are more likely to have a *myocardial infarction* when they are exercising vigorously than when they are not. In general, the benefits of regular physical activity far outweigh risks to the heart and lungs. Rarely, heart problems, such as *arrhythmia*, *sudden cardiac arrest*, or myocardial infarction, occur during physical activity. These events generally happen to people who already have heart conditions. In youth and young adults, the risk for heart problems due to physical activity is higher in people who have underlying *congenital heart problems*. These are heart problems that have been present since birth. Congenital heart problems include hypertrophic cardiomyopathy, congenital heart defects, and myocarditis or inflammation of the myocardium. Individuals who have these conditions should consult with their physician about which physical activities are safe for them. People who already have coronary heart disease are more likely to have a myocardial infarction when they are exercising vigorously than when they are not. The risk for heart problems due to physical activity is related to the fitness level and the intensity of the activity the individual is performing. For example, someone who does not do physical activity regularly is at higher risk for myocardial infarction during vigorous activity than a person who is physically trained and regularly active.

Lack of habitual physical activity is now considered to be a major risk factor for coronary heart disease. *Regular exercise* has numerous *cardiovascular benefits* and has been associated with improved cardiovascular and *all-cause mortality* [11]. Vigorous exertion has been demonstrated to simultaneously trigger and transiently increase the risk of ventricular arrhythmias. Therefore, the first component of this issue that needs attention is whether exercise and *sudden cardiac death* (SCD) are causally related. Although the overall population of athletes is at generally low risk for sudden death [12], a number of largely congenital but clinically unsuspected cardiovascular diseases have been causally linked to sudden cardiac death in young trained athletes, usually in association with physical exertion [12].

The impact of physical effort on sudden cardiac death is somewhat controversial. On one hand, *vigorous exercise* can trigger *sudden cardiac death* and acute *myocardial infarction* [13], in part by increasing *platelet adhesiveness* and aggregability. On the other hand, *moderate physical activity* may be beneficial by decreasing platelet adhesiveness and aggregability [14]. The evidence is clear that regular exercise acts against the development, especially, of coronary atherosclerosis, but it does not provide total immunity. There is also no evidence that exercise accelerates the progression of these other potentially lethal cardiac conditions. Thus far, it is apparent that exercise protects against sudden cardiac death [15] and is associated with a lower risk of cardiovascular events [16]. Although exertion-related sudden cardiac deaths in young athletes are relatively rare compared with other health outcomes, these deaths usually occur in an unexpected fashion among those who appear quite healthy [17]. It is defined as death occurring from a cardiac cause within 1 hour of the onset of symptoms. The overriding conclusion from a large number of studies of sudden cardiac death, including sudden cardiac deaths that occur during exercise, has shown that virtually all individuals who die suddenly during exercise have a serious disease, usually of the heart, that adequately explains the cause of death. *Sudden cardiac death* may occur even in a grossly normal heart. Sudden cardiac death most commonly results from *cardiac arrest* due to a *lethal arrhythmia* and usually occurs in the background of structural heart disease or coronary artery disease [18]. Athletes should not assume that completing a competition will ensure total immunity from coronary heart disease or that reattainment of that event after a heart attack will prevent progression of that disease. Athletes should seek medical advice and not force themselves when exertional symptoms develop. Therefore, professionals should not exclude the possibility of coronary or other life-threatening heart diseases such as *hypertrophic cardiomyopathy*, simply because the athlete is physically well trained.

In *cardiac rehabilitation* programs, *cardiac arrests* occur at a rate of 1 in 12,000–15,000 participants, and during stress testing, cardiac arrest occurs in 0.0005% of the tested population, at least six times greater than the general incidence of sudden cardiac death for patients known to have heart disease. Experimentally, it appears that regular exercise in dogs prevents ischemia-induced ventricular fibrillation and death by increasing vagal activity [19]. Thus, it may be that regular exercise decreases cardiovascular morbidity and mortality, while vigorous exercise, particularly in untrained individuals, may have an adverse effect. The annual incidence of sudden cardiac death during exercise is 1 per 200,000–250,000 healthy young people [20], whereas in competitive athletes participating in individual or collective sports as well as training programs of systematic and regular competitions, sudden cardiac death is very rare [21]. Studies on recreational runners indicate approximately one fatality for every one million man- or woman-hours exercise per year, or roughly 1 death per 10,000 per year. Sedentary individuals who suddenly engage in vigorous exercise are at particular risk for sudden cardiac death. Among men, it has been estimated that approximately 6–17% of all sudden cardiac deaths occur in association with acute exertion [16].

Effect of Exercise on Risk of Sudden Death

Regular physical activity is beneficial because it is associated with a 40% reduction in the risk of death or myocardial infarction. However, sport momentarily increases the risk of adverse cardiovascular events during the sporting activity. Regular physical activity provides a variety of health benefits. In general, physical activity has an acceptable risk-benefit ratio where benefits far outweigh risks to the heart and lungs. Rarely, heart problems occur as a result of physical activity. It includes improvement in cardiopulmonary or metabolic status, reduction of the risk of coronary artery disease or stroke, prevention of cancer, and decrease in total mortality. However, vigorous physical exercise may precipitate acute fatalities in both adults and young competitive athletes with concealed heart diseases. But, the risk-benefit ratio of physical exercise differs among these two age groups. In sedentary adults, vigorous exertion increases the incidence of acute coronary events, whereas trained adults have reduced overall risk of *myocardial infarction* and sudden coronary death. In adolescents and young adults, strenuous sports activity is associated with a significant increase of the risk of sudden death [22].

Exercise-related cardiac events are occasionally reported during highly competitive sports activity or vigorous exercises among individuals with both diagnosed and *occult heart disease*. Though, the risk of sudden death is extremely low during vigorous exercise, and habitual vigorous exercise actually decreases the risk of sudden death during exercise [5]. Therefore, physical activity and exercise training have risks that must be considered when recommending regular physical activity for the general population and for individuals with cardiovascular disease [23]. The incidence of sudden cardiac death, serious arrhythmias, and myocardial infarction in connection with both recreational and rehabilitative physical activity is small. However, the incidence of sudden cardiac death is several times higher in exercise than at other times. This relative risk is highest in middle-aged men and higher in strenuous than in submaximal exercise. The cause of sudden death is ischemic in older subjects (≥35 years old), while cardiomyopathies or genetic ion channel diseases are important underlying pathology in younger (<35 years old) victims [5].

Individuals who are more physically active appear to have lower rates *of all-cause mortality* probably due to a decrease in *chronic diseases* including coronary artery disease. Part of persons who die suddenly during exercise frequently have warning symptoms of heart disease which they ignored, choosing to continue exercising rather than to seek medical advice. Not all episodes of sudden cardiac arrest are preventable because many of the individuals do not have symptoms until they have the episode. In 80% of those cases [24], there are absolutely no symptoms to warn that the cardiac arrest might occur. *Sudden cardiac arrest* has warning signs and symptoms that can go unnoticed. Once coronary artery disease has become manifest, exercise training can clearly improve the functional capacity of patients and reduce overall *mortality* by decreasing the risk of sudden cardiac death [25]. This may result from an improvement in cardiovascular risk factors in addition to enhanced *fibrinolysis*, improved *endothelial function*, decreased sympathetic tone, and other yet undetermined factors [26]. However, athletes who die suddenly have advanced cardiac disease; they are at high risk of dying suddenly, whether or not they exercise. Hence, physical fitness, more than the absence of other factors, is the major determinant of cardiovascular and metabolic risk. This increased risk is higher in the less accomplished athlete and in those with cardiovascular risk factors.

Levels of Physical Fitness

Epidemiologic studies have established that physical activity is associated with substantial improvements in cardiovascular prognosis. Limited data are available on the relation between physical fitness and mortality from cardiovascular disease. In addition, partial information is available about the role of *cardiorespiratory* fitness in the prediction of sudden cardiac death [27]. Few studies exist to show if the prognostic value of VO_2peak for fatal and nonfatal coronary events is different among men with low and high pretest probability for cardiovascular disease. This question was studied in 4,276 men, 30–69 years of age, who were followed for an average of 8.5 years. It was concluded that a lower level of physical fitness is associated with a higher risk of death from coronary heart disease and cardiovascular disease in clinically healthy men, independent of conventional coronary risk factors [28].

Cardiopulmonary fitness was found to be a predictor of *sudden cardiac death* in addition to that predicted by conventional risk factors. *Exercise stress testing* in healthy subjects shows that in the lowest quintile of fitness distribution, cardiovascular morbidity and mortality are greatly increased [29]. There was a slight improvement in the level of discrimination, although the net reclassification index did not change while using cardiopulmonary fitness with conventional risk factors. Minkkinen et al. [30] suggested that reduced exercise capacity, particularly in combination with heightened T-wave alterations, indicating enhanced cardiac electrical instability, powerfully predicts risk for sudden cardiac death in patients referred for exercise testing. Laukkanen et al. [31] suggested that VO_2peak was predictive of nonfatal and fatal cardiac events among men with or without known risk factors. In subjects with or without common risk factors, one MET (3.5 $mLO_2 \cdot kg^{-1} \cdot min^{-1}$) increment amounted to an average decrease of 17–29% in nonfatal and 28–51% in fatal cardiac events after adjustment for age. VO_2peak represented two strong independent and consistent risk predictors. Prognosis improves significantly when reaching a higher level of fitness, where the strength of evidence is best for intensive activity. This increase in cardiorespiratory fitness by one MET brings along a risk reduction of approximately 20% [29].

Physical activity exerts beneficial effects on cardiovascular risk factors and on subclinical atherosclerosis: endothelial function, progression of atherosclerotic plaques and it reduces cardiovascular endpoints. It is important to stress that severe heart disease may be present even in persons who are extremely physically fit. For example are the cases of long-distance runners who completed the run few weeks before their subsequent deaths from severe advanced coronary artery disease, in some cases with associated hypertrophic cardiomyopathy and complete occlusion of one major coronary artery and 75% narrowing, with atherosclerosis, of the other two. To conclude, physical exertion itself is associated with an increased risk of sudden cardiac death, which is alleviated, however, by regular training. All in all, the risk-benefit relation is very favorable and better than most other interventions [29].

Causes of Sudden Cardiac Death

Up to 80% of sudden cardiac death in the young has been attributed to a *heart's structural abnormality*, the most common cause being *hypertrophic cardiomyopathy* (HCM) [18]. The specter of *sudden cardiac death* has been intertwined with the diagnosis of hypertrophic cardiomyopathy which is now regarded as the most common cause of these events in young people, including competitive athletes [32]. In contrast, *arrhythmogenic disorders* of the heart with no evidence of structural abnormalities at postmortem have been reported to account for less than 10% of all sudden cardiac deaths in the young. These primary arrhythmogenic disorders include LQTs, arrhythmogenic right *ventricular dysplasia*, idiopathic *ventricular fibrillation*, and *Brugada syndrome*. Sudden cardiac death can broadly be categorized into disorders which predominantly affect the structure of the heart as well as those which affect mainly the cardiac conduction system or arrhythmogenic disorders. The specific diseases which cause sudden cardiac death within the structural and arrhythmogenic areas are summarized in Table 9.1.

Sudden cardiac death is a heterogeneous condition where causes of sudden death may be caused by *acute ischemia*, structural defects, myocardial scar, and/or genetic mutations. Other less common causes of sudden death during exercise include *congenital anomalies* of the coronary arteries, right ventricular dysplasia, *aortic rupture* associated with *Marfanâs syndrome*, coronary artery dissection, *myocarditis*, and ill-defined conduction disturbances presumed to be related to pathological changes found in the conduction

Table 9.1 Sudden cardiac death causes due to structural abnormalities and arrhythmogenic disorders

Structural changes	Arrhythmogenic disorders
Hypertrophic cardiomyopathy	Long QTS syndrome
Coronary anomalies	Brugada syndrome
Myocarditis	Catecholaminergic tachycardia
Right ventricle dysplasia	Ventricular tachyarrhythmias
Congenital heart disease	Ventricular fibrillation
Coronary artery disease	
Commotio cordis	

pathways at autopsy [18]. Such anomalies may have important clinical implications during intense athletic activity [33]. Thus, sudden cardiac death may include structural abnormalities and/or primary arrhythmias. But the more important point is that none of these conditions is caused by exercise.

While a large number of cardiac conditions have been associated with sudden cardiac death during exercise, in athletes aged 35 years or older, the major risk factor for sudden cardiac death is typically caused by *coronary artery disease* usually in the setting of reduced *ejection fraction*; occasionally, hypertrophic cardiomyopathy, *mitral valve prolapse*, or acquired valvular disease is involved. In other conditions, underlying sudden death in athletes can be asthma, heatstroke, and illicit or performance-enhancing drug-related complications; ventricular tachycardia or fibrillation is a terminal, not a primary, event [34]. Many athletes over the age of 35 years experience warning signs that they ignored prior to their fatal event. The accumulation of *atherosclerotic plaques* within a coronary artery eventually can close up blood flow to the myocardium, resulting in a *myocardial infarction* or sudden death. Globally, the incidence is expected to rise sharply as the prevalence of coronary artery disease and heart failure continues to increase.

Athletes below the age of 35 years who die suddenly during exercise are more likely to have undetected hypertrophic cardiomyopathy which has consistently been the single most common cardiovascular cause of sudden death, accounting for about 48% of these events in prior reports [35]. The association of unsuspected cardiovascular disease and sudden death in young athletes is not coincidental, since participation in competitive sports itself substantially increases the likelihood of sudden death [18].

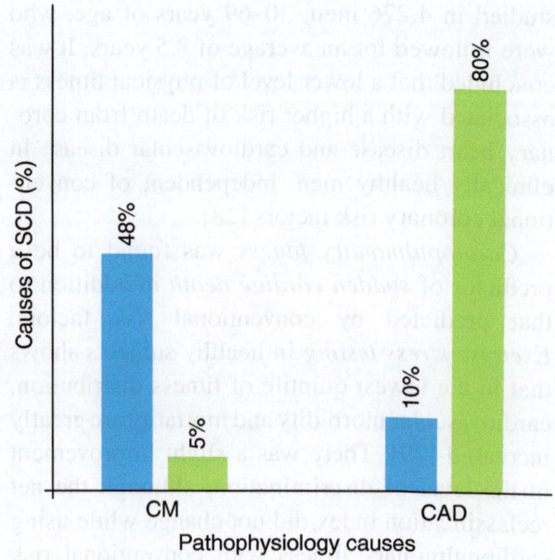

Fig. 9.1 The two main causes of sudden cardiac death in competitive athletes below 35 years (*blue*) and above 35 years (*green*). Majority of deaths caused by cardiovascular disease in athletes younger than 35 years old is hypertrophic cardiomyopathy (48%). Athletes older than 35 years may die due to complications of coronary heart disease often caused by atherosclerosis. Myocardial ischemia and myocardial infarction are responsible for most of sudden cardiac death above this age (80%). *SCD* sudden cardiac death, *CM* cardiomyopathy, *CAD* coronary artery disease

In addition, below age 35 years, the problem is usually a *structural abnormality* in the heart muscle, *valves*, or coronary arteries. In some individuals, it was found to have an anomalous origin in one of their coronary arteries, an exceptionally rare congenital abnormality that completely closes up blood flow to the myocardium. These conditions are usually congenital and are difficult to detect. However, some young athletes who die suddenly during exercise are likely to have severe coronary artery disease as a result of familial hypercholesterolemia (inherited high level of blood cholesterol). Data (Fig. 9.1) suggest that in young athletes, sudden cardiac death most often occurs from hypertrophic cardiomyopathy, and, in older athletes, from coronary heart disease [35].

Interestingly, *arrhythmogenic right ventricular dysplasia*, possibly *commotio cordis* congenital, is the predominant anatomic finding in athletes with sudden cardiac death; that is, concussion of the heart from nonpenetrating blunt trauma to the anterior chest can lead to fatal cardiac arrest due to either myocardial trauma or the mechanoelectrical triggering of a *ventricular tachyarrhythmia* during the vulnerable period of the T wave [36]. As with some other *risk factors*, the overall impact of activity on sudden cardiac death may be small. In the Maastricht Sudden Death study, 67% of the sudden death victims were physically inactive at the time of the event [37]. High percentage of individuals who suffer sudden cardiac death have coronary heart disease, particularly in patients with advanced age in men and women, whites and nonwhites. Epidemiological data on the prevalence of ischemic or *left ventricular dysfunction* that causes sudden cardiac death to a great extent parallels that of coronary heart disease [38].

Coronary artery disease is present in 65–70% of all sudden cardiac deaths. *Sudden cardiac death* has a much higher incidence in men than women [15], probably because young women have lower rates of participation in certain sports. This reflects *sex differences* in the incidence of coronary heart disease as well and suggests that women may have a lower risk of exertion-related sudden cardiac death. *Men* account for approximately 75% of all sudden cardiac deaths [38] and, compared to *women*, have a 50% higher age-adjusted rate of sudden cardiac death. *Blacks* have higher age-adjusted mortality rates for sudden cardiac death than *whites*.

These are potent risk factors that increase the relative risk of sudden cardiac death, but the contribution of sudden cardiac death in those with such risk factors to the cumulative rate of sudden cardiac death is relatively low. Most cases of sudden cardiac death occur in the general population, typically without a known history of heart disease, followed by patients who are at high risk for coronary artery disease or have established coronary artery disease [34]. Patients with *inherited ion channel* or *myocardial defects*, such as a long QT syndrome or hypertrophic cardiomyopathy, are at highest risk for early sudden cardiac death.

Although rare, sudden cardiac death also occurs in athletes. In an autopsy study of 158 American athletes with sudden cardiac death, 36% of subjects had hypertrophic cardiomyopathy, and 13% had *anomalous coronary* circulation [39]. An additional 10% had increased *cardiac mass*, consistent with possible cardiomyopathy, and autopsies were negative in only 3% of cases. A similar Italian study demonstrated a 20% prevalence of coronary disease followed by right ventricular cardiomyopathy/dysplasia in 10% of cases [40].

Pathophysiology

Several mechanisms are proposed, myocardial ischemia and repolarization due to potassium channel downregulation, which may also be explained by the presence of multiple factors such as cardiac hypertrophy (athlete's heart) and/or hypertrophic cardiomyopathy, increased *sympathetic tone*, *genetic defects*, drugs, doping agents, or food ingredients. These factors together may increase the *repolarization homogeneity* which sometimes leads to risk of arrhythmias and sudden cardiac death [41]. Sudden death is probably a consequence of an electrically unstable and unpredictable myocardial substrate with reentrant *ventricular tachyarrhythmias*, as evidenced by the presence of *histopathological markers* of disorganized myocardial architecture and replacement scarring which is the consequence of microvascular abnormalities and myocardial ischemia [42]. There are multiple factors at the organ involved in generation of ventricular tachycardia or *ventricular fibrillation* in different conditions: imbalance of autonomic tone, tissue reentry, wave break, and *action potential* duration alternant (tissue), cellularly triggered activity, and subcellular abnormal activation or *deactivation of ion channels* (automaticity level). At present, the exact mechanism causing exercise-related sudden death in individuals with established disease, especially of the coronary arteries, is not known. Whereas plaque rupture or *thromboses are* present in up to 95% of sudden cardiac deaths in the general population, the incidence seems to be lower in exercise-related deaths. Thus, *exercise-induced ischemia* or *coronary spasm* may be involved in exercise-related deaths.

The most common electrophysiologic mechanisms leading to sudden cardiac death are tachyarrhythmias such as *ventricular fibrillation* (VF) or *ventricular tachycardia* (VT). At the ventricle subcellular level especially in ischemia, altered *intracellular* Ca^{++} currents, altered *intracellular* K^{+} currents, or mutations resulting in dysfunction of a *sodium channel* (Na_{+} channelopathy) can increase the likelihood of ventricular tachycardia and ventricular.

Other causes include inherited arrhythmia syndromes, that is, commotio cordis, long QT syndrome, catecholaminergic polymorphic ventricular tachycardia, and Brugada syndrome. Some young athletes die of *aortic aneurysm* rupture such as in Marfan syndrome.

Commotio Cordis

Sudden death due to nonpenetrating chest wall impact in the absence of injury to the ribs, sternum, and heart is known as *commotio cordis. Athletes* with thin, compliant chest walls are at risk of sudden ventricular tachycardia or fibrillation after a blow to the precordium even when no cardiovascular disorder is present. *Nonpenetrating trauma* of the chest can cause sudden death as a result of a blunt, often innocent-appearing chest wall blow, with increasing frequency, in individuals without known cardiac disease. The clinical spectrum is diverse; however, a substantial number of cases occur in youth athletics. In events that occur during sport, victims are struck by projectiles regarded as standard implements of the game [43]. Sudden death in commotio cordis is due to ventricular fibrillation. The timing of the blow must be during the electric vulnerable period of the electrocardiograph cycles, 10–40 ms before the peak of the T wave (Fig. 9.2).

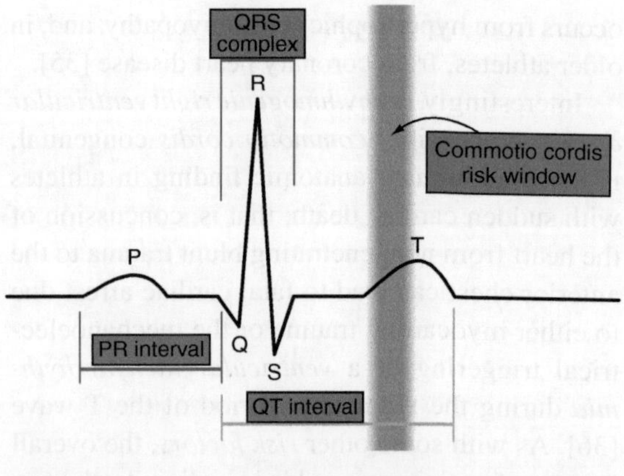

Fig. 9.2 Electrocardiogram schematic tracing showing the period of vulnerability to stretch-induced ventricular fibrillation which occurs in athletes with thin, compliant chest walls who are at risk of sudden ventricular tachycardia or fibrillation after a blow to the precordium (commotio cordis)

Before the peak of the T wave, rapid *left ventricular pressure* rise following chest impact likely results in activation of ion channels via *mechano-electric* coupling. The generation of inward current via *mechanosensitive ion channels* likely results in augmentation of repolarization and non-uniform myocardial activation and is the cause of premature ventricular depolarization that is a trigger of ventricular fibrillation [44]. Thus, peak left ventricular pressure generated by the *chest wall* blow correlated with the risk of ventricular fibrillation. Activation of the ATP-sensitive potassium channel (K_{ATP}) is a likely cause of the ventricular fibrillation produced by chest wall blows. The risk of arrhythmia increases progressively, until a velocity of 64 km·h^{-1}, and at higher velocities, the risk of ventricular fibrillation begins to diminish. The location of the impact must be directly over the cardiac silhouette. Autopsy is notable for the absence of any significant cardiac or thoracic injury [43]. The blow may involve a moderate–force projectile (e.g., baseball, hockey puck, lacrosse ball) or impact with another player during a vulnerable phase of myocardial repolarization. Energy of the impact object was also found to be a critical variable with 64 km·h^{-1} baseballs more likely to cause *ventricular fibrillation* than velocities less or greater than 64 km·h^{-1} [45].

Long QT Syndrome

Long QT (LQTs) is a heterogeneous disease that may be acquired or congenital. Both types may have a genetic basis. *Long QT syndrome* is a familial electrical disorder of *ventricular repolarization* characteristic of electrocardiograph abnormality (prolonged Q-T interval), polymorphic ventricular tachycardia (torsade de pointes), and sudden cardiac death. Not everyone with this disorder will have symptoms. Reentrant excitation caused by increased heterogeneity of *action potential* repolarization by inherited abnormalities affecting cardiac ion channels is the mechanism of torsades.

This form of polymorphic ventricular tachycardia can lead to syncope, seizures, and sudden death [46]. When the episodes are prolonged, circulatory failure due to *arrhythmia* may result in sudden death. Acquired *long QTs* usually result from electrolyte imbalances or drug therapy. Intracellular deficiencies of potassium and magnesium prolong *myocardial repolarization.* This may be clinically recognized by serum hypokalemia, hypomagnesia, and progressive prolongation of the QT interval (Fig. 9.3).

The majority of LQT patients who are genotype positive have abnormalities in genes encoding for potassium and *sodium ion channels.* The genes involved in long QTs have been numbered long QT1–9. *Exercise* is a common trigger in long QT1 [34]. Almost all drugs implicated in long QTS act on the *potassium ion channels* encoded by the *HERG* gene by blocking rapidly activating component (I_{Kr}) current, which is important in myocyte repolarization [34].

Catecholaminergic Polymorphic Ventricular Tachycardia

Catecholaminergic polymorphic ventricular tachycardia is a bidirectional or polymorphic ventricular tachycardia induced by adrenergic stimuli. Catecholamine explosively augments oxidative metabolism much more than cardiac work is generally underappreciated. Thus, adrenergic actions alone are likely to be more prone to cause *cardiac ischemia* than reduced coronary blood flow per se. Actually, all the signs and symptoms of ischemic heart disease reflect autonomic nervous system imbalance, particularly adrenergic hyperactivity, which may by itself cause ischemia as in rest angina. Adrenergic activity causing ischemia tends to induce arrhythmogenic with a continuously varying *QRS morphology* and axis and

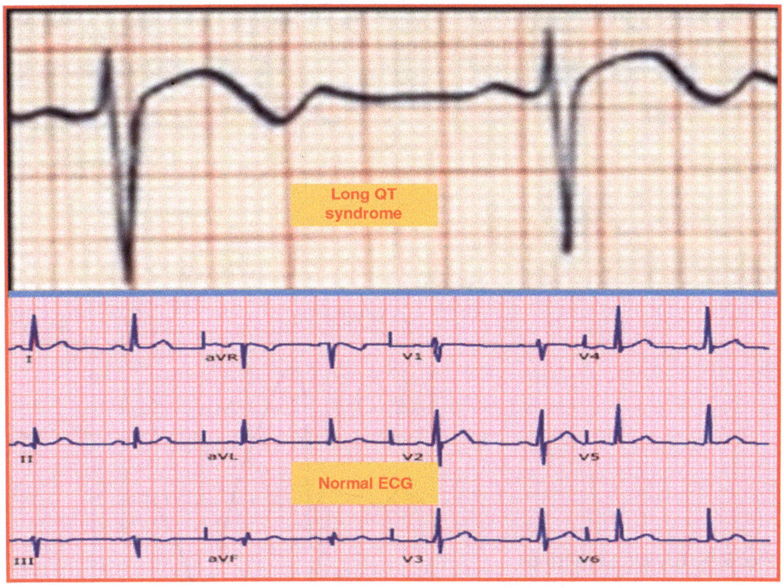

Fig. 9.3 Electrocardiographs showing normal sinus rhythm at a rate of 71 beats·min^{-1}, a P wave axis of 45°, and a PR interval of 0.15 s (Courtesy of Morton Arnsdorf, M.D.) and electrocardiographic strip showing long QT syndrome

necrotizing ischemic actions on the cardiovascular system. This may result in ischemia-induced metabolic *myocardiopathy* not unlike that caused by anatomic or *spasmogenic coronary obstruction* [47]. Catecholaminergic polymorphic ventricular tachycardia is caused by autosomal dominant mutation in the ryanodine type 2 receptor (RYR2) or recessive mutation in calsequestrin 2 (CASQ2) [48].

Brugada Syndrome

Brugada syndrome is an *autosomal* dominant inherited disorder that can lead to spontaneous lethal ventricular arrhythmias. *Brugada syndrome* is a congenital abnormality in the heart's electrical system. The *sudden cardiac death* in Brugada syndrome is uncommonly related to *exercise.* However, there is some evidence that *hyperthermia* during long-lasting exercise may make arrhythmias more likely with Brugada syndrome. *Idiopathic ventricular fibrillation* in a structurally normal heart with electrocardiograph evidence of right ventricular conduction delay is consistent with the Brugada syndrome. The Brugada syndrome is now recognized as a primary, genetically determined [49], electrical disease with a high risk of sudden cardiac death. The electrocardiogram of athletes at rest, especially in those that are endurance-trained, frequently shows *ST-segment* elevation, mainly in precordial leads (Fig. 9.4).

This condition, named early repolarization, is considered a benign electrocardiographic change due to athletic conditioning [50]. The syndrome has been linked to mutations in the SCN5A gene, which encodes the alpha-subunit of the *cardiac sodium channel*, resulting in loss of function. However, the SCN5A gene is affected less than 30% of the time in pedigrees with the Brugada pattern, highlighting the genetic heterogeneity of the Brugada phenotype.

Individuals with the Brugada syndrome classically have an incomplete right bundle branch block pattern characterized by ST elevation in right precordial leads (V1–V3), with or without a delay in right ventricular activation. The relationship between impaired sodium channel function and precordial ST changes is poorly understood. Mutations in the same gene are also associated with other congenital arrhythmias, for example, a gain of function mutation in SCN5A is associated with long QT3. Brugada and long QT3 syndromes are two allelic diseases caused by different mutations in SCN5A gene inherited by an autosomal dominant pattern with variable penetrance. The prevalence of *ventricular fibrillation* in such patients has been estimated as high as 40–60% [51], while the incidence of Brugada syndrome is estimated to be 5 in 10,000.

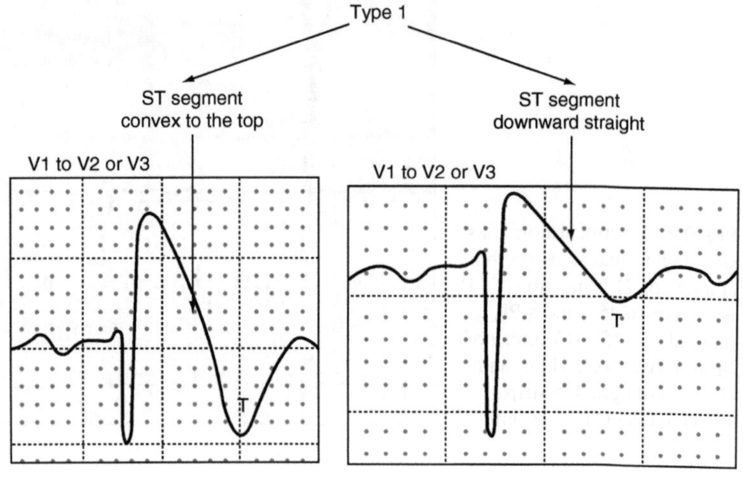

Fig. 9.4 Brugada syndrome electrocardiographic signature/phenotype

Hypertrophic Cardiomyopathy

Hypertrophic cardiomyopathy (HCM) is the most common monogenically inherited form of heart disease, characterized by thickening of the left ventricular wall, contractile dysfunction, and potentially fatal arrhythmias [52].

Individuals with *hypertrophic cardiomyopathy* have some degree of left ventricular hypertrophy.

Right ventricular involvement is usually less evident. Usually, this is an *asymmetric hypertrophy*, involving the interventricular septum, and is known as *asymmetric septal hypertrophy*. *Diastolic dysfunction* is common to most such patients irrespective of the presence or absence of outflow obstruction [53]. This is in contrast to the *concentric hypertrophy* seen in *aortic stenosis* or *hypertension*. About two thirds of individuals with hypertrophic cardiomyopathy have asymmetric septal hypertrophy (Fig. 9.5).

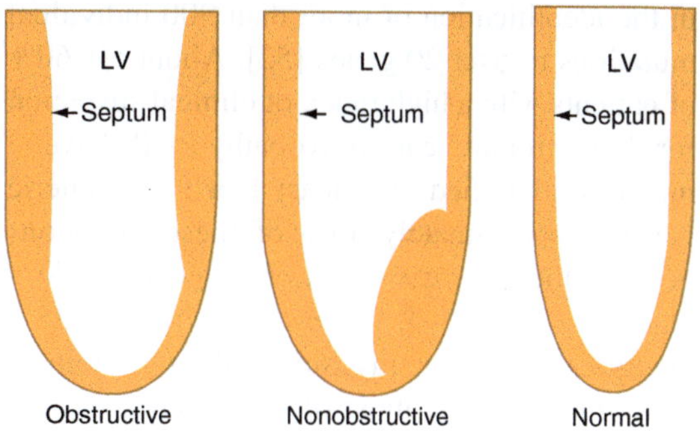

Fig. 9.5 On the *right*, left ventricle walls and axis are normal (*LV*). In the *middle*, left ventricle walls and axis are abnormal, and the form is spade shape, considered as a nonobstructive hypertrophic cardiomyopathy. On the *left side*, left ventricle walls and axis are also abnormal, and the shape is of an obstructive hypertrophic cardiomyopathy. Hypertrophic cardiomyopathy is the thickening of the muscles that make up the left ventricle and may interfere with the normal functioning of the ventricle

Although rare in the general population, this is the most common cause of sudden cardiac death in young athletes. It is inherited, and 60% of individuals with this have an affected first-degree relative. The prevalence of hypertrophic cardiomyopathy is about 0.2–0.5% of the general population. Hypertrophic cardiomyopathy, characterized by an asymmetrically hypertrophied and nondilated left ventricle, is a relatively common genetic cardiac disease with an incidence of 1 in 500 individuals in the general population, with heterogeneous clinical, morphologic, and *genetic expression* [42].

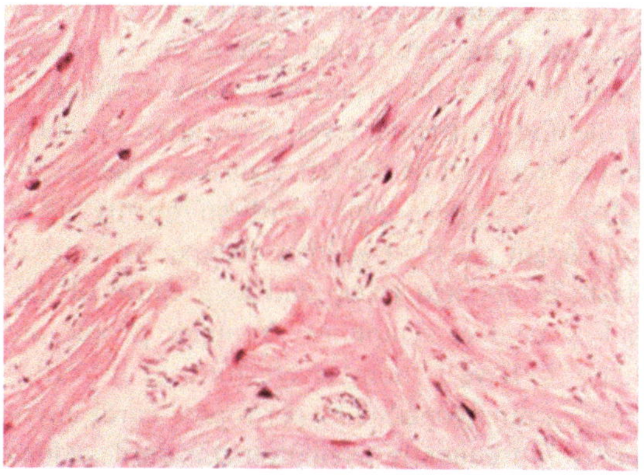

Fig. 9.6 Array of hypertrophied abnormally branching myocytes with connective tissue deposition

A *cardiomyopathy* is a primary disease that affects the *myocardium*. With hypertrophic cardiomyopathy, histological features of *myocyte hypertrophy*, myofibril disarray, and *interstitial fibrosis* occur. In hypertrophic cardiomyopathy – *myofiber disarray* – not all fibers are pulling in the same direction. Thus, the contraction is ineffective. However, the cardiac conduction system can have these same problems, which might cause arrhythmias and sudden cardiac death (Fig. 9.6). In addition, the contractile elements in the myocardium replicate, causing heart muscle cells to increase in size, which results in the thickening of the heart myocardium. Hypertrophic cardiomyopathy is inherited as an autosomal dominant trait and is attributed to *mutations* in one of a number of genes that encode for one of the *sarcomere proteins*. Thus, hypertrophic cardiomyopathy is most commonly due to a mutation in one of nine *sarcomeric genes* that involve genes encoding cardiac sarcomeric protein. This results in a mutated protein in the sarcomere, the primary component of the *myocyte*. Hypertrophic cardiomyopathy also causes disruptions of the electrical functions of the heart. Much progress has been made in the elucidation of the genetic basis of hypertrophic cardiomyopathy, resulting in the identification of more than 900 individual mutations in over 20 genes [52]. About 50–60% of patients with a high index of clinical suspicion for hypertrophic cardiomyopathy will have a mutation identified in at least 1 of 9 sarcomeric genes. Approximately 45% of these mutations occur in the *β myosin heavy chain* gene on *chromosome* 14 q11.2–3, while approximately 35% involve the cardiac myosin binding protein C gene. Interestingly, most of these genes encode sarcomeric proteins, such as myosin-7 also known as cardiac muscle β-myosin heavy chain (MYH7), cardiac myosin-binding protein C (MYBPC3), and myocardium troponin T (TNNT2). However, the molecular events that ultimately lead to the clinical phenotype of hypertrophic cardiomyopathy are still unclear [52].

Hypertrophic cardiomyopathy is a disease of the myocardium in which a portion of the myocardium is thickened without any obvious cause [54]. If asymmetric, the hypertrophy is usually greatest in the ventricular septum, but variations occur in which the hypertrophy may be maximal at the mid-ventricular level, at the apex, or rarely, in the free wall of the left ventricle. The occurrence of hypertrophic cardiomyopathy is a significant cause of sudden unexpected cardiac death in any age group and as a cause of disabling cardiac symptoms. Younger people are likely to have a more severe form of hypertrophic cardiomyopathy. Hypertrophic cardiomyopathy is frequently asymptomatic until sudden cardiac death happens, and for this reason, some suggest routinely screening certain populations for this disease.

Sudden cardiac death in individuals with hypertrophic cardiomyopathy is primary due to ventricular arrhythmias secondary to *intrinsic abnormalities* in the myocytes or can occur due to dynamic *outflow tract obstruction* during exercise. Depending on whether the distortion of normal heart anatomy causes an obstruction of the outflow of blood from the left ventricle of the heart, hypertrophic cardiomyopathy can be defined as obstructive or nonobstructive.

Atrial and *ventricular arrhythmias* are responsible for a significant proportion of the *morbidity* and *mortality*, and their prevalence appears to depend on the presence of obstruction and the extent of hypertrophy. Thus, the major manifestations of hypertrophic cardiomyopathy in systole and diastole, as well as the disturbances in rhythm, appear to be related to the site and/or extent of the hypertrophic process [53].

Septal hypercontractility is thought to be the principal cause of significant left ventricular outflow tract obstruction and *systolic anterior motion* of the *mitral valve* by making the distance between the mitral valve and papillary muscle shorter [55]. Systolic anterior motion occurs as the result of the *Venturi forces* created by the rapid ejection of blood through an outflow tract that is narrowed by upper septal hypertrophy, drawing the mitral leaflets anteriorly. The obstructive variant of hypertrophic cardiomyopathy, hypertrophic obstructive cardiomyopathy, may be idiopathic hypertrophic subaortic stenosis and asymmetric septal hypertrophy. The principal abnormality in systole is the obstruction to left ventricular outflow caused by systolic anterior motion of the anterior or posterior mitral leaflets with mitral leaflet-septal contact. About 25% of individuals with hypertrophic cardiomyopathy demonstrate an obstruction to the outflow of blood from the left ventricle during rest. In other individuals, obstruction only occurs under certain conditions. The principal abnormality in systole is the obstruction to left ventricular outflow caused by systolic anterior motion of the anterior or posterior mitral leaflets with mitral leaflet-septal contact [53]. This is known as *dynamic outflow obstruction*, because the degree of obstruction is variable and is dependent on the amount of blood in the ventricle immediately before ventricle systole. Mitral regurgitation invariably accompanies the obstruction to outflow. Another nonobstructive variant of hypertrophic cardiomyopathy is *apical hypertrophic cardiomyopathy* [56], also called *Yamaguchi syndrome* or Yamaguchi hypertrophy, first described in individuals of Japanese descent.

The cardiac renin-angiotensin system has been suggested to be involved in the development of left ventricular hypertrophy. Some of the components of the renin-angiotensin system have been reported to be synthesized in the ventricle of the heart [57]. In humans, a strong correlation has been found between plasma angiotensin I-converting enzyme activity and the insertion/deletion (I/D) polymorphism of the angiotensin converting enzyme gene, which has been reported to be associated with myocardial infarction, ischemic and idiopathic dilated cardiomyopathy, sudden death in hypertrophic cardiomyopathy, and restenosis after percutaneous transluminal coronary angioplasty. In the present study, we examined the possibility that the genotype of the angiotensin converting enzyme gene might influence the development of left ventricular hypertrophy. An insertion/deletion polymorphism in the gene encoding for angiotensin converting enzyme (ACE) alters the clinical phenotype of the disease. The D/D (deletion/deletion) genotype of angiotensin converting enzyme is associated with more marked hypertrophy of the left ventricle and may be associated with higher risk of adverse outcomes [58]. In humans, the plasma level of angiotensin converting enzyme is determined genetically. The angiotensin converting enzyme gene, which has been mapped to human chromosome 17q23, has insertion/deletion (I/D) polymorphism in intron. The angiotensin converting enzyme genotype with two deletion alleles (DD genotype) has been reported to be associated with higher plasma angiotensin converting enzyme activity, probably due to tight linkage to another locus that is important in regulation of this gene [59]. These findings suggest that intracardiac formation of angiotensin II independent of the circulating renin-angiotensin system may play a key role in the development of left ventricular hypertrophy.

Coronary Artery Anomalies

A variety of inherited coronary artery abnormalities combine to represent the second leading cause of sudden cardiac death in young athletes, the most frequent cardiovascular cause of sudden cardiac death in young athletes in the United States [39]. Only about one third of affected individuals are thought to be symptomatic, experiencing angina, syncope, or shortness of breath with exercise before sudden death. It is a *congenital coronary-artery anomaly* in which the artery arises from the wrong aortic sinus most commonly. The most common coronary anatomy associated with risk of sudden cardiac death is the left main coronary arising from the right sinus of Valsalva with an intra-arterial course between the aorta and pulmonary artery [60]. The mechanism of sudden cardiac death in all cases here is thought to be an arrhythmia triggered by heart tissue ischemia or infarction. These anomalies, which are not usually associated with coronary-artery atherosclerosis, may be more common than previously thought. Their diagnosis requires a high index of suspicion and is particularly important, since surgical correction is feasible. The echocardiography is the method to be utilized in order to detect the existence of anomalous coronary arteries. It is difficult to distinguish anomalous coronary arteries by methods of electrocardiograph since resting electrocardiographs are typically normal and exercise stress testing may be negative. Although some cases may be suspected on echocardiography, a definitive diagnosis is made by coronary angiography, computed tomography, or magnetic resonance imaging.

Mechanism of Ventricular Tachycardia

Ventricular tachyarrhythmias include a number of different rhythms, which arise in a number of different clinical situations. The ventricular tachyarrhythmias are fast heart rhythms that arise entirely from the ventricles. They are faster than 100 beats $\cdot$ min^{-1} by definition. Faster rates >180 beats $\cdot$ min^{-1} may cause drops in arterial pressure and produce syncope. Very fast rates >220 beats $\cdot$ min^{-1} are imminently dangerous because they rarely terminate spontaneously and invariably cause drops in *blood pressure* and low *cardiac output*. Generally, the tachyarrhythmias can be characterized as either monomorphic ventricular tachycardia (Fig. 9.7) or polymorphic ventricular tachycardia. *Monomorphic ventricular tachycardia* would

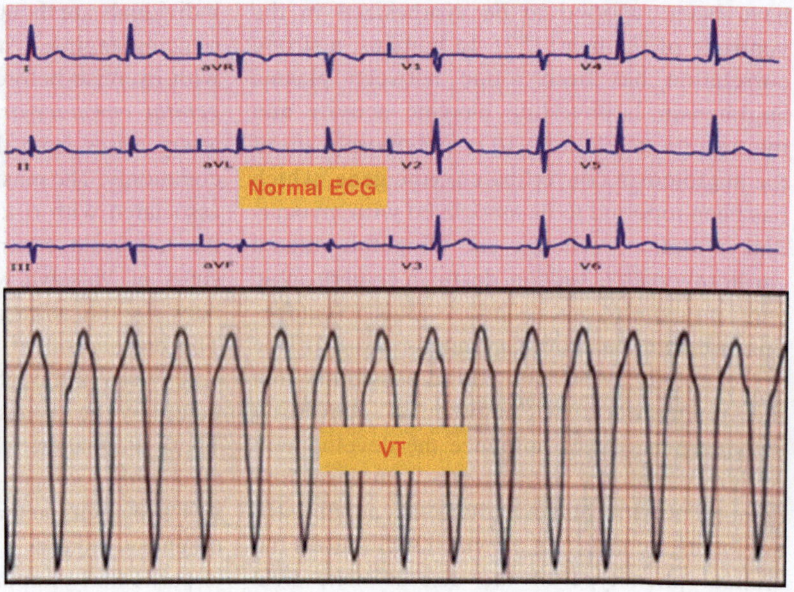

Fig. 9.7 Electrocardiographs showing normal sinus rhythm at a rate of 71 beats·min^{-1}, a P wave axis of 45°, and a PR interval of 0.15 s (Courtesy of Morton Arnsdorf, M.D.) and electrocardiographic strip showing monomorphic ventricular tachycardia

appear on an electrocardiograph record with a regular rate and rhythm and fixed shape or morphology of the electrocardiograph trace. Each beat of the tachycardia would look the same, hence the designation monomorphic. *Polymorphic ventricular tachycardia* typically is irregular in rate and rhythm and has varying shapes or morphologies on the electrocardiograph.

A problem that starts as a monomorphic ventricular tachycardia may deteriorate into polymorphic ventricular tachycardia. The most dangerous rhythm is a form of polymorphic ventricular tachycardia called *ventricular fibrillation*. The electrocardiograph rhythm is extremely disorganized and most often leads to death if not corrected very quickly.

Ventricular tachycardia degenerating into ventricular fibrillation is the most common electrical sequence of events in sudden cardiac death [35]. With faster heart rates and underlying heart disease, loss of consciousness (syncope) or sudden cardiac death may occur. An anatomical or a functional block in the course of impulse propagation may create a circuit with the wave front circling around it and resulting in ventricular tachycardia. *Electrical reentry* forms the basis of the majority of both ventricular tachycardia and ventricular fibrillation. In diseased substrate (myocardial infarction, hypertrophy, myocarditis, and interstitial fibrosis), scar tissue will not conduct or propagate *electrical impulses*. The scar border zone comprises islands of viable *myocardium embedded* in scar tissue and forms the anatomic substrate for ventricular tachycardia. In these areas, conduction is slowed and discontinuous, and dispersion of repolarization exists due to abnormalities in gap junction function and distribution. This heterogeneity in electrophysiologic properties prevents the electrical impulse from traveling across the myocardium in a single uniform wave front. In sustained monomorphic ventricular tachycardia, there is a single reentrant circuit with a single exit from the circuit. Monomorphic ventricular tachycardia may be quite stable and can last minutes, hours, or longer in the absence of hemodynamic or ischemic compromise. Multiple morphologies of monomorphic ventricular tachycardia usually occur in the setting of multiple areas of patchy scar, resulting in changes in rotation of a single circuit, small differences in the reentrant circuit, or multiple reentrant circuits. Scar-related monomorphic ventricular tachycardia may have complex impulse propagation and reentry patterns. This is in contrast to the mechanism for polymorphic ventricular tachycardia, which is dependent on long–short conduction sequences, long QTs intervals, and early after *depolarizations*. Patients with polymorphic ventricular tachycardia appear to have more complex circuits, which appear to rotate around the mid-myocardial cells because they have longer refractory periods.

Mechanism of Ventricular Fibrillation

Ventricular fibrillation results when multiple sites in the ventricles fire impulses very rapidly in an uncoordinated fashion (Fig. 9.8). Although this general scheme appears correct, the exact mechanisms of ventricular fibrillation remain unknown.

Mechanisms such as wave break and collisions are involved in generating ventricular fibrillation from ventricular tachycardia. The development of primary ventricular fibrillation is usually from simultaneous ventricular activation by multiple localized areas of *micro-reentry circuits*. Although this general scheme appears correct, the exact mechanisms of *ventricular fibrillation* remain unknown. The major pathogenic mechanism triggering ventricular fibrillation is *autonomic imbalance*. This includes a wide range of reflex changes in the ratio of *sympathetic* to *vagal* ventricular activation over time, occurring immediately after *coronary artery occlusion* at the onset of acute *myocardial infarction*. Another trigger of ventricular fibrillation is *autonomic disturbance* due to emotional stress [61]. The underlying diffuse myocardial disease forms the substrate, supporting the mechanism of rotating spiral waves. While at the tissue level reentry and wave break mechanisms are the most important known mechanisms of ventricular fibrillation and ventricular tachycardia, at the cellular level, increased excitation or decreased repolarization reserve of *cardiomyocytes* may result in ectopic activity, that is, automaticity, triggered activity, contributing to ventricular fibrillation and *ventricular tachycardia* initiation. The disordered nature of *myocardial depolarization* in ventricular fibrillation results in a lack of organized ventricular contraction and thus no meaningful *cardiac output*.

Arrhythmogenic Right Ventricular Dysplasia

It is a chronic disease of progressive fibrofatty infiltration of the right ventricle that is commonly associated with ventricular arrhythmias.

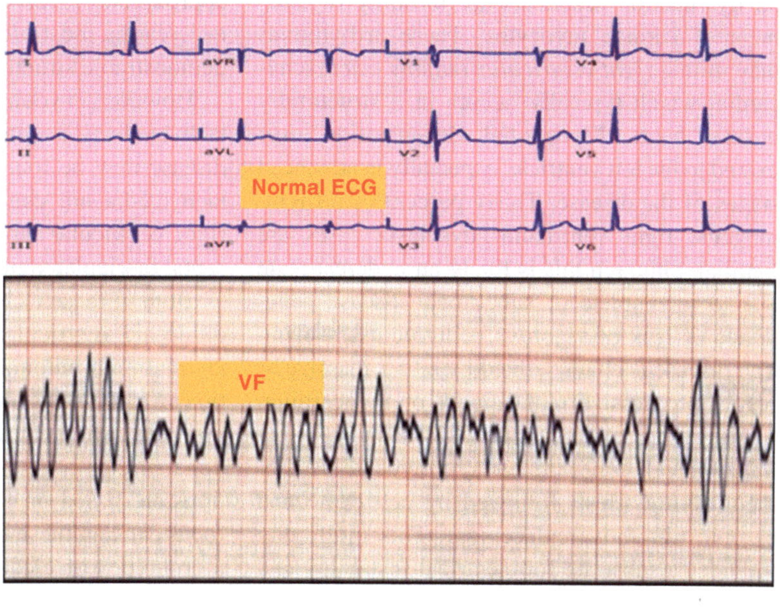

Fig. 9.8 Electrocardiographs showing normal sinus rhythm at a rate of 71 beats·min^{-1}, a P wave axis of 45°, and a PR interval of 0.15 s, and ventricular fibrillation (*VF*) with multiple sites and in an uncoordinated fashion (Courtesy of Morton Arnsdorf, M.D.)

Arrhythmogenic right ventricular dysplasia (ARVD) is a heart muscle disorder of unknown cause that is characterized pathologically by *fibrofatty* replacement of the right ventricular myocardium [62]. *Right ventricular dysplasia* is a rare condition with unclear etiology that produces ventricular tachycardia. It is most frequently found in young adult males, but can be seen in both sexes and at any age without overt heart disease. Symptoms vary from *palpitations* to *syncope*. Some individuals who are considered normal on physical examination may experience malaise or abrupt extreme weakness. This temporary incapacitation could lead to create major risk for themselves and others. This ventricular tachycardia, more common than thought, is emerging as a cause of sudden cardiac death in young otherwise healthy adults. The clinical and phenotypic profile is variable but includes structural and functional abnormalities of the right ventricle, ventricular and *supraventricular arrhythmias*, familial occurrence, and the risk for sudden cardiac death [62].

Arrhythmogenic right ventricular dysplasia, also called *arrhythmogenic right ventricular cardiomyopathy*, is characterized by ventricular arrhythmias and progressive structural abnormalities of the *right ventricle* [63]. Arrhythmogenic right ventricular cardiomyopathy is an inherited cardiomyopathy distinguished by right ventricular dysfunction secondary to fibrofatty replacement of cardiac myocytes. These arrhythmias may mimic *right ventricular outflow tract* tachycardia, which typically occurs in a structurally normal heart. Myocardial degeneration may extend to the left ventricle, especially in advanced stages of the disease. Thirty percent of arrhythmogenic right ventricular dysplasia cases are familial, although this is likely an underestimate due to incomplete or subclinical disease penetrance or lack of vigorous pedigree assessment. The disease is characterized by either massive or partial progressive replacement of myocardium by fatty or fibrofatty tissue. It is postulated that impaired cell adhesion leads to myocyte detachment during stress, followed by cell death and chronic fibrofatty replacement. This infiltration provides a substrate for electrical instability and leads to ventricular arrhythmias ranging from isolated premature ventricular contractions (PVC) to sustained ventricular tachycardias or ventricular fibrillation [64]. The most common arrhythmia is sustained or nonsustained ventricular tachycardia originating from the right ventricle, typically with a left bundle branch block pattern and inferior axis (Figs. 9.9 and 9.10). Prevalence estimates vary by country but are estimated at 1 per 1,000 individuals, with 80% of cases diagnosed in individuals under 40 years of age. The most common mutant gene identified with arrhythmogenic right ventricular dysplasia is the plakophilin mutant, and this is found in approximately 25% of patients. Ventricular tachycardia most often occurs in the presence of demonstrable structural heart disease.

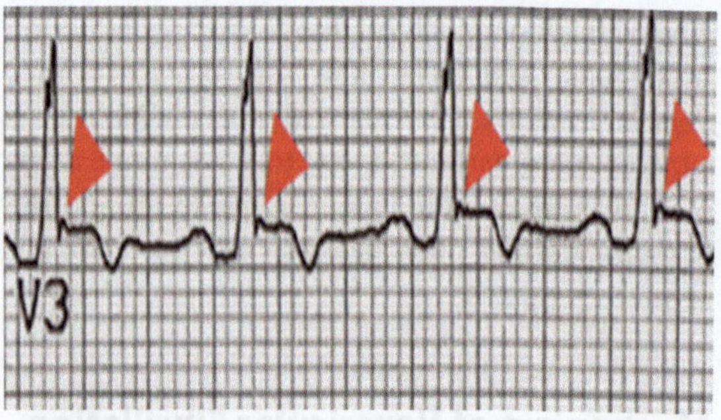

Fig. 9.9 The epsilon wave (*marked by red triangle*) seen in *right* ventricular dysplasia. Monomorphic ventricular tachycardia originating from the right ventricular outflow tract

However, in young individuals with ventricular tachycardia, it is common that no structural heart disease may be found. Two forms of ventricular tachycardia are commonly found, and they are right ventricular outflow tract and left posterior septal fascicular ventricular tachycardia.

Both of these tachycardias are repetitive monomorphic ventricular tachycardias likely due to an abnormal automatic focus amenable to ablation. Ablation is a technique used to treat abnormal heart rhythms, or arrhythmias, and can be done surgically or nonsurgically. These distinctions are based on the location of the abnormal focus causing these tachycardia and the resulting morphology on electrocardiography.

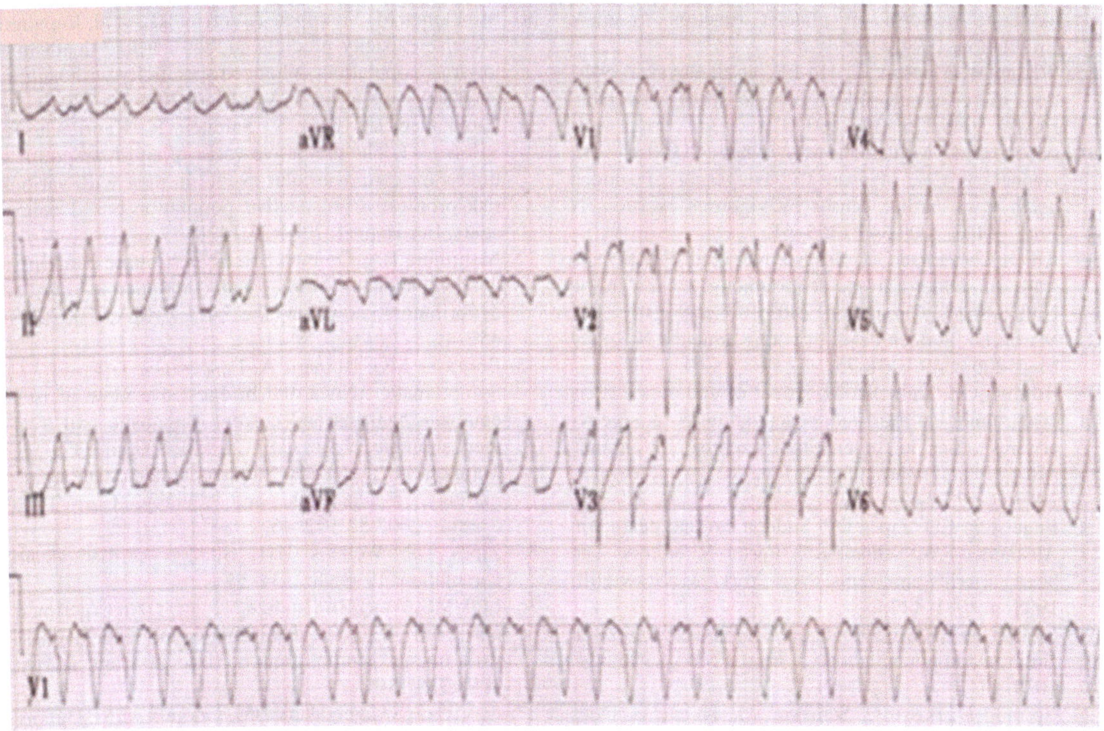

Fig. 9.10 Electrocardiogram of ventricular tachyarrhythmias arising from right ventricle

References

1. Paffenbarger Jr RS, Hyde RT, Wing AL, et al. A natural history of athleticism and cardiovascular health. JAMA. 1984;252:491–5.
2. Ivy JL. Role of exercise training in the prevention and treatment of insulin resistance and non-insulin-dependent diabetes mellitus. Sports Med. 1997;24:321–36.
3. Jayalakshmi MK, Prabhu RN, Shanmukhappa NJ, Smilee JS. Effect of sedentary life style on anthropometric and cardiovascular parameters. Int J Biol Med Res. 2011;2:846–51.
4. Sattelmair J, Pertman J, Ding FL, Kohl 3rd HW, Haskell W, Lee IM. Dose response between physical activity and risk of coronary heart disease a meta-analysis. Circulation. 2011;124:789–95.
5. Nam GB. Exercise, heart and health. Korean Circ J. 2011;41:113–21.
6. Bertrais S, Beyeme-Ondoua JP, Czernichow S, Galan P, Hercberg S, Oppert JM. Sedentary behaviours, physical activity and metabolic syndrome in middle aged French subjects. Obes Res. 2005;13:936–44.
7. Rainwater DL, McMahan CA, Malcom GT, et al. Lipid and apolipoprotein predictors of atherosclerosis in youth: apolipoprotein concentrations do not materially improve prediction of arterial lesions in PDAY subjects. The PDAY Research Group. Arterioscler Thromb Vasc Biol. 1999;19:753–61.
8. Vanhecke TE, Miller WM, Franklin BA, Weber JE, McCullough PA. Awareness, knowledge, and perception of heart disease among adolescents. Eur J Cardiovasc Prev Rehabil. 2006;13:718–23.
9. Highlander P, Shaw GP. Current pharmacotherapeutic concepts for the treatment of cardiovascular disease in diabetics. Ther Adv Cardiovasc Dis. 2010;4:43–54.
10. Kvan E, Pettersen KI, Sandvik L, Reikvam A. High mortality in diabetic patient with acute myocardial infarction: cardiovascular co-morbidities contribute most to the high risk. Int J Cardiol. 2007;121:184–8.
11. Hu FB, Willett WC, Li T, Stampfer MJ, Colditz GA, Manson JE. Adiposity as compared with physical activity in predicting mortality among women. N Engl J Med. 2004;351:2694–703.
12. Maron BJ, Gohman TE, Aeppli D. Prevalence of sudden cardiac death during competitive sports activities in Minnesota high school athletes. J Am Coll Cardiol. 1998;32:1881–4.
13. Neuspiel DR, Kuller LH. Sudden and unexpected natural death in childhood and adolescence. JAMA. 1985;254:1321–5.
14. Wang JS, Jen CJ, Kung HC, Lin LJ, Hsiue TR, Chen HI. Different effects of strenuous exercise and

moderate exercise on platelet function in men. Circulation. 1994;90:2877–85.
15. Whang W, Manson JE, Hu FB, et al. Physical exertion, exercise, and sudden cardiac death in women. JAMA. 2006;295:1399–403.
16. Albert CM, Mittleman MA, Chae CU, Lee IM, Hennekens CH, Manson JE. Triggering of sudden death from cardiac causes by vigorous exertion. N Engl J Med. 2000;343:1355–61.
17. Albert CM, Chae CU, Grodstein F, et al. Prospective study of sudden cardiac death among women in the United States. Circulation. 2003;107:2096–101.
18. Maron BJ. Sudden death in young athletes. N Engl J Med. 2003;349:1064–75.
19. Billman GE, Kukielka M. Effect of endurance exercise training on heart rate onset and heart rate recovery responses to submaximal exercise in animals susceptible to ventricular fibrillation. J Appl Physiol. 2007;102:231–40.
20. Engelstein ED, Zipes DP. Sudden cardiac death. In: Alexander RW, Schlant RC, Fuster V, editors. The heart, arteries and veins. New York: McGraw-Hill; 1998. p. 1081–112.
21. Liberthson RR. Sudden death from cardiac causes in children and young adults. N Engl J Med. 1996;334:1039–44.
22. Corrado D, Basso C, Schiavon M, Thiene G. Does sports activity enhance the risk of sudden cardiac death? J Cardiovasc Med (Hagerstown). 2006;7:228–33.
23. Thompson PD, Buchner D, Pina IL, et al. Exercise and physical activity in the prevention and treatment of atherosclerotic cardiovascular disease: a statement from the council on clinical cardiology (subcommittee on exercise, rehabilitation, and prevention) and the council on nutrition, physical activity, and metabolism (subcommittee on physical activity). Circulation. 2003;107:3109–16.
24. Corrado D, Drezner J, Basso C, Pelliccia A, Thiene G. Strategies for the prevention of sudden cardiac death during sports. Eur J Cardiovasc Prev Rehabil. 2011;18:197–208.
25. Prasad DS, Das BC. Physical inactivity: a cardiovascular risk factor. Indian J Med Sci. 2009;63:33–42.
26. Adamu B, Sani MU, Abdu A. Physical exercise and health: a review. Niger J Med. 2006;15:190–6.
27. Laukkanen JA, Mäkikallio TH, Rauramaa R, Kiviniemi V, Ronkainen K, Kurl S. Cardiorespiratory fitness is related to the risk of sudden cardiac death: a population-based follow-up study. J Am Coll Cardiol. 2010;56:1476–83.
28. Ekelund LG, Haskell WL, Johnson JL, Whaley FS, Criqui MH, Sheps DS. Physical fitness as a predictor of cardiovascular mortality in asymptomatic North American men. The lipid research clinics mortality follow-up study. N Engl J Med. 1988;319:1379–84.
29. Schmermund A. Cardiorespiratory fitness. Importance of sports for health. Herz. 2004;29:365–72 [Article in German].
30. Minkkinen M, Nieminen T, Verrier RL, et al. Impaired exercise capacity predicts sudden cardiac death in a low-risk population: enhanced specificity with heightened T-wave alternans. Ann Med. 2009;41:380–9.
31. Laukkanen JA, Kurl S, Salonen R, Rauramaa R, Salonen JT. The predictive value of cardiorespiratory fitness for cardiovascular events in men with various risk profiles: a prospective population-based cohort study. Eur Heart J. 2004;25:1428–37.
32. Nishimura RA, Ommen SR. Hypertrophic cardiomyopathy, sudden death, and implantable cardiac defibrillators: how low the bar? JAMA. 2007;298:452–4.
33. Bourassa MG, Butnaru A, Lespérance J, Tardif J-C. Symptomatic myocardial bridges: overview of ischemic mechanisms and current diagnostic and treatment strategies. J Am Coll Cardiol. 2003;41:351–9.
34. Turakhia M, Tseng ZH. Sudden cardiac death: epidemiology, mechanisms, and therapy. Curr Probl Cardiol. 2007;32:501–46.
35. Zipes DP, Wellens HJJ. Sudden cardiac death. Circulation. 1998;98:2334–51.
36. Link MS, Wang PJ, Pandian NG, et al. An experimental model of sudden death due to low-energy chest-wall impact (commotion cordis). N Engl J Med. 1998;338:1805–11.
37. de Vreede Swagemakers JJM, Gorgels APM, Dubois-Arbouw WI, van Ree JW, Daemen MJAP, Houben LGE, Wellens HJJ. Out-of-hospital cardiac arrest in the 1990's: a population-based study in the Maastricht area on incidence, characteristics and survival. J Am Coll Cardiol. 1997;30:1500–5.
38. Kannel WB, Thomas Jr HE. Sudden coronary death: the Framingham Study. Ann N Y Acad Sci. 1982;382:3–21.
39. Maron BJ, Shirani J, Poliac LC, Mathenge R, Roberts WC, Mueller FO. Sudden death in young competitive athletes clinical, demographic, and pathological profiles. JAMA. 1996;276:199–204.
40. Corrado D, Basso DC, Thiene G. Sudden cardiac death in young people with apparently normal heart. Cardiovasc Res. 2001;50:399–408.
41. Varro A, Baczko I. Possible mechanisms of sudden cardiac death in top athletes: a basic cardiac electrophysiological point of view. Pflugers Arch. 2010;460:31–40.
42. Maron BJ. Hypertrophic cardiomyopathy: a systematic review. JAMA. 2002;287:1308–20.
43. Madias C, Maron BJ, Weinstock J, Estes 3rd NA, Link MS. Commotio cordis sudden cardiac death with chest wall impact. J Cardiovasc Electrophysiol. 2007;18:115–22.
44. Link MS, Maron BJ, Wang PJ, Pandian NG, VanderBrink BA, Estes 3rd NA. Reduced risk of sudden death from chest wall blows (commotio cordis) with safety baseballs. Pediatrics. 2002;109:873–7.
45. Link MS. Mechanically induced sudden death in chest wall impact (commotio cordis). Prog Biophys Mol Biol. 2003;82:175–86.

46. Garson Jr A, Fournier A. The long QT syndrome in children. An international study of 287 patients. Circulation. 1993;87:1866–72.
47. Bacaner M, Brietenbucher J, LaBree J. Prevention of ventricular fibrillation, acute myocardial infarction (myocardial necrosis), heart failure, and mortality by bretylium: is ischemic heart disease primarily adrenergic cardiovascular disease? Am J Ther. 2004;11:366–411.
48. Laitinen PJ, Brown KM, Piippo K, et al. Mutations of the cardiac ryanodine receptor (RyR2) gene in familial polymorphic ventricular tachycardia. Circulation. 2001;103:485–90.
49. Gussak I, Antzelevitch C, Bjerregaard P, Towbin JA, Chaitman BR. The Brugada syndrome: clinical, electrophysiologic and genetic aspects. J Am Coll Cardiol. 1999;33:5–15.
50. Chen Q, Kirsch GE, Zhang D, et al. Genetic basis and molecular mechanisms for idiopathic ventricular fibrillation. Nature. 1998;392:293–6.
51. Brugada P, Brugada R, Brugada J, Geelen P. Use of the prophylactic implantable cardioverter defibrillator for patients with normal hearts. Am J Cardiol. 1999;83:98D–100.
52. Frey N, Luedde M, Katus HA. Mechanisms of disease: hypertrophic cardiomyopathy. Nat Rev Cardiol. 2011;9(2):91–100.
53. Sasson Z, Rakowski H, Wigle ED. Hypertrophic cardiomyopathy. Cardiol Clin. 1988;6:233–88.
54. Wigle ED, Rakowski H, Kimball BP, Williams WG. Hypertrophic cardiomyopathy. Clinical spectrum and treatment. Circulation. 1995;92:1680–92.
55. Kazui T, Niinuma H, Yamasaki M, Abe K, Watanabe S, Kawazoe K. Septal myectomy and myotomy attenuate left ventricular hyper-contractility in a child with hypertrophic obstructive cardiomyopathy. Ann Thorac Cardiovasc Surg. 2011; [Epub ahead of print].
56. Goldhammer E, Sagiv M, Abinader G. Asymptomatic hypertrophic apical cardiomyopathy in a world-class athlete. J Cardiopulm Rehabil. 1987;7:303–6.
57. Schunkert H, Jackson B, Tang SS, Schoen FJ, Smits JFM, Apstein CS, Lorell BH. Distribution and functional significance of cardiac angiotensin converting enzyme in hypertrophied hearts. Circulation. 1993;87:1328–39.
58. Iwai N, Ohmichi N, Nakamura Y, Kinoshita M. DD genotype of the angiotensin-converting enzyme gene is a risk factor for left. Circulation. 1994;90:2622–8.
59. Rigat B, Hubert C, Alhenc-Gelas F, Cambien F, Corvol P, Soubrier F. An insertion/deletion polymorphism in the angiotensin I-converting enzyme gene accounting for half the variance of serum enzyme levels. J Clin Invest. 1990;86:1343–6.
60. Basso C, Maron BJ, Corrado D, Thiene G. Clinical profile of congenital coronary artery anomalies with origin from the wrong aortic sinus leading to sudden death in young competitive athletes. J Am Coll Cardiol. 2000;35:1493–501.
61. Pokorný J, Staněk V, Vrána M. Sudden cardiac death thirty years ago and at present. The role of autonomic disturbances in acute myocardial infarction revisited. Physiol Res. 2011;60:715–28.
62. McKenna WJ, Thiene G, Nava A, et al. On behalf of the task force of the working group myocardial and pericardial disease of the European society of cardiology and of the scientific council on cardiomyopathies of the international society and federation of cardiology. Diagnosis of arrhythmogenic right ventricular dysplasia/cardiomyopathy. Br Heart J. 1994;71:215–8.
63. Capulzini L, Brugada P, Brugada J, Brugada R. Arrhythmia and right heart disease: from genetic basis to clinical practice. Rev Esp Cardiol. 2010;63:963–83.
64. Thiene G, Basso C. Arrhythmogenic right ventricular cardiomyopathy: an update. Cardiovasc Pathol. 2001;10:109–17.

Cardiac Rehabilitation

10

Program's Aims

Physical activity is the cornerstone of a good *cardiac rehabilitation program*. Therefore, counseling patients to undertake physical activity to prevent chronic health conditions becomes a primary prevention modality. A structured or prescribed *aerobic program*, regularly followed, has been shown to reduce the incidence of coronary heart disease, increase the quality of living, and probably reduce the incidence of further *myocardial infarctions* in the postcoronary patient. New data suggest an increased life expectancy for those who exercise regularly. Ideally, a program to prevent cardiac heart disease should be started during childhood. Although cardiac rehabilitation/secondary prevention programs are recognized as integral to the comprehensive care of patients with cardiovascular disease [1], and as such are recommended as useful and effective (class I) by the American Heart Association and the American College of Cardiology in the treatment of patients with coronary artery disease and chronic heart failure [2], this chapter will focus on the physiological and *pathophysiological factors* responsible for the decline in *work capacity* and cardiovascular function. In addition, the effects of different modes of exercise as medical approach for cardiac rehabilitation are discussed.

Cardiac rehabilitation programs have been consistently shown to improve objective measures of exercise tolerance and psychosocial well-being without increasing the risk of significant complications. Traditionally, cardiac rehabilitation has been provided to somewhat lower-risk patients who could exercise without getting into trouble. However, surprisingly rapid evolution in the management of coronary artery disease also known as *atherosclerotic heart disease* has now changed the demographics of the patients who can be candidates for rehabilitation training. Coronary artery disease is almost always due to atheromatous narrowing and subsequent occlusion of the vessel. Early *atheroma* is present from young adulthood onward [3]. Lack of physical activity is among the risk factors that are considered to have adverse effects on the progression of *coronary atherosclerosis*. Numerous observational studies in both *men* and *women* have demonstrated that both *regular exercise* and *physical fitness* are associated with a reduced risk of coronary events and coronary death.

Cardiac rehabilitation phase II is designed primarily for patients with a diagnosis of coronary artery disease, open-heart surgery, recent myocardial infarction, angioplasty, stent, or stable angina. Based upon observations and the demonstrated benefit of risk factor reduction, cardiac rehabilitation programs have been developed to provide exercise training and counseling on risk factor modification for the secondary prevention of coronary heart disease [4]. This comprehensive program offers prescribed cardiovascular exercise, risk factor modification, education, ongoing nursing assessment and referral to nutritionist and behavioral intervention based on individual need. This multifaceted program is designed to limit the adverse physiological and

M.S. Sagiv, *Exercise Cardiopulmonary Function in Cardiac Patients*,
DOI 10.1007/978-1-4471-2888-5_10, © Springer-Verlag London 2012

psychological effects of cardiac illness, reduce risk of sudden cardiac death or reinfarction, control cardiac symptoms, stabilize the atherosclerotic process, and enhance the patient's psychosocial and vocational status. Cardiac rehabilitation includes provision of comprehensive long-term services involving the following core components: medical evaluation, *prescribed exercise*, and coronary risk factor reduction/secondary prevention [1].

Coronary artery disease is a chronic process that begins during adolescence and slowly progresses throughout life. Independent risk factors include a family history of premature coronary artery disease, cigarette smoking, diabetes mellitus, hypertension, hyperlipidemia, sedentary lifestyle, and obesity. These *risk factors* accelerate or modify a complex and chronic inflammatory process that ultimately manifests as fibrous atherosclerotic plaque. Prevention of coronary artery disease involves modifying atherosclerosis risk factors smoking cessation, weight loss, a healthful diet, regular exercise, modification of serum lipid levels, and control of hypertension and diabetes.

Although regular *physical activity* is beneficial for many clinical conditions, an acute bout of exercise might increase the risk of an adverse clinical event, such as *sudden cardiac death* or myocardial infarction, particularly in vulnerable individuals. The effects of exercise training on *morbidity* and *mortality* in patients after myocardial infarction were summarized in meta-analysis studies [5], concluding that regular physical exertion favorably influenced mortality but not reinfarction. Possibly even more important, increased occupational or recreational physical activity reduces the risk of cardiac death in individuals who have not yet shown manifestations of *coronary artery disease*, that is, primary prevention [6].

Since it is also known that the incidence of these events peaks in the morning and that some cardiac patients prefer to schedule leisure-time physical activity before lunch, the question arises as to whether *morning exercise* is essentially more risky than physical activity performed at other times of day. The observation that an increase in physical activity can alter *circadian pacemakers* in small mammals [7] raises the possibility that alternations in human metabolic rate could have effects on human circadian rhythms. Under these conditions, *circadian rhythms* may play a key role in changing cardiovascular variable values such as systolic and diastolic *blood pressures* which have been shown to be subject to wide fluctuations chiefly due to the *autonomic nervous system* rhythmic discharge, and thus to affect athleticism [8]. As physical exercise is recommended for both primary [9] and secondary [10] prevention of cardiovascular disease and since the exercise training workload for cardiac patients is determined from the *peak heart rate* achieved safely during a stress test, and because circadian rhythms may play a key role in changing physiological responses to the stress test, it is important to keep in mind these changes when prescribing training heart rate to coronary artery disease patients [8].

Cardiovascular disorders are the leading cause of mortality and morbidity in the industrialized countries. Following the industrialization physical inactivity rose in the general population; however, longevity also increased along with the rate of coronary heart disease. Although coronary artery disease is the most common cause of coronary heart disease, it is not the only one. Considerable data show that atherosclerosis and coronary artery disease are preventable diseases. The progression of coronary artery disease has objective reasons including genetics and parts are subjective such as behavioral. It is possible to influence the rate of *coronary stenosis* by modifying behavioral factors linked to cardiac risk factors: smoking, diet, physical inactivity, and sometimes by seeking help through medications. *Cardiac rehabilitation aims* to reverse limitations experienced by patients who have suffered the adverse pathophysiological consequences of cardiac events. While the symptoms and signs of coronary artery disease are noted in the advanced state of disease, most individuals with coronary artery disease show no evidence of disease for decades as the disease progresses before the first onset of symptoms, often as sudden myocardial infarction, finally arises. After decades of progression, some of these atheromatous plaques may rupture along with the activation of the blood clotting system and start limiting blood flow to the myocardium. The current data support the beneficial effects of cardiac rehabilitation and exercise training in the cardiac patients mainly coronary artery disease patients, including modest improvements in cardiac risk factors, and marked improvements in *exercise capacity*. In fact, cardiac patients had greater improvements than younger patients in both exercise capacity after cardiac rehabilitation. These indicate that coronary artery disease patients should be routinely referred to and vigorously encouraged to pursue formal outpatient cardiac rehabilitation and exercise training programs after major cardiac events [11].

Before any enrollment in a cardiac rehabilitation program, there is a need to evaluate individual's work capacity and to define the health status. These cannot be achieved under resting conditions or based on the individual's daily activity. Therefore, there is a need for an assessment of functional capacity, typically performed on a motorized treadmill or a stationary cycle ergometer.

All Causes Mortality

The importance of physical activity as a tool to reduce the risk of various chronic degenerative diseases has been conclusively established in recent years. The American Heart Association stated that regular aerobic exercise plays a primary role in prevention of cardiovascular disease [12]. However, Morris [13] noted as early as in the 1950s of the connection between a *sedentary lifestyle* and onset of coronary heart disease. While addressing two different occupation populations which differ mainly by their physical activity required at work, Morris and Heady [14] demonstrated that the active population, bus conductors and postal workers, had less incidence of coronary heart disease compared to the sedentary population, the bus drivers and civil servants.

In agreement with Morris and Heady's findings [14], two decades later, Paffenbarger et al. [15] illustrated the phenomenon in 22-year follow-up of 3,686 San Francisco longshoremen, a cohort analysis assessed job activity via energy expenditure and risk factors for heart disease mortality and morbidity. The risk factors included cigarette smoking, blood pressure, blood cholesterol level, obesity, and glucose metabolism in relation to fatal myocardial infarction. The study demonstrated an inverse relationship between *energy expenditure* and *fatal myocardial infarction*, which was most evident in the younger and middle-aged cohorts. Furthermore, the role of energy expenditure was still manifested when viewed against the influence of the other risk factors [15]. Along with the increased evidence associating lower level of physical activity with higher risk of death from heart disease, data from longitudinal studies [16] have emerged, indicating the influence of physical activity on longevity and mortality from other chronic diseases such as cancer, diabetes, hypertension, and osteoporosis.

Higher levels of fitness are associated with reduced risk of a wide variety of illnesses and chronic conditions. For cardiovascular disease and many metabolic conditions, the fitness-morbidity/mortality curve is not linear but curvilinear, with lower levels of fitness being associated with significantly higher levels of risk compared to moderate and high levels of fitness [17]. Physical fitness is composed of various components such as cardiovascular-respiratory fitness, body composition, flexibility muscular strength, and endurance. These variables and their adaptive response to regular physical activity result in an enhanced fitness level. Higher fitness achieved over 10 years of regular exercise training in older adults was associated with reduced development of *metabolic risk factors* for cardiovascular disease, fewer exercise-induced cardiac abnormalities, and reduced morbidity [18]. Thus, high level of physical activity, as measured via physical fitness level, may delay *all-cause mortality* primarily due to lowered rates of cardiovascular disease and cancer. Apor [19] has suggested that the qualities of fitness – aerobic capacity, maximal endurance performance or highly related physiological parameters, or physical activity improving fitness – show a tight, reverse correlation to the all-cause and to the cardiovascular mortality within. In most trained individuals, one-third of them expect a 30–40%

smaller chance for cardiovascular events, compared to the untrained subjects. Low fitness level is just as a threatening risk factor as the traditional ones; its detection calls out for simple interventions to improve fitness: proper physical exercise. However, fitness level alone is not the only indicator of future risk of coronary heart disease.

Fitness level is composed of both *genetic factors* and *environmental factors*. The association of sport and leisure physical activity with lower *adiposity* is due, in part, to a common genetic inheritance of both reduced adiposity and the predisposition to engage in more physical activity [20]. Being highly trained individual yet inactivity does not provide any protection against coronary artery disease. Furthermore, untrained individual however is an active men have a lower risk for coronary artery disease than untrained but sedentary men [20]. Hence, physical activity is the key for enhance health status, rather than the fitness level by itself. Particularly, the present status of physical activity should be considered the tool for primary prevention of chronic disease. Blair et al. [21] suggested that men who improved their physical fitness level category from sedentary to a good fitness level over a 5-year span had a 44% reduction in mortality risk. Previously, Paffenbarger et al. [22] demonstrated among Harvard alumni body of former students that a change in lifestyle through increased physical activity level resulted in a favorable effect on mortality rate; also, individuals who were sedentary as college students but adopted more active lifestyle had the same low risk as their classmates who had been vigorously active all along. On the other hand, former athletes who abandoned their sports activities had higher disease and death rates compared to their peers that continued to exercise. Consequently, only the current activity level is associated with the lower rate of death from coronary artery disease.

Physiology and Pathophysiology

In order to understand the use of physical activity as a medical tool for the treatment of coronary artery disease, there is a need to be aware of the

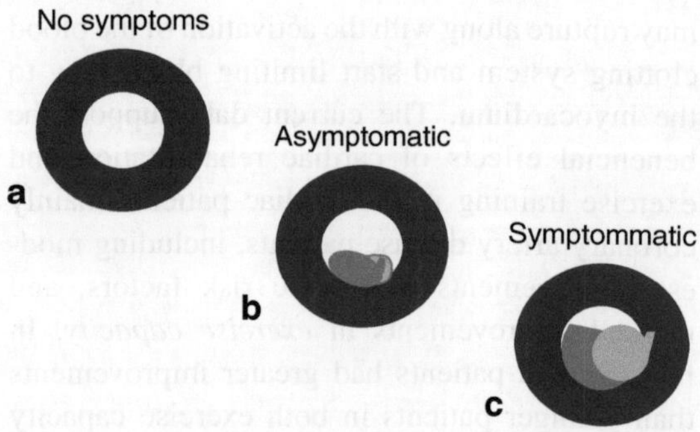

Fig. 10.1 (a) Normal artery, (b) LDL cholesterol accumulates in the arterial wall, the earliest stage of atherosclerosis plaque, and (c) the plaque continues to grow and forms a fibrous cap

linear relationship between the physiology of the coronary arteries and *coronary blood flow*. When *atherosclerosis* is present in the coronary arteries, it narrows the coronary arteries. Nearly three quarters of all cardiovascular disease deaths are caused by the buildup of fatty deposits on the arteries. Coronary atherosclerosis is often irregularly distributed in different vessels but typically occurs at points of turbulence. Inflammation is a key factor in the development of atherosclerosis. As lipids and cholesterol accumulate in the arterial wall, they undergo chemical changes and signal to *endothelial cells* to latch onto white blood cells circulating in the blood. These immune cells penetrate the intima and trigger an inflammatory response, devouring lipids to become fat-laden "foam cells" and from a fatty streak, the earliest stage of atherosclerosis plaque. The plaque continues to grow and forms a fibrous cap. Substance released by foam cells can eventually destabilize the cap, allowing it to rupture, causing a blood clot which can block blood flow and trigger a heart attack (Fig. 10.1).

Certain bacterial products influence *arterial endothelium* by augmenting the expression of adhesion molecules that promote the sticking of blood leukocytes to the inner surface of the arterial wall or risk factors such as diverse dyslipidemia, vasoconstrictor hormones along with hypertension [23]. Additionally, *coronary inflammation* also participates in the local, myocardial, and systemic complications of atherosclerosis.

Atherogenesis depends on mediators of coronary inflammation and immunity, including small molecules that include *lipid mediators* such as prostanoids and other derivatives of arachidonic acid, that is, the leukotrienes [23]. As the atheromatous plaque grows, the arterial lumen progressively narrows, resulting in ischemia often causing angina pectoris. The degree of *stenosis* required to produce ischemia varies with oxygen demand.

As the atheromatous plaque grows, the arterial lumen progressively narrows. When a plaque produces a >50% diameter stenosis, reduced *blood flow* through the coronary artery during exertion may lead to ischemia often causing angina pectoris.

Ischemia results from an imbalance between myocardial *oxygen demand* and *oxygen supply* [24]. The degree of stenosis required to produce ischemia varies with oxygen demand. A distinction should be made between myocardial ischemia and *myocardial infarction*. Ischemia means that the amount of blood supplied to the tissue is inadequate to supply the needs of the myocardium. When the myocardium becomes ischemic, it does not function optimally. The reduction in *coronary artery blood flow* may be symptomatic or asymptomatic, occur with exertion or at rest, and culminate in a myocardial infarction, depending on obstruction severity and the rapidity of development. When large areas of the myocardium become ischemic, there can be impairment in the relaxation and contraction of the *left ventricular*. If the blood flow to the tissue is improved, myocardial ischemia can be reversed. *Infarction* means that the tissue has undergone irreversible death due to lack of sufficient oxygen-rich blood.

A mature *plaque* is composed of two constituents, lipid which migrates into the intima and ingest lipids and *connective tissue matrix* forming a fibrous capsule around the lipid core. Ischemia is generally defined as oxygen deprivation due to reduced perfusion. ST-segment depression is regard as a common electrocardiographic sign of myocardial ischemia during exercise testing [25]. A considerable increase of aerobic glycolysis within the myocardium as a result of the imbalance between myocardial oxygen demand and oxygen supply is of special importance in this process. However, the exact relationship of the ischemic definition to *ST-segment depression* remains unclear.

The most widely accepted theory of atherosclerosis states that the process represents an attempt at healing in response to *endothelial injury*. Coronary artery disease is characterized by *atherosclerosis* in the epicardial coronary arteries. The first step in the atherosclerotic process is the development of fatty streaks, which contain atherogenic lipoproteins and macrophage foam cells. As the degree of coronary artery disease progresses, there may be near-complete obstruction of the lumen of the coronary artery, severely restricting the flow of oxygen-carrying blood to the myocardium. Individuals with this degree of coronary artery disease typically have suffered from one or more myocardial infarctions, and may have signs and symptoms of chronic coronary ischemia, including symptoms of angina at rest and flash pulmonary edema. An individual may develop a rupture of an atheromatous plaque at any stage of the spectrum of coronary artery disease. The acute rupture of a plaque may lead to an acute myocardial infarction.

Factors Determining Myocardial Oxygen Demand

When the myocardium oxygen demand is met, probably coronary artery stenosis is small, and so, coronary artery disease does not exist. Myocardial *oxygen supply* is a very important factor that by increasing its supply it may keep up with the new demand. On the other hand, any reduction in myocardium demand will alleviate the need to increase supply. Myocardial oxygen demand is influenced by the following factors which are the main determinants of myocardial oxygen demand: heart rate and ventricular wall tension. Ventricular wall stress is influenced by all of the following: increased pressure by increased contractility via increased afterload, increased radius via increased preload or ventricular filling, wall.

Each ventricular contraction consumes oxygen. Therefore, high *heart rates* result in a higher VO_2 and therefore increased oxygen demand. The concept of *wall tension* in the ventricle is important but sometimes difficult to conceptualize. Basic principles are as follows: *Wall tension* determines myocardial work, that is, increases in left ventricular work which results in increased VO_2. Wall tension is defined by the *Laplace's law* as (Eq. 9.1):

$$\text{Tension} = P \times R / h \qquad (10.1)$$

where P=pressure, R=radius, h=wall thickness.

In other words, ventricular wall stress is the product of the *left ventricular systolic pressure* and the radius of the left ventricle divided by its *wall thickness*. If there is high pressure inside a circle, it will be more difficult for the circle to contract. Therefore, more *force* will be required to develop within the wall of the circle. Increasing left ventricular *contractility* will increase *ventricular pressure*. Therefore, increased contractility will increase myocardial oxygen demand. *Afterload* will also increase the systolic ventricular pressure and thus increases wall tension [26]. Increased pressure in the ventricle will increase wall tension ending up with increased myocardial oxygen demand.

The total force generated by the contracting wall will be distributed across the width of the wall. The thinner the wall is, the greater the force is per unit of thickness. The thinner wall will experience more force and thus have higher tension. Hypertrophy therefore decreases wall tension. However, a thick-walled ventricle will also have more muscle mass and therefore consume more oxygen, so this factor encounters wall thickness as a factor for myocardial VO_2. As a wall sphere increases in size, the volume increases by the radius cubed (R^3), but the circumference increases linearly with the radius (R). Therefore, the volume grows much faster than the size of the small diameter. The bigger the circle is, the more work will be required to reduce it. Therefore, increasing the preload increases the *left ventricular end-diastolic volume*, and therefore increases wall tension. Thus, increased preload will augment wall tension again bringing to an increased *myocardial oxygen demand.*

Myocardial oxygen supply depends on the following factors: coronary anatomy, left main, left anterior descending (LAD), circumflex, right coronary, posterior descending, coronary dominance (right vs. left); supply to right ventricle, left ventricle anterior, left ventricle lateral, left ventricle posterior, left ventricle inferior; supply to AV node and SA node, the coronary perfusion gradient, the heart rate factor often overlooked, and oxygen carrying capacity of blood or the hemoglobin level. The coronary perfusion gradient is the pressure gradient in which the myocardium is perfused. In order to achieve forward blood flow, there is a need to set up a pressure gradient so that a high pressure from the aorta drains into a low pressure in the myocardium. Therefore, the perfusion gradient will be (Eq. 9.2):

$$\text{Perfusion gradient} = \text{Aortic pressure} - \text{Myocardium pressure}. \qquad (10.2)$$

Although the myocardium is perfused and not the left ventricle chamber, it cannot easily measure the pressure inside the myocardium. However, the myocardium pressure is very close to the left ventricle chamber pressure, so it is possible to measure the left ventricle chamber pressure with a catheter and use it as an estimate for the myocardial pressure. Thus, left ventricular ejects the blood into the aorta increasing aortic pressure. The aorta supplies blood to the myocardium via the epicardial coronary on to perforating coronary branches and finally to the myocardium. During systole, the coronary perfusion gradient is zero and there is no flow, therefore myocardial perfusion must occur *during diastole*. In normal individuals, when the left ventricular is *relaxed during diastole*, it has a pressure of about 10–12 mmHg. However, the aortic valve closes and the aorta maintains a pressure of about 80 mmHg which is the diastolic blood pressure against the left ventricular has to eject. So if the aortic *diastolic pressure* is 80 and the left ventricular diastolic ventricular diastolic pressure is 10, then the gradient is −70 mmHg, therefore no flow occurs. So the conclusion is that the myocardium is only perfused during diastole. Oxygen supply is determined also by *cardiac output* which is very tide to *heart rate*. Consequently, heart rate is a factor in determining oxygen demand and oxygen supply. In addition, when heart rate is low, there are larger intervals of time in between heartbeats lengthening *diastolic time*. In conclusion, low heart rates increase *myocardial perfusion* by increasing diastolic time.

The myocardium can have good flow rates of blood, but if the blood does not carry much oxygen, it means that to perfuse the myocardium with significant higher flow rate to get a normal amount of oxygen delivered. This depends on the hemoglobin levels in the blood. Usually coronary artery disease patients have normal levels of hemoglobin. A drop in hemoglobin level might be significant enough to cause the oxygen supply to be less than the myocardial oxygen demand, and ischemia could result.

Cardiovascular Benefits of Exercise

Regular aerobic physical activity increases exercise capacity and plays a role in both primary and secondary prevention of cardiovascular disease [27]. *Aerobic exercise training* prevents cardiovascular risks and promotes functional and structural adaptations that are associated with several cardiovascular benefits. Swimming training in rats increases *coronary blood flow*, number of cardiac capillaries, and adenine nucleotide hydrolysis. Increased adenosine production may be an important contributor to the enhanced coronary blood flow and *angiogenesis* that were observed in the exercise-trained rats; collectively, these results suggest improved myocardial perfusion [28]. Older coronary patients suffer from a low *functional capacity* and high rates of disability. Supervised exercise programs improve aerobic capacity in middle-aged coronary patients by improving both cardiac output and *peripheral extraction* of oxygen. Physiological adaptations to aerobic conditioning, however, have not been well studied in older coronary patients. Older coronary patients successfully improve peak aerobic capacity after 3 and 12 months of supervised aerobic conditioning compared with control subjects. The mechanism of the increase in peak aerobic capacity is associated almost exclusively with peripheral skeletal muscle adaptations, with no discernible improvements in *cardiac output* [29]. In addition, following exercise training, cardiac patients improve their decreased submaximal *rate-pressure product*, improve *blood pressure*, decrease risk of coronary artery disease, decrease *all-cause mortality* and morbidity, lower *heart rate* at a specific task, lower blood pressure at a specific task, lower rate and depth of breathing required, greater efficiency and less *perceived effort*, more appropriate peripheral blood distribution and return, enhanced blood volume and red blood cell mass, less tendency for hemoconcentration, stimulus for increased arterial size, and stimulus for collateral vessels to bypass obstruction. Physical training improves also *biochemical benefits*: reduction in low-density lipoprotein cholesterol, increase in high-density lipoprotein cholesterol, reduced total serum cholesterol, reduced serum triglycerides, increased electiveness of insulin, reduced platelet adhesiveness, increased fibrinolysis (early dissolution), decreased inappropriate catecholamine responses to stress, and decreased vulnerability or susceptibility to cardiac dysrhythmia.

Impact of Exercise on Functional Capacity

With the progression of the coronary artery disease and aging, *skeletal muscle mass* is lost. Consequently, the physical inactivity may result in a 25–30% decrement in skeletal muscle mass [30]. The decrease in muscle mass observed in the elderly and cardiac patients appears to be comparable to the *atrophy* associated with the decrease in physical activity. Reduced VO_{2max} seen in highly trained older *men* and *women* relative to their younger counterparts is due, in part, to a reduced aerobic capacity per kilogram of active muscle independent of age-associated changes in *body composition*, that is, replacement of muscle tissue by fat. Skeletal muscle adaptations to endurance training can be well maintained in older subjects and coronary artery disease patients; the reduced aerobic capacity per kilogram of muscle likely results from age-associated and health status reductions in maximal oxygen delivery mainly cardiac output and/or muscle blood flow [31]. Also, the loss of muscle mass through intrinsic changes such as decrease in muscle *fiber diameter*, decreased proportion of *fast twist fiber* and selective atrophy of fast twist fibers, and increased amount of connective tissue can explain the decrease in *muscle strength* [32]. It has been reported that maximal strength peaks at approximately 30 years of age, plateaus, and remains relatively stable for the next 20 years, with an age-related decline in strength becoming significant after the age of 50 years. Much of the research attributes this decrease in peak force to age-associated reductions in muscle mass, with a selective atrophy and reduction in fast twist fiber area and number being the primary factors. The influence that chronic endurance training has upon age-associated changes in muscular strength and muscle morphology has been largely undetermined. However, chronic endurance training can delay the age of significant decline in peak torque and changes in muscle morphology [32].

Evidence from the literature demonstrates that the muscle's ability to adapt to stressors does not diminish with *coronary artery disease* and aging. The management of the contractile machinery gathered inside *myofibers* is strictly linked to the activity of the myonuclei, mitochondria, and the system of *T tubules* and *sarcoplasmic reticulum* [33]. Alterations in cell energy metabolism occur in many pathophysiological of functional and structural diversity of mammalian skeletal muscles. Energy metabolism plays a critical role in muscle function [34], ATP production from oxidation phosphorylations of fat and glucose takes place in slow fibers which the myocardium is mainly composed of it, oxidative fibers and cardiac muscle oxidize fatty acids and lactate, while glycolytic fibers mainly use glucose as substrate [35]. In rats, the mitochondrial gene expression and enzyme activity for the oxidative capacity in myocardium are quite high compared to those in skeletal muscle; therefore, adaptation to the training in *myocardium* is attained by increasing the muscle mass, but not *mitochondrial gene expression* [36]. Under nonischemic conditions, almost all (>95%) of ATP formation in the myocardium comes from *oxidative phosphorylation* in the mitochondria. Aerobic exercise training enhances muscle mitochondrial transcription factors, mtDNA abundance, mitochondria-related *gene transcript* levels, and mitochondrial function, and this enhancement in *mitochondrial function* occurs in association with increased spontaneous physical activity [37]. In humans, *physical inactivity* results in decline of mitochondrial ATP production and *insulin resistance* [38], due to damage and decreased mtDNA abundance [39]. Aerobic exercise partially reverses the typical inactivity-associated decline in muscle function. Six-week-old rats subjected to a 12-week treadmill exercise training program have shown increased skeletal muscle *cytochrome c* in the mitochondrial oxidative capacity. Chronic aerobic exercise has been shown to stimulate *5′-AMP-activated protein kinase* (AMPK) activity with subsequent increases in fatty acid oxidation and glucose uptake in skeletal muscle. In addition, there is also evidence that chronic chemical activation of 5′-AMP-activated protein kinase increases mitochondrial enzyme activity in selected skeletal muscle, suggesting a possible role of AMPK in mitochondrial biogenesis. Cytochrome c is an essential component of the electron transport chain, where it carries one electron. Cytochrome c is capable of undergoing oxidation and reduction, but does not bind oxygen. It transfers electrons between complexes III (coenzyme Q–cytochrome c reductase) and IV (cytochrome c oxidase). In humans, cytochrome c is encoded by the CYCS gene [40]. In the well-perfused human heart, almost 90% of the *acetyl-CoA* comes from β-oxidation of fatty acids, and

10% comes from the oxidation of pyruvate [41] that is derived in approximately equal amounts from glycolysis and lactic acid oxidation. In the human myocardium and skeletal muscles, aerobic exercise increases acetyl-CoA formed from decarboxylation of pyruvate and from β-oxidation of fatty acids, accumulation of acetyl-CoA would result in inhibition of pyruvate dehydrogenase enzyme, accumulation of citrate would inhibit phosphofructokinase enzyme, and accumulation of glucose-6-phosphate would reduce hexokinase enzyme activity. Ultimately, this would inhibit *carbohydrate metabolism* with increasing availability and oxidation of *free fatty acids*. Under resting conditions, pyruvate dehydrogenase enzyme activity will be influenced by the availability of fat or carbohydrate fuels acting through changes in the intramuscular acetyl-CoA-to-CoA radical (CoASH) ratio. However, during exercise the activation of pyruvate dehydrogenase activity occur independent of changes in the acetyl-CoA-to-CoASH ratio, suggesting that other factors are more important. The exact mechanism behind the effects of exercise on increasing mitochondrial function, however, remains incompletely defined [42].

The improvement of *exercise capacity* due to exercise training in *cardiac disease patients* has been associated with *peripheral adaptation*, but the contribution of cardiac responses is less clear, although Smart et al. [43] suggested that change in VO_{2peak} following 16 weeks exercise training is related to myocardial function at baseline. Exercise is the most important physiological stimulus for increased *myocardial oxygen demand*. The requirement of exercising muscle for increased blood flow necessitates an increase in *cardiac output*. Previous investigations have suggested that the immediate beneficial effects of physical conditioning on symptoms related to chronic coronary artery disease could be explained by hemodynamic alterations which reduce myocardial pressure work. Following aerobic training attained a significant decrease in systemic vessel resistance and significant increases in VO_2 and cardiac output at peak exercise. Changes in reactive hyperemic calf blood flow were significantly correlated with the changes in cardiac output, systemic vascular resistance, and the kinetics of VO_2 during warm-up exercise. By improving the peripheral vasodilatory capacity in these patients, short-term, moderate-intensity physical training was found to improve the cardiovascular adaptation not only at peak exercise, but also during the onset of exercise [44].

Cardiac Biomarkers

Cardiac biomarkers are substances that are released into the blood when the heart is damaged. Measurements of these biomarkers are used to help diagnose, evaluate, and monitor patients with suspected acute coronary syndrome. The symptoms of acute coronary syndrome include chest pain, pressure, nausea, and/or shortness of breath. These symptoms are associated with heart attacks and angina, but they may also be seen with non-heart-related conditions. Increases in one or more cardiac biomarkers can identify patients with acute coronary syndrome, allowing rapid diagnosis and appropriate treatment of their condition. Acute coronary syndrome is caused by a sudden decrease in the amount of blood and oxygen reaching the heart. This decrease, also termed ischemia, is usually due to severe narrowing of the coronary arteries or a sudden blockage of blood flow through these arteries. A decrease in the supply of blood to the heart can cause angina (chest pain). When blood flow to the heart is blocked or significantly reduced, it can cause myocardial cells to die, triggering an acute myocardial infarction. This can lead to death of the affected heart muscle and to permanent damage and scarring of the heart.

Diseases of the heart such as *myocardial ischemia and reperfusion injury* remain the major cause of death in the industrialized world. The extent of ischemia-reperfusion injury is dependent on the interactions of several events, including energy depletion, metabolite accumulation, oxidant stress, and calcium overload. Myocardial ischemia-reperfusion injury is the major event contributing to the morbidity and mortality associated with coronary artery disease. Although several factors contribute to ischemia-reperfusion-mediated myocardial injury, compelling evidence indicates that generation of radicals and other reactive oxygen species are important mediators of this type of cardiac damage. Additionally, it is also related to some metabolic diseases such as *diabetes* and to some side effects of drug treatments. Therefore, developing a pragmatic countermeasure to reduce myocardial ischemia-reperfusion injury is vital. In this regard, an excess of evidence indicates that *regular exercise* has been confirmed as a pragmatic countermeasure to protect against cardiac injury; hence, it can protect the myocardium during an ischemia-reperfusion insult, that is, *cardioprotection* [45]. Lifelong physical activity and endurance exercise training have been proven to provide cardioprotection against cardiac insults in both young and old animals. In addition, long-term (months) endurance exercise training and not short-term exercise training provides cardioprotection against ischemia-reperfusion-induced injury. It is suggested that the beneficial effects resulting from increased *physical activity* efforts occur at different levels of cellular organization, being mitochondria preferential target organelles; however, the adaptations within the myocardium that provide the protection are still in doubt [46].

Proposed mechanisms to explain the cardioprotective effects of exercise are mediated, at least partially, by *redox changes* and include alterations in coronary circulation, expression of endoplasmic reticulum stress proteins, increased cyclooxygenase-2 activity, induction of myocardial *heat shock proteins 72* (HSP72), increase in cardiac antioxidant capacity, anatomical and physiological changes in the coronary arteries, changes in *nitric oxide* production, adaptation changes in *cardiac mitochondria*, increased *autophagy*, and/or elevation of ATP-sensitive potassium channels on both the sarcolemmal and the mitochondrial inner membranes [47, 48]. The exercise-induced cardioprotective phenotype is likely to include additional cytoprotective proteins beyond antioxidant enzymes or heat shock proteins [46].

Some redox-based mechanisms behind the cross-tolerance effects particularly induced by endurance training, against certain stressors responsible for the impairments in cardiac homeostasis caused by aging, diabetes, drug administration, or ischemia-reperfusion, are also outlined [49]. Moreover, it seems possible that other, yet to be defined, mechanisms of exercise-induced cardioprotection may also exist. Of the known putative cardioprotective mechanisms, current evidence suggests that elevated myocardial levels of antioxidants and increased expression of *sarcolemmal ATP-sensitive potassium channels* (K_{ATP}) are both contributors to exercise-induced cardioprotection against ischemia-reperfusion injury [48].

Exercise training has been shown to confer sustainable protection against myocardial infarction in animal models and has been associated with improved survival following a myocardial infarction in humans. It is still unclear how exercise training is able to protect the heart, but some studies have suggested that it increases a number of classical signaling molecules. For instance, exercise can increase components of the endogenous antioxidant defenses, that is, superoxide dismutase and catalase, increase the expression of heat shock proteins, activate ATP-sensitive potassium channels, and increase the expression and activity of endothelial nitric oxide synthase resulting in an increase in nitric oxide levels [50].

Data suggest that these positive modulator effects occur at different levels of cellular organization, being mitochondria fundamental organelles that are sensitive to disturbances imposed by exercise on basal homeostasis [49]. The most compelling evidence for exercise-induced cardioprotection is the fact that exercise training upregulates key antioxidant enzymes that have been shown to promote cardioprotection. Data suggest that exercise duration should last for 60 min and exercise intensity should be performed at about 75% VO_2max. Both duration and intensity are important factors in achieving a cardioprotective phenotype. Furthermore, exercise-induced cardioprotection against myocardial can persist for at least 9 days following the cessation of exercise training, but is lost 18 days after exercise [45].

Malfunction of the endoplasmic reticulum during an ischemia-reperfusion-induced injury event can lead to both mitochondrial-dependent and mitochondrial-independent cell death due to disruption of calcium homeostasis and/or impaired protein folding [47]. The mechanisms responsible for exercise-induced cardioprotection are not well understood. Emerging evidence indicates that a family of cardioprotective protein collectively called *endoplasmic reticulum stress proteins* contributes to ischemia-reperfusion-induced myocardial injury. During a cardiac ischemia-reperfusion insult, the endoplasmic reticulum helps cellular homeostasis by maintaining intracellular calcium regulation and protein folding. It follows that exercise-induced expression of endoplasmic reticulum stress proteins could serve as the mediators of exercise-induced cardioprotection against *ischemia-reperfusion-induced* injury [51].

Cyclooxygenase (COX) is an enzyme that is responsible for formation of important biological mediators called prostanoids, including prostaglandins, prostacyclin, and thromboxane. Currently three COX isoenzymes are known: COX-1, COX-2, and COX-3. Different tissues express varying levels of COX-1 and COX-2. Pharmacological inhibition of COX can provide relief from the symptoms of inflammation and pain. Cyclooxygenase (COX) is a key regulatory enzyme in eicosanoid metabolism, converting free arachidonic acid to prostaglandin H2 (PGH2), from which a number of prostanoids, including PGE2, PGI2, PGD2, and thromboxane, are produced [52]. The *prostanoids* are important mediators in the control of normal tissue homeostasis and regulate inflammation in response to trauma or infection [53]. Reduce COX-2 activity has proven beneficial in attenuating chronic inflammatory conditions. *Intense exercise* causes oxygen free radical generation and oxidative stress, which can lead to injuries and chronic fatigue as well as inflammation. A single bout of exercise induces COX-2 expression and DNA-binding activity of NF-kappaB in human peripheral blood mononuclear cells, and both COX-2 expression and DNA-binding activity of NF-kappaB were dependent on exercise intensity. Nuclear factor-kappaB (NF-kappaB) is a major transcription factor involved in regulation of COX-2 gene expression [54].

A class of functionally related proteins whose expression is increased when cells are exposed to elevated temperatures or other stress [55]. The dramatic upregulation of the *heat shock proteins* is a key part of the heat shock response and is induced primarily by heat shock factor. Heat shock proteins are quintessential intracellular proteins present in the cells of all living organisms, where their primary function is to interact with denatured and naïve proteins, preventing the aggregation of aberrantly folded proteins, and aiding naïve proteins in reaching their native state [56]. Data demonstrate that the human brain is able to release heat shock proteins 72 in vivo in response to a physical stressor such as exercise.

Intracellular and *extracellular heat shock proteins 72* have different functions. An intracellular heat shock protein 72 confers cellular protection from subsequent stressors, while an extracellular heat shock protein 72 has a whole-body systemic role in antigen presentation and immunity. An *acute exercise* bout stimulates an increase in both extracellular and *intracellular heat shock proteins 72*. Long-term training and improved fitness increases the rate of availability of intracellular heat shock proteins 72 in response to stress. Other factors that affect heat shock proteins 72 production include environmental factors, *exercise mode*, *duration* and *intensity*, age, estrogen, and antioxidant and glycogen availability. The functions and roles of heat shock proteins 72 also depend on the tissue of origin [57]. Production of high levels of heat shock proteins can also be triggered by exposure to different kinds of environmental stress conditions, such as infection, inflammation, exercise, exposure of the cell to toxins starvation and *hypoxia*. Consequently, the heat shock proteins are also referred to as stress proteins, and their upregulation is sometimes described more generally as part of the stress response. The heat shock response is a common cellular reaction to external stimuli such as *ischemia*, hypoxia, *acidosis*, oxidative stress, protein degradation, increased intracellular calcium, and energy depletion [47]. Therefore, heat shock protein 72 and heat shock protein 73 are suggested to play an important role in the cardioprotection against stress-induced functional damage.

Myocardial tolerance against ischemia-reperfusion-induced myocardial infarction is increased when myocardial heat shock protein 72 is accumulated after an exposure of normal animals to heat shock. However, the role of heat shock protein 72 and heat shock protein 73 in the failing heart following acute myocardial infarction remains unclear [57]. In transgenic mice that overexpress heat shock proteins 72 provide convincing evidence that heat shock proteins 72 imparts cardioprotection. Indeed, compared with wild type, these transgenic animals possess a cardioprotective phenotype as illustrated by improved postischemic contractile function and decreased infarction size [58]. Although heat shock proteins 72 has cardioprotective properties, results reveal that increased myocardial levels of heat shock proteins 72 above control are not essential for *exercise-induced protection* against ischemia-reperfusion-induced myocardial infarction and apoptosis. Therefore, other cytoprotective molecules are responsible for providing protection during ischemia-reperfusion [59].

Nitric oxide plays a fundamental role in protecting the heart against ischemia-reperfusion injury. The heart is able to produce and store nitric oxide as an important way exercise protects the myocardium from injury. *Nitric oxide*, a short-lived gas generated within the body, turns on chemical pathways that relax blood vessels to increase blood flow and activate survival pathways. Both the chemical nitrite and nitrosothiols, where nitric oxide is attached to proteins via sulfur, appear to act as convertible reservoirs for nitric oxide in situations where the body needs it, such as a lack of blood flow or oxygen. Increased production of nitric oxide by polymorphic variant eNOS alleles is an important trigger in the late phase of ischemia and exercise-induced preconditioning, and enhanced NO production by polymorphic variant eNOS alleles is mandatory in the mediation of the antistunning and anti-infarct actions of late preconditioning [60]. Exercise training is able to protect the heart, by increasing the expression and activity of endothelial nitric oxide synthase resulting in an increase in nitric oxide levels. Stable nitric oxide metabolite, nitrite, may play a major role in mediating these cardioprotective effects. Exercise training attenuates left ventricular dysfunction after myocardial infarction. This attenuation following exercise training is mediated by increased endothelial nitric oxide synthase activity. Suggested mechanisms of action for nitric oxide include inhibition of calcium influx into myocytes, antagonism of β-adrenergic stimulation, reduction in cardiac oxygen consumption, and actions on sarcolemmal ATP-sensitive potassium channels [47]. This protection is aminoguanidine sensitive, suggesting a role for nitric oxide in this exercise-induced delayed antiarrhythmic effect. Nitric oxide is both the trigger and the mediator of this delayed protection against ischemia- and reperfusion-induced arrhythmias [61]. The beneficial effects of exercise after MI on LV remodeling and dysfunction depend critically on endogenous polymorphic variant eNOS alleles. The observation that the lack of one eNOS allele is sufficient to negate all beneficial effects of exercise strongly suggests that exercise depends on full polymorphic variant eNOS alleles availability and activity.

Brain natriuretic peptide (BNP) is a 32 amino acid polypeptide secreted by the ventricles of the heart in response to excessive stretching of the myocardium cells (cardiomyocytes). Brain natriuretic peptide is named as such because it was originally identified in extracts of porcine brain, although in humans it is produced mainly in the cardiac ventricles. Brain natriuretic peptide is co-secreted along with a 76 amino acid N-terminal fragment (NT-proBNP) which is biologically inactive. Brain natriuretic peptide binds to and activates the atrial natriuretic factor receptor-A (NPRA), and to a lesser extent natriuretic factor receptors-B, in a fashion similar to atrial natriuretic peptide (ANP) but with tenfold lower affinity. The physiological actions of brain natriuretic peptide are similar to atrial natriuretic peptide and include decrease in systemic vascular resistance and central venous pressure as well as an increase in natriuresis. Thus, the net effect of brain natriuretic peptide and atrial natriuretic peptide is an increase in cardiac output and a decrease in blood volume. Brain-type natriuretic peptide belongs to cardiac-derived mediators; it reflects myocardial wall stress [62]. By affecting both blood volume and pressure, it plays a key role in cardiovascular homeostasis. Its measurement is used as a biological hormonal marker and independent predictor of cardiac survival in the diagnosis and prognosis of ischemic cardiac dysfunction and heart failure [63]. *Prolonged exercise* such as marathons can increase cardiac biomarkers such as troponin-T, *brain-type natriuretic peptide*, and ischemia-modified albumin. Brain natriuretic peptide levels are high in patients with cardiovascular disease. It has been shown that brain natriuretic peptide values after exercise are significantly elevated compared with resting values and that the brain natriuretic peptide levels both at rest and after exercise have a significant negative correlation with left ventricular ejection fraction [64]. If cardiac drift or myocardial injury after exhaustive exercise does occur, even at subclinical levels, plasma brain natriuretic peptide should increase after such exercise. Also, brain natriuretic peptide should more sensitively respond to cardiac dysfunction or myocardial cell necrosis than atrial natriuretic peptide. This hormone is composed of 28 amino acid residues and is released by muscle cells of upper chamber of heart when blood pressure rises to a high level. *Atrial natriuretic peptide* is a potent vasodilator and a protein: it regulates atrial blood pressure; it stimulates vasodilation, fluid egress, increased glomerular filtration, and salt and water excretion; and it blocks the release and/or actions of several hormones, including angiotensin II, aldosterone, and vasopressin. This can be misinterpreted by medical personnel as signs of myocardial ischemia or cardiac dysfunction. Although it is clear that exercise promotes a cardioprotective phenotype, a detailed understanding of the cellular mechanisms responsible for this cardioprotection remains incomplete. The plasma level of brain natriuretic peptide at rest in normal individuals is lower than that of atrial natriuretic peptide. On the other hand, plasma levels of atrial natriuretic peptide and brain natriuretic peptide markedly increase in patients with heart failure in proportion to its severity [64].

The *cytoprotective mechanisms* that have garnered most attention are inducible heat shock proteins and antioxidant enzymes, especially superoxide dismutase [58]. However, there are numerous clues suggesting that other mechanisms may also be part of exercise-induced cardioprotective phenotype, and they may have significant roles in the protective process. Improving our understanding of the molecular basis for exercise-induced cardioprotection will play an important role in developing optimal exercise interventions for primary and secondary prophylaxis.

Increasing evidence demonstrates that *atherosclerosis* is an immunologically mediated disease in which the secretion of atherogenic and atheroprotective cytokines, by infiltrating blood mononuclear cells, plays an important role. It is not known whether long-term exercise alters this atherogenic and atheroprotective activity directly [65]. Atherosclerosis is characterized by the accumulation of lipids and fibrous elements in the large arteries; lately, there has been much focus on the role of inflammation in the pathogenesis of atherosclerosis [66]. Inflammation is an important factor in the pathogenesis of atherosclerosis, and several markers of inflammation have been associated with an increased risk of cardiovascular events [67]. Furthermore, inflammation has been suggested to be a key factor in insulin resistance [68]. An association between low-grade systemic inflammation on one hand and the metabolic syndrome, type 2 diabetes, and atherosclerosis on the other hand [69] is reflected by increased *C-reactive protein* (CRP) concentrations and increased systemic levels of some cytokines [70].

C-reactive protein is a protein found in the blood in response to inflammation and is synthesized by the liver in response to factors released by fat cells (adipocytes). C-reactive protein levels rise dramatically during inflammatory processes occurring in the body. This increment is due to a rise in the plasma concentration of interleukin-6, which is produced predominantly by macrophages. C-reactive protein binds to phosphocholine on microbes. It is thought to assist in complement binding to foreign and damaged cells and enhances phagocytosis by macrophages. Interleukin-6 is a pleiotropic hormone that has both proinflammatory (cytokine) and anti-inflammatory actions. Interleukin-6 is synthesized and released from skeletal muscle in large amounts during exercise; interleukin-6 correlates temporally with increases in AMP-activated protein kinase activity in multiple tissues. Interleukin-6 increases AMP-activated protein kinase activity both in muscle and adipose tissue in vivo and in incubated muscles and cultured adipocytes. Interleukin-6 has a wide range of biological activities including immune regulation, hematopoiesis, inflammation, and oncogenesis. Numerous stimuli have been shown to activate AMPK including exercise, glucose deprivation, and hypoxia. Once it is activated, AMPK generates ATP by enhancing fatty acid oxidation.

Nonspecific markers of inflammation such as C-reactive protein are recognized as major risk factors for cardiovascular events. The acute phase reactant C-reactive protein is sensitive marker on inflammation. Elevated levels of C-reactive protein are independently associated with increased risk of cardiovascular disease mortality and morbidity as well as acute coronary events in both men and women [71]. Several roles have been postulated for C-reactive protein, including binding to phospholipids of damaged cells to activate complement and enhance uptake of these cells by macrophages, as well as activating endothelial cells to express adhesion molecules and decreasing the expression and bioavailability of endothelial nitric oxide synthase [72]. Many studies have demonstrated that elevated C-reactive protein levels have an increased risk of cardiovascular events. The JUPITER study showed that reducing C-reactive protein levels can mitigate this risk [73]. General population studies have reported an inverse association between serum C-reactive protein levels and physical fitness [74]. Studies suggested that regular physical exercise might lower C-reactive protein levels by an anti-inflammatory action [75].

High level of C-reactive protein increases the risk of thrombotic cardiovascular events. Data suggest that long-term exercise decreases the atherogenic activity of blood mononuclear cells in persons at risk of developing ischemic heart disease. This may be a mechanism whereby physical activity protects against ischemic heart disease [65].

Smith et al. [65] reported a trend for C-reactive protein reduction following 6 months of aerobic exercise training in individuals at high risk for ischemic heart disease, as well as a decrease production of proinflammatory, atherogenic cytokines interleukin-1β (IL-1β), tumor necrosis factor-α (TNF-α) and interferon γ (INF γ) and an increased production of anti-inflammatory, atheroprotective cytokine, interleukin-10. Physical activity induces also a subclinical inflammatory response, mediated in part by leukocytes, and manifested by elevated concentrations of circulating proinflammatory cytokines interleukin-6. However, the source of the cytokines that appears during exercise remains unknown.

Tumor necrosis factor-α is a cytokine involved in systemic inflammation and is a member of a group of cytokines that all stimulate the acute phase reaction; tumor necrosis factor-α is a pleiotropic proinflammatory cytokine and contributes to many kinds of cardiovascular diseases via its receptors (tumor necrosis factor-α R1/INF R2). Adipose tissue contributes to the production of tumor necrosis factor-α, which is reflected by elevated levels of soluble tumor necrosis factor-α receptors, interleukin-6 and interleukin-1 receptor antagonist, and C-reactive protein. Elevated tumor necrosis factor-α in the plasma and left atrial tissue had positive correlation with proximal left anterior descending artery in patients of chronic atrial fibrillation. Tumor necrosis factor-α might involve in the pathogenesis of chronic atrial fibrillation [76]. The primary role of tumor necrosis factor-α is in the regulation of immune cells. Tumor necrosis factor-α is also able to induce apoptotic cell death, to induce inflammation, and to inhibit tumorigenesis and viral replication [77]. Regular exercise induces suppression of tumor necrosis factor-α and thereby offers protection against tumor necrosis factor-α-induced insulin resistance.

Recently, *interleukin-6* was introduced as the first myokine, defined as a cytokine that is produced and released by contracting skeletal muscle fibers, exerting its effects in other organs of the body. This suggests that myokines may be involved in mediating the health-beneficial effects of exercise and that these in particular are involved in the protection against chronic diseases associated with low-grade inflammation such as diabetes and cardiovascular diseases [77]. High levels of interleukin-6 and tumor necrosis factor-α in patients with the metabolic syndrome are associated with truncal fat mass, and both tumor necrosis factor-α and interleukin-6 are produced in adipose tissue. Given the different biological profiles of *tumor necrosis factor-α* and interleukin-6 and given that tumor necrosis factor-α can trigger interleukin-6 release, one theory holds that it is *adipose tissue*-derived tumor necrosis factor-α that actually is the cause behind the metabolic syndrome and that locally produced tumor necrosis factor-α causes increased systemic levels of interleukin-6.

Cardiac biomarker tests are ordered to help detect the presence of acute coronary syndrome and to evaluate its severity as soon as possible so that appropriate therapy can be initiated. It is important to distinguish heart attack from angina, heart failure, or another condition because the treatments and monitoring requirements are different. For heart attacks, prompt medical intervention is crucial to minimize heart damage and future complications. Only a few cardiac biomarker tests are routinely used by physicians. The current biomarker test of choice for detecting heart damage is troponin; other cardiac biomarkers are less specific for the heart.

How Much Exercise Is Enough?

No reviews have quantified the specific amounts of physical activity required for lower risks of coronary heart disease when assessing the dose–response relation. Instead, previous reviews have used qualitative estimates such as *low physical activity*, *moderate efforts*, and *vigorous exercise*. Findings provide quantitative data supporting US physical activity guidelines that stipulate that some physical activity is better than none and additional benefits occur with more physical activity. Exercise training increases *cardiovascular functional capacity* and decreases *myocardial oxygen demand* at any level of physical activity in apparently healthy persons as well as in most subjects with cardiovascular disease. Regular physical activity is required to maintain these training effects. Since the early 1980s, ample amounts of data have been accumulated, indicating a definite distinction between the amounts of physical activity required for cardiovascular benefits versus the amount needed to evoke fitness benefits. Samitz et al. [78] demonstrated an inverse association between *energy expenditure* and reduction in *cardiovascular risk factors*. It is apparent that there is a minimum physical activity threshold which results in cardiovascular benefits.

Moderate-intensity activities of daily living were to a lesser extent beneficial in reducing mortality. Study by Tully et al. [79] on the effects of 30 min of self-paced, non-supervised, brisk walking, 5 days/week on the health and fitness of people aged 50–65 years provided evidence of benefit fitness and cardiovascular risk from exercising at a level below that currently recommended in healthy sedentary adults. Risk reduction per unit of time increase is largest for *vigorous exercise*. The dose–response relation between physical activity and all-cause mortality is not well defined at present. Higher levels of total and domain-specific physical activity are associated with reduced all-cause mortality [81]. Paffenbarger et al. [80] previously showed also an inverse association between energy expenditure and *all-cause death rate* in Harvard alumni. Men whose weekly energy output in various physical activities summed to 2,000 or more kcal per week had a 28% lower *all-cause mortality* rate compared to less active men. Furthermore, a trend was shown toward lower death rate as physical activity increased from less than 500–2,000 or more kcal per week. Thus, the total amount or volume of work performed is the key factor positively changing the risk profile for coronary heart disease and other chronic diseases. Studies have shown that a lower exercise intensity performed for longer duration is associated with increased health benefits, lower rates of orthopedic injuries, and higher adherence to training program [81].

Physical inactivity is a waste of human potential for health and well-being, and its high prevalence is a cause for concern. Its potential contribution to positive health, not merely the absence of disease but associated with a capacity to enjoy life and to withstand challenges [82], is considerable. The effective dose of exercise needed to elicit effects likely to be of clinical importance must be defined, and this information translated into practical advice readily understood by the population at risk [81]. Evaluating the relation between coronary heart disease and overall mortality in middle-age men and the amount of leisure-time physical activity reveals that habitual *moderate physical activity* has significantly inverse relation with acute coronary events [83]. Moreover, death rate following an acute cardiac event is significantly higher in the least active individuals. Yet, more *vigorous exercise* did not provide any additional protection from coronary heart disease than did moderate-intensity activities.

What Is Moderate Intensity?

The next obvious question to be asked is: How hard is moderate intensity? Intensity is the amount of physical power, expressed as a percentage of maximum work capacity. Moderate cardiovascular exercise comes in many forms. It is often difficult for the novice exerciser to determine how hard to train during exercise. There are several ways to measure exercise intensity. One common method measures the amount of oxygen consumed by the body as an activity is performed. This method is expressed in studies as the percentage of VO_2max. However, the VO_2 method is used most often in a research setting [84]. Morris [85] defines the following intensity levels adjusted to the average middle-age male and coronary artery disease patients weighing 70 kg by METs (metabolic equivalents):

1. Light = below 3 METs, equivalent to strolling, that is, less than 5 km · h^{-1}.
2. Moderate = 3–6 METs, walking 5–6.5 km · h^{-1}, a common average pace.
3. Vigorous = above 6 METS, walking more than 6.5 km · h^{-1}, a brisk fast pace.

The most common method used to express intensity relatively to one's capacity is by the rating of perceived exertion [86]. The method was developed by Borg and has 15-grade levels ranging from 6 to 20, with verbal description at every odd number (Table 10.1).

The American College of Sports Medicine [87] defines exercise intensity by percentage of maximum heart rate, rate of perceived exertion, and METs. Moderate activity has been defined as 55–69% of maximum heart rate. The American College of Sports Medicine defines hard exercise at 70–89% of maximal heart rate, and "very hard" at 90% and above, with 100% being maximal exertion.

The last measure METs refers to metabolic equivalents. One MET is equivalent to your resting metabolic rate, 2 METs is any activity that requires two times the metabolic rate, etc. This measure is determined by the amount of oxygen consumed, which indicates the level of intensity a person is working. At 1 MET, an average man would be consuming 3.5 $mLO_2 \cdot kg^{-1} \cdot min^{-1}$. Assigning a MET equivalent can give us an idea as to how intense an activity is (see Chap. 1). The American College of Sports Medicine rates moderate intensity using METs as decreasing with age (Table 10.2). For men, moderate intensity by age is:

Table 10.1 The Borg's rating of perceived exertion levels

Perceived exertion	Intensity level
6	No exertion at all
7	Extremely light
8	
9	Very light – easy, slowly walking
10	
11	Light
12	
13	Somewhat hard, feel tired
14	
15	Hard (heavy)
16	
17	Very hard, very strenuous, very fatigued
18	
19	Extremely hard, cannot last for long time
20	Maximal exertion

Table 10.2 Physical activity intensities (METs) decrease with aging

Age (years)	METs (moderate)	METs (hard)	METs (very hard)
20–39	4.8–7.1	7.2–10.1	>10.2
40–64	4.0–5.9	6.0–8.4	>8.5
65–70	3.2–4.7	4.8–6.7	>6.8
80 and over	2.0–2.9	3.0–4.25	>4.25

Table 10.3 Exercise intensities as related to METs

METs	Activity
1	Resting
3	Level walking at 4 km · h^{-1}
5	Walking at 4 km · h^{-1} and 5% elevation
5.5	Walking at 4 km · h^{-1} and 10% elevation
9.5	Jogging at 9 km · h^{-1}
12.5	Running 12 km · h^{-1}
15.3	Competitive runner (15 km · h^{-1})
20	Marathon runner (20 km · h^{-1})

For women, mean values are 1–2 METs lower than for men.

Table 10.3 shows some examples of how METs are associated with activity.

Along with the increasing scientific evidence illustrating the impact of an active lifestyle and its importance on one's health, the Center for Disease Control and Prevention and the American College of Sports Medicine published in 1998 a statement recommending the amounts and modes of exercise needed by adults for good health [87]. For the first time, short bouts of daily *moderate exercise intensity* lasting 30 min were recommended. The impact of such training for the same level of external work performed, can be demonstrated by a decrease in the product of heart rate · systolic arterial blood pressure an index of myocardial oxygen demand [88].

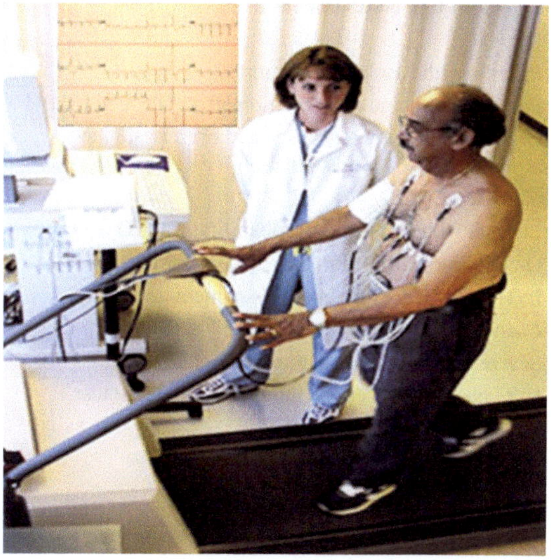

Fig. 10.2 Exercise tests serve as diagnostic tool for diagnose of coronary artery disease, evaluation of the training level, exercise control after cardiac rehabilitation intervention, blood pressure, and control evaluation of exercise-induced arrhythmias

Exercise Stress Test in Coronary Artery Disease

Exercise testing is a cardiovascular stress test using treadmill or bicycle exercise with electrocardiogram (ECG) and blood pressure monitoring [89]. *Exercise stress testing* is a well-established procedure that has been in widespread clinical use for decades, and, although it is generally a safe procedure, both myocardial infarction and death have been reported and can be expected to occur at a rate of 1 incident per 2,500 tests [12]. Cardiovascular *exercise stress testing* in conjunction with an electrocardiogram has been established as one of the focal points in the diagnosis and prognosis of cardiovascular disease, specifically *coronary artery disease*. Exercise stress testing (Fig. 10.2) is a cardiovascular stress test using treadmill or bicycle exercise with *electrocardiogram* and *blood pressure monitoring*, which has to evaluate the current status of coronary artery disease, screen for exercise-related cardiac dysrhythmias and to predict all-cause mortality. Table 10.4 lists the ACC/AHA guidelines [12] indications for exercise stress test. Class I indications are those for which there is evidence or agreement that the test is of value. Class IIa indications are

Table 10.4 Indications for exercise stress test

Class I
Adults with intermediate CAD risk and symptoms
Initial workup of suspected or known CAD
Known CAD with change in clinical status
Submaximal EST, 4–7 days post-MI followed by symptom-limited EST at 3–6 weeks
Symptom-limited EST at 14–21 days post-MI
Class IIa
Patients with vasospastic angina
For post-discharge rehabilitation after PTCA or CABG
Evaluation of known or suspected exercise-related arrhythmia, pre- or post-ablation
Class IIb
Patients with high or low probability of CAD
On digoxin with ≤1 mm ST-segment depression
LVH by EKG with ≤1 mm ST-segment depression
Class III
Severe comorbidity obviating revascularization
EKG changes preventing interpretation of the test

Table 10.5 Contraindications

Absolute
Acute MI within 2 days
Unstable angina not yet stabilized medically
Uncontrolled cardiac arrhythmias causing symptoms or hemodynamic compromise
Severe symptomatic aortic stenosis
Uncontrolled congestive heart failure
Acute pulmonary embolism or pulmonary infarction
Acute myocarditis or pericarditis
Acute aortic dissection
Relative
Left main coronary artery stenosis
Moderate stenotic valvular heart disease
Electrolyte abnormalities
Severe arterial hypertension
Tachyarrhythmia or bradyarrhythmia
Obstructive cardiomyopathy or outflow obstruction
Mental or physical inability to perform the test
High-degree A-V block

those in which evidence/opinion is generally favorable. Class IIb are indications less well established. Class III are indications for which there is evidence/agreement that the test is not useful and/or may be harmful. Table 10.5 lists contraindications.

Electrocardiogram is usually the first and most simple test used to look for any coronary artery disease signs unless the patient is actively having a *myocardial infarction* which is often seen as an electrical change in the heart rhythm as ST-segment elevation; the electrocardiogram may show electrical changes such as ST depressions or Q waves that suggest the patient has coronary artery disease or coronary artery disease with signs of a previous myocardial infarction [90].

Exercise stress testing is now widely available at a relatively low cost and is currently used most frequently to estimate prognosis and determine functional capacity, to assess the probability and extent of coronary disease, and to assess the effects of therapy. An *electrocardiogram* often encourages the physician to proceed with initial screening test(s). Ancillary techniques, such as metabolic gas analysis, *radionuclide imaging*, and *echocardiography*, can provide further information that may be needed in selected patients, such as those with moderate or prior risk. In many patients, the first symptom of coronary artery disease is myocardial infarction or *sudden cardiac death*, with no preceding chest pain as a warning. For this reason, there is a need to perform *screening tests* to detect signs of coronary artery disease before serious medical events occur so the tests are designed to detect plaque before a coronary artery becomes completely blocked. The American College of Sports Medicine recommends exercise stress testing for all sedentary or minimally active older adults who plan to begin exercising at a vigorous intensity. Most elderly patients, however, can safely begin a moderate aerobic and resistance training program without stress testing if they begin slowly and gradually increase their level of activity. However, a stage is reach where a performance of a stress test is needed. A community-based walking program in Massachusetts involving almost 8,000 elderly patients reported no incidence of myocardial infarction or other adverse cardiac events during exercise over an 8-year period. Patients should be counseled to discontinue exercise and seek medical advice if they experience major warning signs or symptoms, that is, chest pain, palpitations, or light-headedness. However, sometimes the ability of stress testing to predict coronary artery disease is limited in a heterogeneous population in which the prevalence of disease can be estimated through classification of chest pain and the sex of the patient.

Initial screening for coronary artery disease commonly involves stressing the heart under controlled conditions. These stress tests are able to detect the presence of flow-limiting blockages in the coronary arteries, generally in the range of at least a 50% reduction in the diameter of at least one of the three major coronary arteries. There are two basic types of stress tests: those that involve exercising the patient to stress the heart (physiological exercise stress tests); and those that involve *pharmacological stress testing* stimulating the heart directly to mimic the stress of exercise. Pharmacological stress testing, established after exercise testing, is a diagnostic procedure in which cardiovascular stress induced by pharmacological agents is demonstrated in patients with decreased functional capacity or in patients who cannot exercise. Exercise stress testing can also be used to determine a patient's fitness level, generally expressed as metabolic equivalents (METs), and to define an appropriate range of exercise intensity.

The long-standing use of exercise stress testing in the diagnostic and prognostic evaluation of patients with suspected or known coronary artery disease has provided a large body of data on the utility of functional capacity assessment in such populations. For this reason, screening tests are performed to detect signs of coronary artery disease before serious medical events occur. The reader is referred to the American College of Cardiology (ACC)/American Heart Association (AHA) guidelines for exercise stress testing regarding the appropriate use of testing in the diagnosis, prognosis, and treatment of patients with known or probable cardiovascular disease [12].

Exercise stress testing is currently used most frequently to *estimate prognosis* and determine *functional capacity*, to assess the probability and extent of coronary disease, and to assess the effects of therapy. An *electrocardiogram* is usually the first and most simple test used to look for any coronary artery disease signs [91].

Exercise Prescription in Coronary Heart Disease

Aerobic exercise such as walking, jogging, cycling, swimming, rowing, stair climbing, and *resistance training* such as hand weights, elastic bands, weight machines, and calisthenics are recommended for cardiac patients. The *duration session* recommended for *aerobic exercise* is at least 20–30 min preferably 45–60 min and for the *resistance training* 10–15 repetitions; 1–3 sets of 8–10 different exercises for both upper and lower body. *Frequency of training for* aerobic exercise is most days at least 5 days per week and preferably 6–7 walking days per week; for *resistance training*, the recommendation is 2–3 nonconsecutive sessions weekly. With regard to the *exercise training intensity* during aerobic exercise, the recommendation is 65–80% of VO_2peak or in any case above the anaerobic threshold, which usually corresponds with 60–70% of heart rate reserve when *maximal heart rate* is defined following exercise stress test. Thus, calculated training heart rate utilizing the Karvonen equation will be as follows (Eqs. 10.1 and 10.2):

$$\text{HRR} = \text{MHR attained} - \text{RHR} \qquad (10.3)$$

where HRR = heart rate reserve also can be maximal work capacity, MHR = maximal heart rate attained at peak stress test, and RHR = resting heart rate.

$$\text{THR} = \left[(\text{HRR}\cdot\%\ \text{intensity})/100\right] + \text{RHR} \qquad (10.4)$$

where THR = training heart rate, RHR = resting heart rate.

As an example, a patient had a resting heart rate of 60 beats · min^{-1} and attained a maximal heart rate of 155 beats · min^{-1} at peak stress test.

As a beginner, workload for this patient should be 65% of his/her maximal work capacity. Calculating maximal work capacity, that is, heart rate reserve, will be as follows (Eq. 10.3):

$$\mathrm{HRR} = 155\ \text{beats}\cdot\text{min}^{-1} - 60\ \text{beats}\cdot\text{min}^{-1} = 95\ \text{beats}\cdot\text{min}^{-1} \quad (10.5)$$

Calculating patients training heart rate will be as follows (Eq. 10.4):

$$\mathrm{THR} = [(95\ \text{beats}\cdot\text{min}^{-1}\cdot 65\%)/100] + 60\ \text{beats}\cdot\text{min}^{-1} = 117\ \text{beats}\cdot \quad (10.6)$$

Exercising at a heart rate of 117 beats · min^{-1} means that the patient's workload intensity is 65% of his/her maximal work capacity.

Cardiac Power Output, Cardiac Reserve, and Circulatory Power

Evidence is emerging that direct measurements of cardiac indices are more powerful predictors of prognosis in cardiac patients. Short- and long-term survival have been shown to be significantly lower in response to exercise in patients with reduced cardiac power output, contractile reserve [92], and circulatory power.

Tan [93] showed, for the first time, that in cardiac patients with severe acute heart failure, survival rate was distinctly worse in patients with lower cardiac power output. These observations have been confirmed in a subsequent study with patients diagnosed with cardiogenic shock [93]. Roul et al. [94] analyzed several invasive hemodynamic parameters at rest and during exercise in 50 patients with cardiac heart failure. They found that hemodynamic parameters at rest had no prognostic value, while cardiac power output of less than 2 W was more effective than any other index at identifying patients with short-term poor prognosis. Later, these findings were replicated by Williams et al. [95, 96] using noninvasive methods to evaluate cardiac function. In this study, the authors employed CO_2 re-breathing techniques for the noninvasive estimation of cardiac output, and derived cardiac power output by multiplying cardiac output and mean arterial blood pressure.

Submaximal exercise testing is routinely performed in patients before hospital discharge after acute myocardial infarction, before participating in cardiac rehabilitation program and for follow-up. Determination of functional capacity in coronary artery disease patients referred for *cardiac rehabilitation* is essential for developing an appropriate exercise prescription and in evaluating the results of training. Serial testing may be useful in revising the exercise prescription, evaluating improvement in aerobic capacity, and providing patient feedback. Meta-analyses of randomized cardiac rehabilitation trials have calculated a 20–25% reduction in cardiovascular deaths in patients enrolled in these exercise programs [97]. Screening tests are of particular importance for patients with risk factors for coronary artery disease. These risk factors include a family history of coronary artery disease at relatively young ages, an abnormal serum cholesterol profile, cigarette smoking, elevated blood pressure (hypertension), and diabetes mellitus. In this population, the MET level or exercise duration achieved is a powerful predictor of future adverse cardiac events; a commonly used marker for increased risk is the failure to achieve 5 METs during treadmill exercise. Initial screening for coronary artery disease commonly involves stressing the heart under controlled conditions. These stress tests are able to detect the presence of flow-limiting blockages in the coronary arteries, generally in the range of at least a 50% reduction in the diameter of at least one of the three major coronary arteries. In postinfarction studies, the highest mortality rate occurs in the subset that is unable to undergo exercise testing [98].

In the Research on Instability in Coronary Artery Disease study, the major predictors of 1-year infarction-free survival in 740 men with unstable angina or non-Q-wave myocardial infarction who underwent predischarge cycle ergometer exercise testing were the number of leads with ischemic ST-segment depression and peak workload (>5 METs) attained [99].

Cardiopulmonary and Ventilator Markers

Cardiopulmonary exercise testing (*CPET*) has become an integral part of the cardiovascular investigation of populations with a variety of conditions, including those with congenital heart defects. Cardiopulmonary exercise testing has been extensively used in cardiology to objectively measure exercise capacity, to assess the results of medical or surgical interventions, and to predict prognosis. Risk stratification is important in the assessment of cardiac patients enrolled in physical activity to ensure that these patients receive the appropriate levels of surveillance and exercise intensity. Risk levels, an estimate of the likelihood of future cardiac events, are indicated as low, moderate, or high. Poor left ventricular function is the most important risk factor for death [100]. The gold standard for assessing left ventricular function is echocardiography, but this is often not available to cardiac rehabilitation coordinators. The additional information provided by ventilator markers might be helpful.

The need to accurately estimate the prognosis of cardiovascular disease patients has led to the identification of several cardiac and respiratory physiological prognostic markers [96], purported to represent the stage of the disease. Nevertheless, invasive evaluations are not promptly available in routine clinical settings. So, efforts should be focused in determining if physiological markers can serve effectively as invasive methods in predicting prognosis in patients with cardiovascular disease.

Because most daily activities do not require maximal effort, a widely used submaximal index of aerobic capacity is the anaerobic threshold, defined by the exercise level at which ventilation begins to increase exponentially for a given increment in oxygen uptake. This increase in ventilation is necessitated to eliminate the excess CO_2 produced in response to a sustained rise in blood lactate. Although the anaerobic threshold usually occurs at 47–64% of VO_2max in healthy untrained subjects [111], it generally occurs at a higher percentage of VO_2max in endurance-trained individuals [120]. Several methods have been proposed for determining anaerobic threshold; however, no universal agreement exists regarding which is best.

The Minute Ventilation to Carbon Dioxide Ratio (V_E/VCO_2)

The rise in minute ventilation and carbon dioxide or the ventilatory equivalent for carbon dioxide with aerobic exercise is tightly coupled as increasing carbon dioxide levels as a consequence of increased metabolism and, at higher exercise intensities, lactic acid buffering drive the ventilatory response. This relationship is most commonly expressed as the minute ventilation/carbon dioxide slope, although the ratio between minute ventilation and carbon dioxide at maximal exercise has also been shown to provide prognostic value [101]. The three most common definitions of anaerobic threshold are these: (a) the point at which a systematic increase in the ventilatory equivalent for oxygen (V_E/VO_2) occurs without an increase in the ventilatory equivalent for carbon dioxide (V_E/VCO_2); (b) the point at which a systematic rise in end-tidal oxygen pressure ($PETO_2$) occurs without a decrease in the end-tidal carbon dioxide pressure ($PETCO_2$); and (c) the departure of carbon dioxide from a line of identity drawn through a plot of carbon dioxide versus oxygen uptake oxygen uptake. The minute ventilation/carbon dioxide slope is a better determinant than minute ventilation/oxygen uptake and $PETCO_2$, in defining the anaerobic threshold and to identify abnormalities.

The minute ventilation/carbon dioxide slope, obtained during exercise testing, possesses prognostic value in cardiovascular disease. The minute ventilation/carbon dioxide slope relationship is generally linear, thereby hypothetically producing similar slope values regardless of the exercise-test time interval used for calculation. The departure of carbon dioxide from a line of identity drawn through a plot of carbon dioxide versus oxygen uptake, often called the V-slope method [102]. Peak exercise oxygen uptake is a widely used prognosticator. Of the many variables currently the focus of active research and currently included in the standard cardiopulmonary exercise testing report, *ventilatory efficiency* (V_E/VCO_2 slope) has gained attention because of its ability to identify abnormalities in the interaction between the lungs and the circulation and also because of its role as a prognostic marker in different cardiovascular conditions affecting the adult as well as the child. Because the relationship between minute ventilation and carbon dioxide is so stable and predictable in normal people, particularly in the range of work intensities between the anaerobic threshold and the ventilatory compensation point, it is being used with increasing frequency as evidence for an inappropriately high ventilatory response due to ventilation-perfusion unevenness. However, this relationship between minute ventilation and carbon dioxide is being calculated in many different ways, sometimes without a physiological rationale [103].

Increased ventilatory drive, reflected by the slope of increase of ventilation relative to carbon dioxide production (V_E/VCO_2 slope), has been shown to have a high prognostic value in patients with cardiovascular diseases. However, there is no consensus on how to calculate it, as the relation between ventilation and carbon dioxide production becomes nonlinear near the end of exercise, when ventilation is driven both by carbon dioxide output and by decrease in plasma pH, and thus influence the results. Maximal exercise testing, whether involving cycling or walking-based protocols, is often not well tolerated in patients with cardiovascular disease. The peak oxygen uptake and the slope of the relation between ventilation and carbon dioxide production are independent predictors of outcome and help risk stratification.

Novel spirometric parameters, less affected by submaximal performance, such as the rate of increase of *minute ventilation* per unit decrease of carbon dioxide production (V_E/VCO_2 slope) and the oxygen uptake efficiency slope have recently been introduce. It is difficult to perform a maximal exercise tolerance test on patients with cardiovascular disease to evaluate their exercise capacity. However, it is possible to assess exercise capacity by the *slope* of the linear regression line between *carbon dioxide productions over minute ventilation* (V_E/VCO_2) at lower exercise level. The slope of this relationship is typically between ratio cutoff point of 20 and 30 in normal subjects, though values above 30 are commonly observed in patients with mild-to-moderate coronary artery disease and heart failure [104]. Several studies have demonstrated that V_E/VCO_2 *slope* is a strong and independent predictor of survival. However, the ratio cutoff points that distinguish survivors from non-survivors vary substantially among studies; Corra et al. [105] found a ratio cutoff point of 35, while other studies [101] found ratio cutoff points from 34 to 44.7. The widely discrepant ratio cutoff points probably are due to study cohorts who differ in their heart failure severity. In addition, it remains unsettled if V_E/VCO_2 slope is more accurate in the prognostic evaluation of cardiovascular disease patients than other cardiopulmonary markers.

The prognostic power of V_E/VCO_2 *slope* was higher than *peak oxygen uptake* in a number of studies [101, 105], but similar [106] and lower in others. These differences may lie in the V_E/VCO_2 slope shape due to the disease severity. Corra et al. [105], for instance, noticed that patients with a V_E/VCO_2 slope ≥35 have increased mortality but slightly lower than patients with a peak oxygen uptake ≤10 mLO_2. kg^{-1}. min^{-1}. Also in another study [107], patients with an abnormally high V_E/VCO_2 slope and high peak oxygen uptake had similar survival rate as patients with low V_E/VCO_2 slope. Therefore, it seems that V_E/VCO_2 is a better predictor than the peak oxygen uptake. However, it is also important to point out that several studies were retrospective and the prognostic value of peak oxygen uptake might have been underestimated; patients with poorer exercise capacity are generally considered for heart transplantation, which may attenuate the relationship between peak oxygen uptake and mortality. It is not clear how V_E/VCO_2 slope relates with mortality and the reasons why it may be prognostically superior to peak oxygen uptake. In contrast to oxygen uptake, linked to cardiac function by the Fick equation, the connection of V_E/VCO_2 slope to cardiac function and prognosis is less straightforward.

The prognostic usefulness of submaximal exercise testing is not clear. The V_E/VCO_2 slope should be calculated from all data points to optimize prognostic sensitivity. Data acquired from the first 50% of exercise and below the ventilatory compensation point provide adequate prognostic surrogates in patients who may not be able to perform efforts at respiratory exchange ratio <1.10 [108]. Therefore, V_E/VCO_2 slope should be computed from all the data points to have its highest prognostic value.

Patients with heart failure exhibit an increased ventilator response to exercise; their slope of the overall ventilation/carbon dioxide production ratio is elevated. This elevation is related to impaired exercise performance and is commonly explained by an increased ventilation/perfusion mismatch. In addition, in patients with heart failure, ventilation during exercise is not only influenced by an increased ventilation-perfusion mismatch but is in part mediated by the responsiveness of the respiratory center, explained by an increase in pulmonary dead space [109]. The increased pulmonary dead space is attributed to a ventilation-perfusion mismatch [110] and rapid shallow breathing due to decreased lung compliance and activation of pulmonary J-receptors [109].

Pulmonary Ventilation-Perfusion Mismatch: During Exercise

Augmentation in *alveolar ventilation* is very important for the diffusion of oxygen from the lung to the blood capillaries while at the same time blood flow to the capillaries is enlarged. Thus, the ratio of *alveolar ventilation* (V_A) over *cardiac output* (Q) or *ventilation/perfusion ratio* (V_A/Q) is increased. At rest, the *dead space/tidal volume ratio* (V_D/V_T) is normally about one-third of the tidal volume. During exercise, in normal subjects, it declines to about one-fifth, the major decrement occurring at the lowest work rates. The dead space/tidal volume ratio is higher when

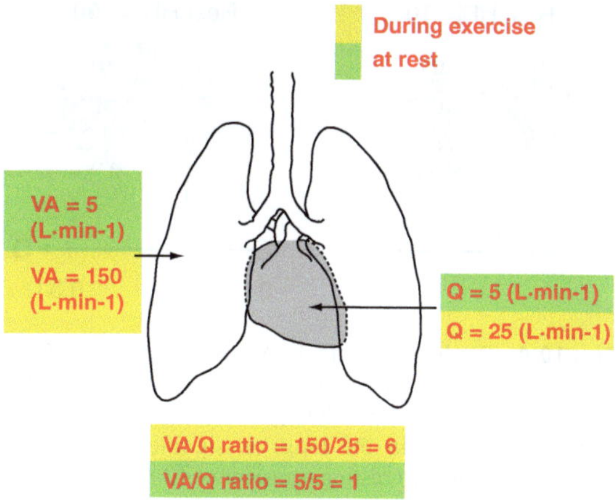

Fig. 10.3 Ventilation/perfusion is a ratio of air volume that reaches the alveoli (V_A) to the blood amount reaching (Q) the alveoli. The ventilation/perfusion ratio during exercise changes from resting ratio of 1 (*green*), a ratio that is increased by sixfold (*yellow*)

alveolar ventilation relative to perfusion is nonuniform. When dead space/tidal volume ratio is increased, minute ventilation is typically inordinately high for the work rate performed. A high minute ventilation at a given exercise carbon dioxide (high V_E/VCO_2) is indicative of either high *dead space/tidal volume ratio* or acute or chronic *hyperventilation* [111].

At rest, *alveolar ventilation* corresponds to 5 L · min^{-1}, and *cardiac output* also equals approximately 5 L · min^{-1}; therefore, the ratio at rest is 1. The increased ventilation/perfusion ratio at maximal oxygen uptake increases alveolar oxygen partial pressure which, in turn, facilitates diffusion capacity in the face of the reduced *red blood cell transit time* in the lung (Fig. 10.3).

This transit time reduction is due to a significant increase in heart rate. *Heavy exercise*, however, may lower the percentage of arterial oxygen bound to hemoglobin saturation by greater than or equal to 5% below resting values in some highly trained endurance athletes [112]. Despite that, none of the athletes showed signs of cyanosis [113]. This reduction of 5% in the arterial *hemoglobin saturation* may be due to the fast velocity of the red blood cells within the pulmonary capillary at high work rates. At rest, as heart rate averages 70 beats · min^{-1}, the red blood cell's transit time in the lung is 0.8 s. During exercise,

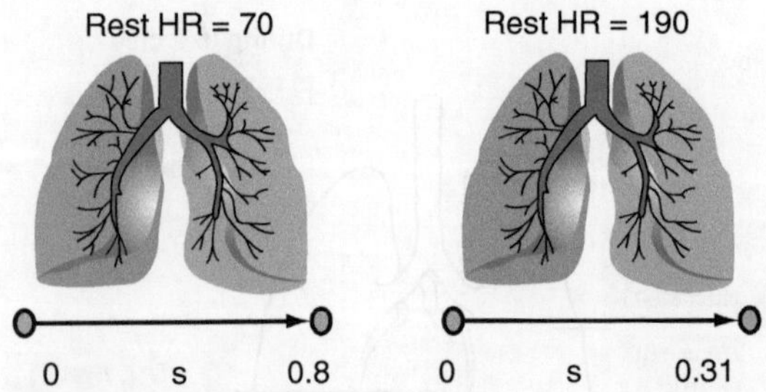

Fig. 10.4 The lung as a clock. At rest, heart rate (*HR*) is 70 beats · min^{-1}, and during exercise, it is increased to 190 beats · min^{-1}. Therefore, during exercise, the red blood cell's transit time in the lungs is significantly shorter (0.31 s) compared to resting transit time (0.8 s)

if heart rate is 190 beats · min^{-1}, transit time in the lung will be 0.31 s. Since it takes 0.25 s for the red blood cell to bond oxygen, it means that during rest, there is enough time for the red blood cell to be oxygenated, while during exercise, there is only one chance for the red blood cell to be oxygenated (Fig. 10.4).

This in turn may create incomplete *ventilation/perfusion ratio* for gas exchange [113]. Gas exchange in the lungs is most efficient when there is a good match between ventilation and perfusion; an imbalance can cause anoxia and cyanosis.

Ventilation/perfusion ratio inequality is the most common clinical cause of arterial hypoxemia. In respiratory physiology, the ventilation/perfusion ratio is a measurement used to assess the efficiency and adequacy of the matching of two variables: It is defined as the ratio of the amount of air reaching the alveoli to the amount of blood reaching the alveoli. Although the ratio *ventilation/perfusion* is higher in elite athletes and even though that they have significantly higher maximal cardiac output than untrained [114], still they are more likely to undergo arterial oxygen desaturation during maximal endurance effort compared to normal subjects [112].

This is due to decreased transit time of the red blood cell in the lung capillaries. Therefore, there is not time enough to saturate the red blood cell with oxygen before it exits the pulmonary capillary [115].

Evidence suggests that increased pulmonary ventilation-perfusion (V_A/Q) mismatch and abnormal control of ventilation are the primary mechanisms for the increased *ventilation* response to exercise in patients with heart failure. The increased ventilation during exercise, which must be related to *exertional dyspnea*, in patients with cardiovascular disease is primarily the consequence of a stimulus to regulate arterial pH [116]. Because blood gases, lung volumes, and respiratory rates are relatively normal in patients with cardiovascular disease, a reduced lung perfusion, as a result of cardiac dysfunction, is the primary mechanism for the pulmonary V_A/Q mismatch during exercise. In addition, hyperventilation response to exercise has been related to abnormal ventilatory control, as indicated by increased chemoreflex activity, and reflects therefore increased sympathetic activity [104]. Thus, data suggest that decreased ventilatory efficiency reflects the severity of the cardiovascular and is related with outcome. However, V_A/Q ratio is increased in cardiovascular disease during exercise compared to resting values although to the lesser extent than normal subjects. This increase in the V_A/Q ratio in cardiovascular helps to oxygenate the blood in the lungs in the face of the increased cardiac output and the short transit time that the red blood cells have to be oxygenated. Thus, reduced V_A/Q ratio is a strong physiological marker for the severity of cardiovascular.

Estimating Stroke Volume

Oxygen pulse is calculated as oxygen uptake divided by heart rate; it is a cardiopulmonary variable which may be used to estimate stroke volume at rest and during aerobic exercise [117]. The exercise stroke volume is one of the most important indices of both the functional state of the heart and the propensity for achieving a high level of physical activity. Consequently, several noninvasive estimators have been developed that obviate the requirements for intravascular catheterization or noninvasive methods such as echo-Doppler which is not commonly available to most laboratories. On the other hand, temporarily disrupt the determination of other ventilatory and gas-exchange variables may allow the stroke volume profile to be estimated. In healthy subjects, the stroke volume estimation relies on the Fick equation where the relationship between heart rate and oxygen uptake is linear.

Cohen-Solal et al. [118] suggested the product of *peak oxygen uptake* and *peak systolic blood pressure*. The circulatory power surpassed peak oxygen uptake by identifying those with particularly poor prognosis, that is, reduced peak oxygen uptake and reduced systolic blood pressure response. However, circulatory power outperforms peak oxygen uptake and V_E/VCO_2 *slope* in the prognosis of patients with cardiovascular disease receiving β-blockers therapy [119]. It should be noted, however, that circulatory power is only an approximation to direct measures of cardiac function. Therefore, researchers have recommended caution in the acceptance of circulatory power when more critical clinical decisions are to be made.

References

1. Wenger NK. Current status of cardiac rehabilitation. J Am Coll Cardiol. 2008;51:1619–31.
2. Balady GJ, Williams MA, Ades PA, et al. Core components of cardiac rehabilitation/secondary prevention programs: 2007 update: a scientific statement from the American Heart Association Exercise, Cardiac Rehabilitation, and Prevention Committee, the Council on Clinical Cardiology; the Councils on Cardiovascular Nursing, Epidemiology and Prevention, and Nutrition, Physical Activity, and Metabolism; and the American Association of Cardiovascular and Pulmonary Rehabilitation. Circulation. 2007;115:2675–82.
3. Grech ED. Pathophysiology and investigation of coronary artery disease. BMJ. 2003;326:1027–30.
4. Ades PA. Cardiac rehabilitation and secondary prevention of coronary heart disease. N Engl J Med. 2001; 345:892–902.
5. Oldridge N, Guyatt G, Fischer M, Rimm AA. Cardiac rehabilitation after myocardial infarction. Combined experience of randomized clinical trials. JAMA. 1998;260:945–50.
6. Atkinson G, Drust B, George K, Reilly T, Waterhouse J. Chronobiological considerations for exercise and heart disease. Sports Med. 2006;36:487–500.
7. Loudon AS, Meng QJ, Maywood ES, Bechtold DA, Boot-Handford RP, Hastings MH. The biology of the circadian Ck1epsilon tau mutation in mice and Syrian hamsters: a tale of two species. Cold Spring Harb Symp Quant Biol. 2007;72:261–71.
8. Sagiv M, Sagiv A, Soudry M, Ben-Sira D, Ben-Gal S, Rudoy J. Influence of the time of day on physical performance in patients with coronary artery disease. Eur J Appl Physiol Occup Physiol. 1995;71:530–4.
9. Grundy SM, Balady GJ, Criqui MH. Primary prevention of coronary heart disease: guidance from Framingham: a statement for healthcare professionals from the AHA task force on risk reduction. Circulation. 1998;97:1876–87.
10. Shephard RJ, Balady GJ. Exercise as cardiovascular therapy. Circulation. 1999;99:963–72.
11. Lavie LJ, Milani RV. Effects of cardiac rehabilitation programs on exercise capacity, coronary risk factors, behavioral characteristics, and quality of life in a large elderly cohort. Am J Cardiol. 1995;76:177–9.
12. Gibbons R, Balady G, Timothybricker J, et al. ACC/AHA 2002 guideline update for exercise testing: summary article. A report of the American College of Cardiology/American Heart Association Task Force on Practice Guidelines. J Am Coll Cardiol. 2002;40: 1531–40.
13. Norris JN, Heady JA, Raffle PA, Roberts CG, Parks JW. Coronary heart disease and physical activity of work. Lancet. 1953;265:1053–7.
14. Norris JN, Heady JA, Raffle PA, Roberts CG, Parks JW. Coronary heart disease and physical activity of work. Lancet. 1953;265:1111–20.
15. Paffenbarger Jr RS, Hale WE, Brand RJ, Hyde RT. Work-energy level, personal characteristics, and fatal heart attack: a birth-cohort effect. Am J Epidemiol. 1977;105:200–13.
16. Powell KE, Blair SN. The public health burdens of sedentary living habits: theoretical but realistic estimates. Med Sci Sports Exerc. 1994;26:851–6.
17. Church T. The low-fitness phenotype as a risk factor: more than just being sedentary? Obesity (Silver Spring). 2009;17 Suppl 3:S39–42.
18. Petrella RJ, Lattanzio CN, Demeray A, Varallo V, Blore R. Can adoption of regular exercise later in life prevent metabolic risk for cardiovascular disease? Diabetes Care. 2005;28:694–701.
19. Apor P. Measure of fitness and physical activity related to cardiovascular diseases and death (Article in Hungarian). Orv Hetil. 2011;152:107–13.
20. Choh AC, Demerath EW, Lee M, et al. Genetic analysis of self-reported physical activity and adiposity: the Southwest Ohio Family Study. Public Health Nutr. 2009;12:1052–60.
21. Blair SN, Kohl 3rd HW, Barlow CE, Paffenbarger Jr RS, Gibbons LW, Macera CA. Changes in physical fitness and all-cause mortality. A prospective study of healthy and unhealthy men. JAMA. 1995;273: 1093–8.
22. Paffenbarger Jr RS, Hyde RT, Wing AL, Lee IM, Jung DL, Kampert JB. The association of changes in physical-activity level and other lifestyle characteristics with mortality among men. N Engl J Med. 1993;328: 538–45.
23. Libby P, Theroux P. Pathophysiology of coronary artery disease. Circulation. 2005;111:3481–8.

24. Kones R. Recent advances in the management of chronic stable angina I: approach to the patient, diagnosis, pathophysiology, risk stratification, and gender disparities. Vasc Health Risk Manag. 2010;6:635–56.
25. Watanabe T, Akutsu Y, Yamanaka H, Michihata T, Okazaki O, Katagiri T, Harumi K. Exercise-induced ST-segment depression: imbalance between myocardial oxygen demand and myocardial blood flow. Acta Cardiol. 2000;55:25–31.
26. Nakamura Y, Iwanaga S, Uno K. Increased protection of the ischemic myocardium by decreased aortic pressure. Jpn Heart J. 1995;36:689–97.
27. Chandrasheckhar Y, Anand IS. Exercise as a coronary protective factor. Am Heart J. 1991;122:1723–39.
28. Roque FR, Soci UP, Angelis KD, et al. Moderate exercise training promotes adaptations in coronary blood flow and adenosine production in normotensive rats. Clinics (Sao Paulo). 2011;66:2105–11.
29. Ades PA, Waldmann ML, Meyer WL, et al. Skeletal muscle and cardiovascular adaptations to exercise conditioning in older coronary patients. Circulation. 1996;94:323–30.
30. Faulkner JA, Larkin LM, Claflin DR, Brooks SV. Age-related changes in the structure and function of skeletal muscles. Clin Exp Pharmacol Physiol. 2007;34:1091–6.
31. Proctor DN, Joyner MJ. Skeletal muscle mass and the reduction of VO_2max in trained older subjects. J Appl Physiol. 1997;82:1411–5.
32. Tarpenning KM, Hamilton-Wessler M, Wiswell RA, Hawkins SA. Endurance training delays age of decline in leg strength and muscle morphology. Med Sci Sports Exerc. 2004;36:74–8.
33. Magaudda L, Di Mauro D, Trimarchi F, Anastasi G. Effects of physical exercise on skeletal muscle fiber ultrastructural and molecular aspects. Basic Appl Myol. 2004;14:17–21.
34. Ventura-Clapier R, Mettauer B, Bigard X. Beneficial effects of endurance training on cardiac and skeletal muscle energy metabolism in heart failure. Cardiovasc Res. 2007;73:10–8.
35. Dyck DJ, Glatz PJ, Keizer GH, et al. Functional differences in lipid metabolism in resting skeletal muscle of various types. Am J Physiol. 1997;272:E340–51.
36. Murakami T, Shimomura Y, Fujitsuka N, Sugiyama S. Differential adaptation to endurance training between heart and gastrocnemius muscle mitochondria in rats. Biochem Mol Biol Int. 1995;36:285–90.
37. Chow LS, Greenlund LJ, Asmann YW, Short KR, McCrady SK, Levine JA, Nair KS. Impact of endurance training on murine spontaneous activity, muscle mitochondrial DNA abundance, gene transcripts, and function. J Appl Physiol. 2007;102:1078–89.
38. Short KR, Vittone JL, Bigelow ML, et al. Impact of aerobic exercise training on age-related changes in insulin sensitivity and muscle oxidative capacity. Diabetes. 2003;52:1888–96.
39. Nair KS. Aging muscle. Am J Clin Nutr. 2005;81: 953–63.
40. Tafani M, Karpinich NO, Hurster KA, Pastorino JG, Schneider T, Russo MA, Farber JL. Cytochrome c release upon Fas receptor activation depends on translocation of full-length bid and the induction of the mitochondrial permeability transition. J Biol Chem. 2002;277:10073–82.
41. Stanley WC, Recchia FA, Lopaschuk GD. Myocardial substrate metabolism in the normal and failing heart. Physiol Rev. 2005;85:1093–129.
42. Jeukendrup AE. Regulation of fat metabolism in skeletal muscle. Ann N Y AcadSci. 2002;967:217–35.
43. Smart N, Haluska B, Jeffriess L, Case C, Marwick TH. Cardiac contributions to exercise training responses in patients with chronic heart failure: a strain imaging study. Echocardiography. 2006;23: 376–82.
44. Akashi YJ, Koike A, Osada N, Omiya K, Itoh H. Short-term physical training improves vasodilatory capacity in cardiac patients. Jpn Heart J. 2002;43: 13–24.
45. Kavazis AN. Exercise preconditioning of the myocardium. Sports Med. 2009;39:923–35.
46. Starnes JW, Taylor RP. Exercise-induced cardioprotection: endogenous mechanisms. Med Sci Sports Exerc. 2007;39:1537–43.
47. Golbidi S, Laher I. Molecular mechanisms in exercise-induced cardioprotection. Cardiol Res Pract. 2011;2011:972807.
48. Powers SK, Quindry JC, Kavazis AN. Exercise-induced cardioprotection against myocardial ischemia-reperfusion injury. Free Radic Biol Med. 2008;44:193–201.
49. Ascensao A, Ferreira R, Magalhaes J. Exercise-induced cardioprotection – biochemical, morphological and functional evidence in whole tissue and isolated mitochondria. Int J Cardiol. 2007;117:16–30.
50. Calvert JW. Cardioprotective effects of nitrite during exercise. Cardiovasc Res. 2011;89:499–506.
51. Murlasits Z, Lee Y, Powers SK. Short-term exercise does not increase ER stress protein expression in cardiac muscle. Med Sci Sports Exerc. 2007;39:1522–8.
52. Papafili A, Hill MR, Brull DJ, McAnulty RJ, Marshall RP, Humphries SE, Laurent GJ. Common promoter variant in cyclooxygenase-2 represses gene expression: evidence of role in acute-phase inflammatory response. Arterioscler Thromb Vasc Biol. 2002;22: 1631–6.
53. DuBois RN, Abramson SB, Crofford L, Gupta RA, Simon LS, Van de Putte LBA, Lipsky PE. Cyclooxygenase in biology and disease. FASEB J. 1998;12:1063–73.
54. Kim SY, Jun TW, Lee YS, Na HK, Surh YJ, Song W. Effects of exercise on cyclooxygenase-2 expression and nuclear factor-kappaB DNA binding in human peripheral blood mononuclear cells. Ann N Y Acad Sci. 2009;1171:464–71.
55. Young JC, Barral JM, Ulrich Hartl F. More than folding: localized functions of cytosolic chaperones. Trends Biochem Sci. 2003;28:541–7.

56. Yamada P, Amorim F, Moseley P, Schneider S. Heat shock protein 72 response to exercise in humans. Sports Med. 2008;38:715–33.
57. Tanonaka K, Toga W, Takeo S. Induction of heat shock protein 70 in failing heart (Article). Nihon Yakurigaku Zasshi. 2004;123:71–6.
58. Lennon SL, Quindry J, Hamilton KL, et al. Loss of exercise-induced cardioprotection after cessation of exercise. J Appl Physiol. 2004;96:1299–305.
59. Quindry JC, Hamilton KL, French JP, Lee Y, Murlasits Z, Tumer N, Powers SK. Exercise-induced HSP-72 elevation and cardioprotection against infarct and apoptosis. J Appl Physiol. 2007;103: 1056–62.
60. Stein AB, Tang XL, Guo Y, Xuan YT, Dawn B, Bolli R. Delayed adaptation of the heart to stress: late preconditioning. Stroke. 2004;35:2676–9.
61. Hajnal A, Nagy O, Litvai A, Papp J, Parratt JR, Vegh A. Nitric oxide involvement in the delayed antiarrhythmic effect of treadmill exercise in dogs. Life Sci. 2005;77:1960–71.
62. Hall C. Essential biochemistry and physiology of (NT-pro) BNP. Eur J Heart Fail. 2004;6:257–60.
63. de Groote P, Dagorn J, Soudan B, Lamblin N, McFadden E, Bauters C. B-type natriuretic peptide and peak exercise oxygen consumption provide independent information for risk stratification in patients with stable congestive heart failure. J Am Coll Cardiol. 2004;43:1584–9.
64. Ohba H, Takada H, Musha H, et al. Effects of prolonged strenuous exercise on plasma levels of atrial natriuretic peptide and brain natriuretic peptide in healthy men. Am Heart J. 2001;141:751–78.
65. Smith JK, Dykes R, Douglas JE, Krishnaswamy G, Berk S. Long-term exercise and atherogenic activity of blood mononuclear cells in persons at risk of developing ischemic heart disease. JAMA. 1999;281:1722–7.
66. Libby P. Inflammation in atherosclerosis. Nature. 2002;420:868–74.
67. Beattie MS, Shlipak MG, Liu H, Browner WS, Schiller NB, Whooley MA. C-reactive protein and ischemia in users and nonusers of beta-blockers and statins: data from the Heart and Soul Study. Circulation. 2003;107:245–50.
68. Dandona P, Aljada A, Bandyopadhyay A. Inflammation: the link between insulin resistance, obesity and diabetes. Trends Immunol. 2004;25:4–7.
69. Duncan BB, Schmidt MI, Pankow JS, et al. Low-grade systemic inflammation and the development of type 2 diabetes: the atherosclerosis risk in communities study. Diabetes. 2003;52:1799–805.
70. Ross R. Atherosclerosis-an inflammatory disease. N Engl J Med. 1999;340:115–26.
71. Goldhammer E, Tanchilevitch A, Maor I, Beniamini Y, Rosenschein U, Sagiv M. Exercise training modulates cytokines activity in coronary heart disease patients. Int J Cardiol. 2005;100:93–9.
72. Verma S, Wang CH, Li SH, et al. A self-fulfilling prophecy: C-reactive protein attenuates nitric oxide production and inhibits angiogenesis. Circulation. 2002;106:913–9.
73. Michigan A, Johnson TV, Master VA. Review of the relationship between C-reactive protein and exercise. Mol Diagn Ther. 2011;15:265–75.
74. Wannamethee SG, Lowe GD, Whincup PH, et al. Physical activity and hemostatic and inflammatory variables in elderly men. Circulation. 2002;105:1785–90.
75. Hammett CJ, Oxenham HC, Baldi JC, et al. Effect of six months' exercise training on C-reactive protein levels in healthy elderly subjects. J Am Coll Cardiol. 2004;44:2411–3.
76. Hachinohe D, Jeong MH, Kim MC, et al. Drug-eluting stent as an option for intractable in-stent coronary restenosis. Korean Circ J. 2011;41:677–80.
77. Moldoveanu AI, Shephard RJ, Shek PN. Exercise elevates plasma levels but not gene expression of IL-1β, IL-6, and TNF-α in blood mononuclear cells. J Appl Physiol. 2000;89:1499–504.
78. Samitz G, Egger M, Zwahlen M. Domains of physical activity and all-cause mortality: systematic review and dose–response meta-analysis of cohort studies. Int J Epidemiol. 2011;40:1382–400.
79. Tully MA, Cupples ME, Hart ND, McEneny J, McGlade KJ, Chan WS, Young IS. Randomised controlled trial of home-based walking programmes at and below current recommended levels of exercise in sedentary adults. J Epidemiol Community Health. 2007;61:778–83.
80. Paffenbarger Jr RS, Hyde RT, Wing AL, Hsieh CC. Physical activity, all-cause mortality, and longevity of college alumni. N Engl J Med. 1986;314:605–13.
81. Hardman AE. Physical activity and health: current issues and research needs. Int J Epidemiol. 2001;30:1193–7.
82. Surgeon General. Physical activity and health. A report of the surgeon general. US departments of health and human services. Centers for disease control and prevention. Atlanta; 1996.
83. Lakka TA, Venalainen JM, Rauramaa R, Salonen R, Tuomilehto J, Salonen JT. Relation of leisure-time physical activity and cardiorespiratory fitness to the risk of acute myocardial infarction in men. N Engl J Med. 1994;330:1549–54.
84. Hiilloskorpi HK, Pasanen ME, Fogelholm MG, Laukkanen RM, Manttari AT. Use of heart rate to predict energy expenditure from low to high activity levels. Int J Sports Med. 2003;24:332–6.
85. Morris JN. Exercise in the prevention of coronary heart disease: today's best buy in public health. Med Sci Sports Exerc. 1994;26:807–14.
86. Dunbar CC, Kalinski MI. Using RPE to regulate exercise intensity during a 20-week training program for postmenopausal women: a pilot study. Percept Mot Skills. 2004;99:688–90.
87. Pollock ML, Gaesser GA, Butcher JD, Després JP, Dishman RK, Franklin BA, Garber CE. ACSM position stand on the recommended quantity and quality of exercise for developing and maintaining

cardiorespiratory and muscular fitness, and flexibility in adults. Med Sci Sports Exerc. 1998;30:975–91.
88. Fletcher GF, Gary Balady G, Blair SN, et al. Statement on exercise: benefits and recommendations for physical activity programs for all Americans. Circulation. 1996;94:857–62.
89. Goraya TY, Jacobsen SJ, Pellikka PA, et al. Prognostic value of treadmill exercise testing in elderly persons. Ann Intern Med. 2000;132:862–70.
90. Ellstead MH. Stress testing: principles and practice. 4th ed. Philadelphia: FA Davis; 1995.
91. Braunwald E, Antman EM, Beasley JW, et al. ACC/AHA 2002 guideline update for the management of patients with unstable angina and non-ST-segment elevation myocardial infarction – summary article: a report of the American College of Cardiology/American Heart Association task force on practice guidelines (Committee on the Management of Patients with Unstable Angina). J Am Coll Cardiol. 2002;40:1366–74.
92. Parameshwar J, Keegan J, Sparrow J, Sutton GC, Poole-Wilson PA. Predictors of prognosis in severe chronic heart failure. Am Heart J. 1992;123:421–6.
93. Tan LB, Littler WA. Measurement of cardiac reserve in cardiogenic shock: implications for prognosis and management. Br Heart J. 1990;64:121–8.
94. Roul G, Moulichon ME, Bareiss P, et al. Prognostic factors of chronic heart failure in NYHA class II or III: value of invasive exercise haemodynamic data. Eur Heart J. 1995;16:1387–98.
95. Williams SG, Cooke GA, Wright DJ, et al. Peak exercise cardiac power output; a direct indicator of cardiac function strongly predictive of prognosis in chronic heart failure. Eur Heart J. 2001;22:1496–503.
96. Goda A, Lang CC, Williams P, Jones M, Farr MJ, Mancini DM. Usefulness of non-invasive measurement of cardiac output during sub-maximal exercise to predict outcome in patients with chronic heart failure. Am J Cardiol. 2009;104:1556–60.
97. Clausen JP, Trap-Jensen J. Heart rate and arterial blood pressure during exercise in patients with angina pectoris: effects of training and of nitroglycerin. Circulation. 1976;53:436–42.
98. Billman GE. Aerobic exercise conditioning: a non-pharmacological antiarrhythmic intervention. J Appl Physiol. 2002;92:446–54.
99. Hamilton KL, Powers SK, Sugiura T, et al. Short-term exercise training can improve myocardial tolerance to I/R without elevation in heat shock proteins. Am J Physiol Heart Circ Physiol. 2001;281:H1346–52.
100. American Association of Cardiovascular and Pulmonary Rehabilitation. Guidelines for cardiac rehabilitation and secondary prevention programs. 4th ed. Champaign: Human Kinetics; 2004.
101. Arena R, Myers J, Aslam S, Varughese EB, Peberdy MA. Prognostic comparison of the V_E/VCO_2 ratio and slope in patients with heart failure. Heart Drug. 2004;4:133–9.
102. Myers JN. Information from ventilatory gas exchange data. In: Myers JW, editor. Essentials of cardiopulmonary exercise testing. Champaign: Human Kinetics; 1996. p. 83–108.
103. Giardini A, Odendaal D, Khambadkone S, Derrick G. Physiologic decrease of ventilatory response to exercise in the second decade of life in healthy children. Am Heart J. 2011;161:1214–9.
104. Myers J, Zaheer N, Quaglietti S, Madhavan R, Froelicher V, Heidenreich P. Association of functional and health status measures in heart failure. J Card Fail. 2006;12:439–45.
105. Corra U, Mezzani A, Bosimini E, Scapellato F, Imparato A, Giannuzzi P. Ventilatory response to exercise improves risk stratification in patients with chronic heart failure and intermediate functional capacity. Am Heart J. 2002;143:418–26.
106. Francis DP, Shamim W, Davies LC, et al. Cardiopulmonary exercise testing for prognosis in chronic heart failure: continuous and independent prognostic value from V_E/VCO(2)slope and peak VO(2). Eur Heart J. 2000;21:154–61.
107. Kleber FX, Vietzke G, Wernecke KD, Bauer U, Opitz C, Wensel R, Sperfeld A, Gläser S. Impairment of ventilatory efficiency in heart failure: prognostic impact. Circulation. 2000;101:2803–9.
108. Ingle L, Goode K, Carroll S, Sloan R, Boyes C, Cleland JG, Clark AL. Prognostic value of the V_E/VCO_2 slope calculated from different time intervals in patients with suspected heart failure. Int J Cardiol. 2007;118:350–5.
109. Wilson JR, Mancini DM. Factors contributing to the exercise limitation of heart failure. J Am Coll Cardiol. 1993;22(Suppl A):93A–8.
110. Andreas S, Morguet AJ, Werner GS, Kreuzer H. Ventilatory response to exercise and to carbon dioxide in patients with heart failure. Eur Heart J. 1996;17:750–5.
111. Wasserman K, Hansen JE, Sue DY, Stringer WW, Whipp BJ. Principles of exercise testing and interpretation including pathophysiology and clinical applications. 4th ed. Philadelphia: Lippincott Williams and Wilkins; 2005.
112. Scrutinio D, Passantino A, Lagioia R, Napoli F, Ricci A, Rizzon P. Percent achieved of predicted peak exercise oxygen uptake and kinetics of recovery of oxygen uptake after exercise for risk stratification in chronic heart failure. Int J Cardiol. 1998;64:117–24.
113. Calbet JA, Rådegran G, Boushel R, Saltin B. On the mechanisms that limit oxygen uptake during exercise in acute and chronic hypoxia: role of muscle mass. J Physiol. 2009;587:477–90.
114. Van de Veirea NR, Van Laethemb C, Philippéc J, De Winterd O, De Backere G, Vanderheyden M, De Suttere J. V_E/VCO_2 slope and oxygen uptake efficiency slope in patients with coronary artery disease and intermediate peakVO_2. Eur J Cardiovasc Prev Rehabil. 2006;13:916–23.
115. Zavorsky GS, Walley KR, Russell JA. Red cell pulmonary transit times through the healthy human lung. Exp Physiol. 2003;88:191–200.

116. Koike A, Hiroe M, Taniguchi K, Marumo F. Respiratory control during exercise in patients with cardiovascular disease. Am Rev Respir Dis. 1993; 147:425–9.
117. Sagiv M, Rotstein A, Ben-Sira D, Grodjinovsky A, Fisher N, Kufmann D. Physiological responses to wrist weights during endurance cycling in normal subjects. Med Sci Sports Exerc. 1991;23:748–51.
118. Cohen-Solal A, Tabet JY, Logeart D, Bourgoin P, Tokmakova M, Dahan M. A non-invasively determined surrogate of cardiac power ('circulatory power') at peak exercise is a powerful prognostic factor in chronic heart failure. Eur Heart J. 2002; 23:806–14.
119. Stager JM, Tanner DA. Swimming. 2nd edition; An International Olympic Committee Publication. Oxford: Blackwell Science Ltd.; 2005.
120. Helgerud J, Ingjer F, Stromme SB. Sex differences in performance-matched marathon runners. Eur J Appl Physiol Occup Physiol. 1990;61:433–9.

Index

A

Aerobic exercise
  benefits, 4
  blood pressure
    diastolic blood pressure, 138
    intense exercise, 138–139
    sympathetic and catecholamine hormone, 138
    systolic and diastolic, 138
    systolic pressure, 138
    TPR, 138
  capacity, 4
  defined, 3
  left ventricular function
    cardiac output, 110
    coronary artery disease patients, 110
    dyskinesia, 110
    echocardiography, 110
    ischemic heart disease, 110
    wall motion abnormalities, 110
  metabolism, 8
  oxygen uptake, 4
  slow twitch fiber muscles, 3–4
Aerobic stress test, 42
Aging
  arteries
    aortic stiffness, 185
    diastolic blood pressure, 185
    genetic factors, 184
    hypertension, 184
    hypertrophic growth, 184
    pulse pressure, 185
    systolic blood pressure, 184
  cardiac output and pulmonary system, 171
  exercise stress, 173
  genetic component, 173
  genetic factors, 171, 172
  heart rate dynamics, 172–173
  maximal stroke volume, 173
  oxygen delivery and extraction, 172
  oxygen uptake
    adolescents, 173
    elite athletes, 174
    maximum heart rate and maximal stoke volume, 174
    Vo_2 max, 173
  peak aerobic capacity, 173
  physical activity, 171
  pulmonary function
    alveolar ventilation, 174
    coronary artery disease, 174
    expiratory airflow, 174
    trained older adults, 174
  trained and untrained individuals, 171, 172
  work capacity, 172
Anaerobic bout
  auscultation *vs.* intra-arterial values, 145
  autonomic nervous system, 145
  cessation, dynamic aerobic exercise, 145
  metabolites, 146
  percentage, maximal workload, 145
  physiological variables relations, 145, 146
Anaerobic exercise
  adenosine monophosphate (AMP), 6
  blood pH, 5
  cardiac output
    adrenergic state, 75
    autoregulation mechanism, 60, 75
    strenuous anaerobic efforts, 74
    stroke volume and Doppler-derived indices, 75
    total peripheral resistance, 74
    vasoconstriction, 75
  energy expenditure, 5
  energy sources, 5
  fast twitch fibers, 5
  lactic acid, 5
  left ventricular function
    EDV and ESV, 111
    hypoxia and acidosis, 111
  metabolism, 4–5
  PC system, 5
Anemia, 52
Arterial baroreceptors, hypertension
  arteriole vasodilatation, 143
  autoregulation mechanism, 143
  baroreflex, 141
  blood pressure, 141
  exercise stimuli, 142–143
  muscle blood flow, 143
  sensitivity and activity, baroreflex, 142
  sympathetic nervous system, 142
  sympatho-sympathetic reflexes, 143
  systolic blood pressure, 143

M.S. Sagiv, *Exercise Cardiopulmonary Function in Cardiac Patients*,
DOI 10.1007/978-1-4471-2888-5, © Springer-Verlag London 2012

Atherosclerosis
aerobic physical exercise, 137
chronic inflammatory disorder, 136
nitric oxide, 137–138
pathogenesis, 137
peroxidation and cardiovascular mortality, 137
pharmacological therapies, 138
physical activity, 137
physical exercise, 136–137
risk factors, 136
Athlete's heart syndrome
cardiovascular adaptations, 125
electrocardiogram (ECG), 126–127
isodynamic exercise, 126
left ventricular hypertrophy, 126
left ventricular wall, 127
morphological cardiac changes, 126
physical and static exercise, 126
strength-trained *vs.* endurance-trained, 127
total peripheral resistance, 126
Atrial filling fraction
blood volume measurement, 121
coronary artery disease hypertensive patients, 122
filling rate, 121

B
Balke and Naughton protocols, 23
Bicycle test, 26–27
Blood flow
exercise
autoregulatory resistance, 87
cellular and molecular mechanisms, 87
endurance training, 87
metabolic requirement, 86
precapillary sphincters, 87
resistance value, 87
myocardial (*see* Myocardial blood flow)
nitric oxide and Kinins influence
ACE splits, 90
endothelial cells, 89
hypoxia and hyperemia, 90
shear stress, 89–90
regulation
metabolic theory, 87–88
myogenic theory, 89
Blood pressure
aerobic exercise, 138–139
anaerobic bout, 145–146
arterial baroreceptors, 141–143
arterials and aortic stiffening
angiotensin-converting enzyme *vs.* bradykinin, 147
cardiovascular disease, 147
coronary blood flow, 147
fitness level, 148
physical activity, 147
atherosclerosis, 136–138
chronic disorders, 135
coronary artery disease, 135
endothelium damage and dysfunction, 135–136
endothelium-dependent vasodilation, 136
flow-mediated dilation and exercise capacity, 136
MABP, 140–141
physical activity, hypertension, 148–150
post-exercise hypotension, 139–140
resistive training, 143–145
total peripheral resistance, 146–147
vascular endothelium, 135
Bruce Test, 23
Brugada syndrome
autosomal dominant inherited disorder, 204
cardiac sodium channel, 204
electrocardiographic signature/phenotype, 204
idiopathic ventricular fibrillation, 204
ventricular fibrillation, 204

C
Cardiac biomarkers
acute coronary syndrome, 223
AMPK, 228
antioxidant enzymes, 224
atherosclerosis, 227
atrial natriuretic peptide (ANP), 227
brain natriuretic peptide (BNP), 226–227
C-reactive protein (CRP), 227
cyclooxygenase (COX), 225
cytoprotective mechanisms, 227
description, 223
diabetes, 224
endoplasmic reticulum stress proteins, 225
exercise-induced cardioprotective phenotype, 224
exercise training, 224
heat shock proteins, 225–226
interleukin-6, 227, 228
JUPITER study, 228
malfunction, endoplasmic reticulum, 224–225
myocardial ischemia and reperfusion injury, 223
myocardial tolerance, 226
nitric oxide, 226
nuclear factor-kappaB (NF-kappaB), 225
prolonged exercise, 227
redox-based mechanisms, 224
regular exercise, 224
tumor necrosis factor-α, 228, 229
Cardiac output. *See also* Redistribution, cardiac output
adolescents, 60
aerobic exercise
coronary artery disease, 81–82
training effect, 78–79
anaerobic exercise, 74–75
atrial filling fraction, 178
cardiopulmonary system, 176
core temperature effect
heat acclimatization, 71
hypohydration, 70
hypothermia, 71
intense exercise, 70

metabolic heat, 70
physiological mechanisms, 71
warm ambient places, 70
coronary artery disease patients, 76–77
description, 59
dynamic aerobic exercise, 59
end-diastolic volume, 177
end-diastolic volume and end-systolic volume, 177–178
Frank-Starling mechanism, 61–62, 177
heart rate and stroke volume
augmented stroke volume, 61
controlling factors, 62–63
endurance training, 63
peak diastolic filling rate, 63
PWC170 test, 61
rate-workload relationship, 62
stages, 61
untrained individuals, 63
heart rate control
aerobic exercise, 67
autonomic nervous system, 65, 66
baroreceptors and chemoreceptor, 66
extrinsic regulation, 65
Karvonen formula, 66
parasympathetic stimulation, 65
rest, 66
true maximum heart rate, 66
vagal and sympathetic nerve, 65
isodynamic exercise, 75–76
isometric exercise, 71–74, 77–78, 178
left ventricular compliance, 177
left ventricular mass, 177
maximal heart rate and stroke volume, 177
oxygen extraction
anaerobic metabolism, 69
cardiac ischemia, 69
oxygen uptake, 59
stroke volume factors, 67–69
stroke volume variation, 59
submaximal dynamic aerobic exercise, 59
supine exercise (*see* Supine exercise)
systolic blood pressure, 177
Cardiac rehabilitation
aims
atheroma, 215
circadian rhythms, 216
coronary stenosis, 216
exercise capacity, 217
morning exercise, 216
phase II, 215
physical activity, 215, 216
risk factors, 216
amount, exercise
inverse association, energy expenditure and risk factors, 229
moderate physical activity, 230
physical inactivity, 229–230
vigorous exercise, 229, 230
benefits, exercise, 221
biomarkers (*see* Cardiac biomarkers)
cardiopulmonary and ventilator markers, 235
coronary artery disease
exercise stress test, 231–233
prescription, exercise, 233–234
exercise, functional capacity
acetyl-CoA formation, 223
activated protein kinase (AMPK) activity, 222
aerobic training, 223
age-associated changes, body, 222
cytochrome c, 222–223
oxidative phosphorylation, 222
peripheral adaptation, 223
skeletal muscle mass, 221
minute ventilation, CO_2 ratio, 235–237
moderate intensity
aging, 231
Borg's rating, 230
exercise intensities, 231
METs, 230
perceived exertion, 230
VO_2 method, 230
mortality
athletes, 218
fitness level, 217–218
genetic and environmental factors, 218
regular aerobic exercise, 217
risk factors, 217
myocardial oxygen demand
diastolic pressure, 220–221
hypertrophy, 220
left ventricular contractility, 220
left ventricular end-diastolic volume, 220
myocardial oxygen supply, 220
oxygen supply, 221
systole, 220
ventricular wall stress, 219
wall tension, 220
physiology and pathophysiology
atherogenesis, 219
atherosclerosis, 218
inflammation, 218
ischemia, 219
plaque, 219
rupture, atheromatous plaque, 219
stenosis, 219
ST-segment depression, 219
power output, reserve and circulatory power, 234–235
pulmonary ventilation-perfusion mismatch, 237–238
stroke volume estimation, 238–239
Cardiac stress test, 25
Cardiopulmonary exercise testing (CPET), 235
Cardiopulmonary function
aerobic exercise capacity, 176
age effect, oxygen uptake, 173–174
aging, 171–173
arteries, aging, 184–185
cardiac changes and output, 176–178

Cardiopulmonary function (*cont.*)
  cardiovascular and physical performance
    aging process, 182
    cardiopulmonary function, 183
    degree, Vo_2 max, 184
    diastolic left ventricular filling, 183
    end-systolic volume and ejection fraction, 183
    peak filling, 183
    total peripheral resistance, 182
  exercise training, CAD, 188
  heart rate, 178
  hypertensive elderly, 188–189
  left ventricular
    aerobic exercise, 179–181
    anaerobic exercise, 181–182
    isometric exercise, 182
  metabolic improvements, 190
  and muscle mass
    aerobic capacity, 174, 175
    aging, 174, 175
    cardiac output, 174
    mitochondrial density, 174
    myocardial oxygen demand, 175
  physical activity
    aerobic capacity and aging, 176
    heart rate, 175–176
    isometric maneuver, 175
    myocardial perfusion, 176
    Vo_2 max, 176
  pulmonary exercise
    aged lung, 189
    alveolar ventilation, 189–190
    breathing efficiency, 190
    expiratory airflow rates, 190
    forced expiratory volume, 189
  stroke volume, 178–179
  stroke volume response, training, 179
  training effect
    aerobic exercise, 186
    cardiac contractile force, 187
    cardiac function, 186
    cardiovascular changes, 186
    dynamic aerobic training, 187
    endurance exercise, 187
    submaximal exercise, 187–188
    ventricular systolic function, 186–187
    veteran athletes, 185
Catecholaminergic polymorphic ventricular tachycardia (CPVT)
  cardiac ischemia, 203
  QRS morphology and myocardiopathy, 203–204
"Chloride shift", 38–39
Commotio cordis
  definition, 202
  electrocardiogram, 202
  mechanosensitive ion channel, 202
  nonpenetrating trauma, 202
Coronary artery disease
  aerobic exercise training
    heart rate and VO_2, 82
    left ventricular stroke volume, 81
    submaximal exercise, 81, 82
    ventricular volume changes, 81
  exercise
    arrhythmias, 19
    atherosclerosis, 19
    left ventricular contractility, 19
    stress test, 231–233
    training, 19
  left ventricular function
    EDV, ESV and stroke volume, 117
    maximal intensity exercise, 117
    supine exercise, 117
CPET. *See* Cardiopulmonary exercise testing (CPET)
CPVT. *See* Catecholaminergic polymorphic ventricular tachycardia (CPVT)

D
Diabetes
  cardiovascular disease, 163
  diagnosis, 163
  exercise effects
    aerobic training, 164
    AMP-activated protein kinase (AMPK) and GLUT4, 165–166
    chronic aerobic activity, 164
    and chronic training, 164
    diagnosis, type 2, 166
    gluconeogenesis, 163
    glucose transportation, 165
    GLUT4, 164
    glycemic control, 166
    heavy-resistance strength training, 166
    physical activity, 166
    skeletal muscle, 165
    therapeutic management, glycemic, 165
    treatment, 166
    type 1 and type 2, 163
    weight and resistance training, 164
  fracture risk, 163
  HbA1c, 162
  insulin secretion, 163
  levels, sugar, 162
  treatment, 163
  type 1 and type 2, 162–163
Doppler indices during systole
  aortic diameter, 117
  cardiac output, 118
  coronary artery disease, 118
  dynamic aerobic exercise, 118
  flow velocity integral, 118

E
Eccentric left ventricular hypertrophy, 2
Electrocardiogram, 232, 233
Excess post-exercise oxygen consumption (EPOC), 14
Exercise electrocardiography test, 25
Exercise physiology
  aerobic exercise, 3–4
  anaerobic exercise, 4–6

cardiovascular system
angiotensin II, 18
cardiac output, 18
hydraulic system, 18
myocardium, 17
coronary artery disease, 19
defined, 2
description, 3
efforts, altitude, 21–22
energy cost
bicycle test, 26–27
metabolic cost calculation, stepping, 26
metabolic equivalent of task (MET), 24
stepwise test, 25
stress tests, 25
energy expenditure
anaerobic and resistive exercises, 8
ATP, 7
balance, measurement, 6
carbohydrates and fatty acids, 7
factors, performance, 8
skeletal muscle, 7
strenuous exercise, 7
VO_2 augmentation, 7
Fick equation, 20–21
gender differences, oxygen extraction
cardiopulmonary responses, 17
in vitro studies, 16–17
left ventricular contractility, 17
mean values, VO_2, 16
skeletal muscle fibers, 16
genetics, 22–23
interplay, aerobic and anaerobic pathways
ATP, 14
EPOC, 14
mitochondrial respiration, 13
sports events, physical stress, 13
steady-state heart rate, 13
isometric exercise, 6
laboratory equipments, 24
lactic acid threshold (*see* Lactic acid threshold)
measurements and metabolic calculations, 23
metabolic demands, 17
metabolism (*see* Metabolism)
mitochondrial changes (*see* Skeletal muscle, mitochondrial changes)
physical activity
aerobic, 1–2
pressure overload, 2
treadmill
running, metabolic cost, 28–29
walking, metabolic cost, 28
work and power, 27
unit measurements, 23–24
Exercise stress test
ACC/AHA guidelines, 231, 232
community-based walking program, 232–233
contraindications, 232
description, 231
electrocardiogram, 232
pharmacological stress testing, 233
prognosis estimation, 233
radionuclide imaging, 232
screening tests, 232

F
Fick equation, 20–21
Frank-Starling mechanism, 61–62, 128, 177

H
HCM. *See* Hypertrophic Cardiomyopathy (HCM)
Heart rate
calculation, 178
chronic exercise, 178
sympathetic and parasympathetic, 178
Hypertension. *See also* Blood pressure
aerobic and isometric exercises, 149
aerobic training, 149
arterial pressure, 149
catecholamine, 149
direct intra arterial method *vs.* indirect conventional sphygmomanometer, 149
exercise program, 149
genetic variance, 148
metaanalysis, 148
norepinephrine, 149
normotensive and hypertensive individuals, 149
sympathetic nervous system, 149
Hypertrophic cardiomyopathy (HCM)
abnormally branching myocytes, 205
angiotensin converting enzyme (ACE), 207
asymmetric septal hypertrophy, 205
atrial and ventricular arrhythmias, 206
cardiomyopathy, 205
diastolic dysfunction, 205
dynamic outflow obstruction, 206
genetic expression, 205
insertion/deletion (I/D) polymorphism, 207
intrinsic abnormalities and outflow tract obstruction, 206
myosin heavy chain, 206
sarcomeric genes, 205
septal hypercontractility, 206
Hypertrophy
concentric
left ventricular wall thickness, 127
pressure overload and isometric exercise, 127
left ventricular
blood pressure, 122
definition, 122
endurance training, 122
rowing and cycling, 123
strength training, 122
pathological
coronary artery disease/hypertensive patients, 128
hypertension, 127
left ventricular filling rate, 128
valvular heart disease, 127

I

Isodynamic exercise, cardiac output
- autoregulation mechanism, 75–76
- blood flow, 75
- ischemic responses, 76
- total peripheral resistance, 76

Isometric exercise
- cardiac output
  - adaptations, 79–80
  - baroreflex sensitivity, 72
  - coronary artery disease patients, 73
  - exercise pressor reflex theory, 72
  - increased ventricular performance, 74
  - isometric handgrip, 72
  - pressor response, 71–72
  - resistive training, 71
  - response, isometric bout, 73
  - voluntary contractions, 73
- coronary artery disease patient, 77–78
- description, 6
- left ventricular function
  - dead lift, 111, 112
  - EDV and ESV, 112
  - end-systolic volume and cardiac output, 112
  - pressor response, 112–113
  - stroke volume, 112
  - total peripheral resistance, 112
  - ventricular contractility, 111

Isotonic exercise, 6

L

Lactic acid threshold
- defined, 14–15
- elimination, 15, 16
- mitochondrial density, 16
- AT and OBLA, 15

Left ventricular ejection fraction (LVEF)
- dead lift, EF, 116, 117
- EDV, ESV and inotropic state, 115
- EF aerobic exercise, 116, 117
- EF calculation, 116
- ejection fraction, 116
- pressure–volume relationship, 116
- stroke volume and EDV, 116

Left ventricular function
- adaptations
  - aerobic, anaerobic and isometric exercise, 129
  - aerobic exercise training, 128
  - aerobic training, 130
  - anatomical changes, 128
  - cardiac output, 129
  - cardiovascular changes, training, 128, 129
  - concentric *vs.* eccentric hypertrophy, 128
  - ejection fraction, 130
  - end-diastolic volume and wall thickness, 128, 129
  - Frank-Starling mechanism, 128
- aerobic exercise
  - autoregulation mechanism, 181
  - ejection fraction, 180
  - end-diastolic and end-systolic volume, 181
  - hypertrophy and contractility, 179–180
  - myocardial perfusion, 180
  - ratio, early and late diastolic filling velocity, 180
  - stroke volume, 180
  - total peripheral resistance, 180
  - velocity, circumferential fiber, 179
  - wall motion abnormalities, 180
- anaerobic exercise
  - end-diastolic and end-systolic volume, 181
  - hypoxia and acidosis, 181
  - systolic function, 181
  - venous filling, 181
- "athlete's heart", 125–127
- atrial filling fraction, 121–122
- concentric hypertrophy, 127
- coronary artery disease, 117
- diastol function, 118
- diastol indices
  - intrinsic and extrinsic, 120
  - mitral peak early diastole, 119
  - mitral valve/presystole, 119
  - myocardial hypertrophy, 120
  - ventricular filling, 120
- diastol ratio, 120–121
- Doppler indices (*see* Doppler indices during systole)
- end-systolic pressure–volume ratio (P/V), 114–115
- exercise mode hypertrophy, 122–123
- genome
  - angiotensin-converting enzyme, 125
  - coronary artery disease and hypertension patients, 125
  - DD, II and ID, 125
  - deoxyribonucleic acid (DNA), 123
  - eccentric *vs.* concentric, 124
  - endurance training, 123
  - left ventricular mass, 124
  - pathological and physiological hypertrophy, 123–124
  - ribonucleic acids (RNA), 123
  - systolic pressure/volume overload, 123
- isometric exercise, 111–113, 182
- LVEF, 115–117
- measurements
  - echocardiography and radionuclide, 109
  - LVEF, 109
  - metaanalysis, 109
  - systolic and diastolic, 109
- pathological left ventricular hypertrophy, 127–128
- systolic
  - afterload, 113
  - diastolic dysfunction, 113–114
  - echocardiography, 114
  - heart rate and stroke volume, 113
  - post and pre-exercise, 114
  - preload/end-diastolic volume, 113
  - Starling's law, 113
  - strength, contraction, 113

Lipoproteins
aerobic exercise
anaerobic training, 156
cardiovascular morbidity and mortality, 155
high and low-density, 155–156
physical training, 155
total cholesterol/triglyceride, 156
aerobic fitness and exercise programs, 155
apolipoproteins, 155, 156
cholesterol synthesis, high-density
acyl transferase, 159
apoprotein AI (Apo AI), 159
arteriovenous, 159
high-density, 158–159
triglyceride hydrolysis, 158
high-density
cycle ergometer training, 158
effect, aerobic exercise, 158
heart disease risk, 158
LVDL, 157
Marathon runners and total cholesterol, 157–158
meta-analysis, 158
physical training, 157
VO_2 max, 157
strength training effect
cholesterol levels, 157
high and low-density, 157
hypercholesterolemic, 157
resistance, 157
Long QT syndrome (LQTs)
arrhythmia, 203
electrocardiographs, 203
sodium and potassium ion channel, 203
ventricular repolarization, 203
LVEF. *See* Left ventricular ejection fraction (LVEF)

M

MABP. *See* Mean arterial blood pressure (MABP)
Mean arterial blood pressure (MABP)
average, systolic and diastolic, 140–141
calculation, 141
cardiac output, 141
total peripheral resistance (TPR), 141
venous return and Starling's Law, 141
Mechanical bicycle ergometry, 27
Metabolic cardiovascular risk factors
aerobic exercise effect, 155–156
cholesterol synthesis, 158–159
diabetes, 162–163
exercise, obesity, 160–161
exercise's effects, diabetes, 163–166
high-density lipoprotein, 157–158
lipoproteins, 155
obesity, 159–160
resistive exercise training, 162
strength training effect, 157
Metabolic theory, blood flow regulation
acid-base balance, 88
vascular responses, 88
Metabolism
aerobic exercise, 8
anaerobic energy systems, 10
ATP molecules, 9, 10
ATP-PC system, 10
carbohydrates, 10–11
fatty acids, 12
glycolysis, 11
Krebs cycle, 11
myocardium, 12
resistance training, 8
respiratory exchange ratio, 12
VCO_2/VO_2, 11
Minute ventilation
aerobic exercise, 36
breathing rate *vs.* tidal volume, 36
chemoreceptors, 36
control mechanisms, exercise, 36
CO_2 ratio
anaerobic threshold, 235
exercise capacity, 236
exercise testing, 235
increased ventilatory drive, 236
patients, heart failure, 237
peak exercise oxygen uptake, 236
prognostic power, 236–237
spirometric parameters, 236
dead space
anatomical, 37
physiological, 37
description, 35
lactic acid production, 37
maximal exercise, 35
maximal voluntary ventilation, 35
oxygen uptake, 37
Motor drive treadmill ergometer, 27
Myocardial blood flow
anaerobic capacity, 92
anemia, 92–93
angina threshold, 95
autoregulation mechanism, 92
cardiac energy metabolism, 92
contractile state, 95
coronary
abnormalities, 96
atherosclerosis, 92
capillaries, 91
vasodilatation, 93
coronary artery disease patients, 94
diastole time, 94
exercise training, 93
hemodynamic alterations, 93
hemoglobin concentration, 93
intramyocardial tension, 95
isodynamic exercise, 92
myocardium, 91
myogenic tone, 93
oxygen extraction, 92, 93
physiological hypertrophy, 94
RPP, 95

Myocardial blood flow (*cont.*)
- variables, oxygen demand-supply, 95
- VO_2, 92, 94

Myogenic theory, blood flow regulation
- circumferential stretch, 89
- endurance exercise, 89
- shear stress, 89

O

Obesity
- arterial pressure and left ventricular hypertrophy, 160
- definition, 159
- exercise
  - anaerobic threshold and lipid utilization, 160
  - appetite suppressant, 161
  - cardiovascular health, 161
  - dieting and increased physical activity, 161
  - fat oxidation, 161
  - free fatty acid (FFA), 160
  - insulin and catecholamine, 160
  - molecular mechanisms, 161
  - oxidative metabolism, fatty acids and carbohydrates, 160
  - physical activity, moderate intensity, 160
  - protein translation rate, 161
  - uncoupling protein (UCP), 161
  - weight loss, 160
- insulin resistance, 159
- moderate aerobic exercise, 160
- overweight and cardiovascular risk profile, 159
- resistive exercise training
  - fat free mass, 162
  - total volume, 162
  - weight loss, 162
- triglycerides and high-density lipoprotein cholesterol, 159
- type 2 diabetes mellitus, 159–160
- weight reduction programs, 159

Onset of blood lactate accumulation (OBLA), 15

Open circuit spirometry, 41

Oxygen uptake (VO_2)
- aerobic metabolism, 40
- cardiopulmonary function and endurance, 40
- factors
  - stroke volume, 43
  - supply, 42
  - variables, 42–43
- gender effect, 44
- genetics role, variability
  - human genomic regions, 43
  - mitochondrial DNA, 43
  - polymorphisms, 43
- hot and cold ambient
  - core temperature, 45
  - heat stress, 45
  - lactic acid levels, 46
  - muscles, 46
  - oxygen delivery, 46
  - rest, 45
- lactic acid threshold, 41
- muscles, 7
- oxygen-carrying and release capacity, blood
  - Bohr effect, 51
  - coronary artery disease patients, 51–52
  - doping, 51
  - 2,3-DPG, 51
  - Haldane effect, 51
  - hemoglobin saturation levels, 50
  - oxyhemoglobin curve, healthy person, 50
- pulmonary artery desaturation, 41
- pulmonary system
  - augmentation, alveolar ventilation, 52
  - dead space/tidal volume ratio, 52
- VO_2max
  - altitude, 46
  - cardiovascular disease patients, 48
  - determination, 41–42
  - following training, 48–49

P

Peak early diastole/presystole maximal velocity ratio
- coronary artery disease and hypertensive patients, 121
- isometric handgrip exercise, 121
- peak early diastole/presystole maximal velocity (E/A), 120, 121

Peak oxygen uptake (VO_{2peak})
- high-intensity aerobic interval exercise, 39
- mortality, 39, 40
- muscle mass, 39–40
- pulmonary and peripheral vascular adaptation, 40

Post-exercise hypotension
- baroreflex, 139
- gender differences, 139
- heavy weight lifting, 140
- isometric contraction, 140
- normotensive humans, 139
- resistive exercise, 139
- single-arm curl, 139–140
- stroke and left ventricular end-diastolic volume, 140
- sympathetic nervous activity, 139

Pressure–volume ratio (P/V), left ventricular end-systolic
- aerobic, anaerobic and isometric exercise, 115
- and blood pressure, 115
- coronary artery disease patient, 115
- ejection fraction, 114
- isometric exercise, 115
- mechanics, contraction, 114
- myocardial fiber shortening, 114
- preload and afterload, heart rate, 114

Pulmonary function
- ACE
  - angiotensin II, 44
  - endurance performance, 44
- altitude
  - breathing frequency, 54
  - hyperventilation, 53–54

hypoxia, 54, 55
minute ventilation, 54
muscular chemoreceptors, 54
anemia, 52
gases
ATPS and ATPD units, 34
oxygen cascade, 35
oxygen partial pressure, 34
STPD and BTPS units, 34
volume, 33
gender effect
lung diffusing capacity, 53
sedentary women, 53
tidal volume, 53
minute ventilation (*see* Minute ventilation)
oxygen and carbon dioxide transport, blood, 38–39
oxygen-carrying and release capacity, blood
oxygen-diffusing capacity
blood flow, 38
capillaries recruitment, 38
description, 37
peripheral *vs.* central theories, 46–48
training effect, pulmonary system, 55
VO_2 (*see* Oxygen uptake (VO_2))
VO_{2peak} (*see* Peak oxygen uptake (VO_{2peak}))
Pulmonary ventilation-perfusion mismatch
augmentation, alveolar ventilation, 237
exertional dyspnea, 238
heavy exercise, 237
hemoglobin saturation, 237
inequality, 238
ventilation/perfusion ratio, 237

R
RAS. *See* Rennin-angiotensin system (RAS)
Redistribution, cardiac output
altitude
coronary artery disease patients, 104
hypoxia, 103
maximal heart rate, 103, 104
oxygen demand, 103
plasma volume, 103
stable angina, 104
stroke volume, 103, 104
submaximal aerobic exercise, 103–104
autoregulation mechanism
anaerobic and isometric exercise, 86
angiogenesis, 86
arterioles, 85
description, 85–86
reduced blood flow curve, 85
blood flow
exercise, 86–87
myocardial, 91–96
nitric oxide (NO) Kinins influence, 89–90
regulation, 87–89
body core temperature regulation, 98
body organs, rest, 97
cold environment, 102
endurance exercise, 97–98
exercise, 96–97
neurotransmitter, 98
RAS, 90–91
respiratory muscle work
cardiovascular disease patients, 98
energy expenditure, 98
maximal aerobic exercise, 99
peak strenuous exercise, 98
peripheral fatigue, 99
warm environments, 99–102
working skeletal muscle, 97
Rennin-angiotensin system (RAS)
A1166C variant, 91
blood pressure and extracellular fluid, 90
functional polymorphism, 90–91
Resistive training, blood pressure
borderline hypertension, 144
circuit weight, 145
intensity, contraction, 144
isometric exercise, 144
maximal voluntary contraction (MVC), 143
mean arterial blood pressure, 143, 144

S
SCD. *See* Sudden cardiac death (SCD)
Skeletal muscle, mitochondrial changes
atrophy, 19
endurance exercise, 19
factors, oxygen transfer, 20
myoglobin, 20
oxygen extraction, 20
Starling's law, 113
Stepwise test
metabolic cost, 26
work and power calculation, 25
Stress test, 25
Stroke volume
cardiac output and physical inactivity, 179
estimation
oxygen pulse, 238
peak oxygen uptake and systolic blood pressure, 239
and heart rate, 61–63
inotropic state, 178
left ventricular end-diastolic volume, 178–179
total peripheral resistance, 179
training
catecholamin, 179
chronic exercise, 179
Sudden cardiac death (SCD)
arrhythmogenic right ventricular dysplasia, 201
athletes, 200
coronary artery disease, 200
hypertrophic cardiomyopathy (HCM), 199
inherited ion channel/myocardial defects, 201
mitral valve prolapse, 200
sex differences, 201

Sudden cardiac death (SCD) (*cont.*)
structural abnormalities and arrhythmogenic disorders, 199, 200
ventricular tachyarrhythmia, 201
Sudden death, exercise and
arrhythmogenic right ventricular dysplasia, 209–211
Brugada syndrome, 204
cardiac arrest, lethal arrhythmia, 197
cardiac rehabilitation, 197
catecholaminergic polymorphic ventricular tachycardia, 203–204
commotio cordis, 202
congenital heart problems, 196
coronary artery anomalies, 207
hypertrophic cardiomyopathy, 205–207
levels, physical fitness
atherosclerosis, 199
cardiopulmonary, 199
cardiorespiratory, 198
exercise stress testing, 199
pathophysiology
exercise induced ischemia/coronary spasm, 202
repolarization homogeneity, 201
ventricular fibrillation (VF), 201
ventricular tachyarrhythmia (VT), 201
physical inactivity and cardiovascular disease
acute thrombotic occlusion, 196
atherosclerosis, 195
coronary artery disease, 195
heart disease, 196
obesity and diabetes mellitus, 196
SCD, 195
QT Syndrome, 203
regular exercise and cardiovascular benefits, 196
risk
of all-cause mortality, 198
fibrinolysis and endothelial function, 198
myocardial infarction, 198
occult heart disease, 198
regular physical activity, 197
sudden cardiac arrest, 198
SCD causes, 199–201
ventricular fibrillation mechanism, 209
ventricular tachycardia mechanism, 209
vigorous exercise and moderate physical activit, 197
Supine exercise
blood pooling, 64
linear regression analysis, 63–64
maximal heart rate, 64
oxygen uptake, 64
sitting dynamic exercise, 64–65

T

Total peripheral resistance (TPR)
aerobic exercise and at rest, 146
anaerobic bout, 146
baroreceptor reflex, 147
equations, 146
left ventricular ejection, 146
mean arterial blood pressure, 147
stroke volume, 146
TPR. *See* Total peripheral resistance (TPR)
Treadmill
metabolic cost
running, 28–29
walking, 28
work and power, 27

V

Ventricular fibrillation (VF)
arrhythmogenic right ventricular cardiomyopathy, 210
arrhythmogenic right ventricular dysplasia (ARVD), 210
coronary artery occlusion, 209
electrocardiogram, 210, 211
electrocardiographs, 209
epsilon wave, 210
micro-reentry circuit, 209
myocardial depolarization, 209
palpitations, 210
Ventricular tachycardia (VT)
blood pressure and low cardiac output, 207
depolarizations, 209
electrical reentry, 208
electrocardiograph, 207, 208
fibrillation, 208
myocardium embedded, 208
VF. *See* Ventricular fibrillation (VF)
VO_2. *See* Oxygen uptake (VO_2)
VT. *See* Ventricular tachycardia (VT)

W

Wall motion abnormalities, 110, 180
Warm environments, cardiac output in
acclimatization, 102
anaerobic metabolism and lactic acid production, 100
blood flow competition, 100
core temperature, 101
dehydration, 101
endurance exercise, 100
heart rate, 101
heat production, 99
heat stress, 99
hemodynamic responses, 102
hyperthermia, 99–100
stroke volume, 101
VO_2, 100

MIX
Papier aus verantwortungsvollen Quellen
Paper from responsible sources
FSC® C105338

If you have any concerns about our products,
you can contact us on
ProductSafety@springernature.com

In case Publisher is established outside the EU,
the EU authorized representative is:
Springer Nature Customer Service Center GmbH
Europaplatz 3, 69115 Heidelberg, Germany

Printed by Libri Plureos GmbH
in Hamburg, Germany